Metabolic Aspects of Alcoholism

Metabolic Aspects of Alcoholism

Edited by

CHARLES S. LIEBER

Chief, Section of Liver Disease, Nutrition and Alcoholism,
Veterans Administration Hospital New York
and Professor of Medicine and Pathology
Mount Sinai School of Medicine (CUNY) New York

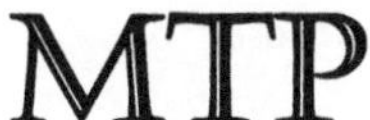

Published by

MTP Press Limited
St. Leonard's House
St. Leonardgate
LANCASTER

Softcover reprint of the hardcover 1st edition 1977

ISBN-13: 978-94-011-6155-8 e-ISBN-13: 978-94-011-6153-4
DOI: 10.1007/ 978-94-011-6153-4

at the Spottiswoode Ballantyne Press
by William Clowes & Sons Limited,
London, Colchester and Beccles

Contents

List of Contributors vii

Introduction ix
C. S. Lieber

1. **Metabolism of Ethanol** 1
   C. S. Lieber

2. **Metabolic Effects of Alcohol on the Liver** 31
   C. S. Lieber and L. M. DeCarli

3. **Metabolic Effects of Alcohol on the Intestine** 81
   E. Baraona and J. Lindenbaum

4. **The Effect of Alcohol on the Heart** 117
   R. J. Bing and H. Tillmanns

5. **Alcohol and Skeletal Disease** 135
   P. D. Saville

6. **Metabolic Aspects of Alcoholism in the Brain** 149
   E. P. Noble and S. Tewari

7. **The Effect of Alcohol on Striated and Smooth Muscle** 187
   S. A. Geller and E. Rubin

8. **Metabolic Effects of Alcohol on the Blood and Bone Marrow** 215
   J. Lindenbaum

9. **Metabolic Effects of Alcohol on the Endocrine System** 249
   G. G. Gordon and A. L. Southren

Index 303

List of Contributors

ENRIQUE BARAONA
Assistant Professor of Medicine,
Mount Sinai School of Medicine (CUNY),
Bronx Veterans Administration Hospital,
Bronx, New York 10468, U.S.A.

RICHARD J. BING
Professor of Medicine,
University of Southern California,
Huntington Memorial Hospital,
Pasadena, California 91105, U.S.A.

LEONORE M. DeCARLI
Research Assistant,
Bronx Veterans Administration Hospital,
Bronx, New York 10468, U.S.A.

STEPHEN A. GELLER
Associate Professor of Pathology,
Mount Sinai School of Medicine (CUNY)
New York, New York 10029, U.S.A.

GARY G. GORDON
Professor of Medicine,
Endocrine Section, Department of Medicine,
New York Medical College,
Flower and Fifth Avenue Hospitals,
New York, New York 10029, U.S.A.

CHARLES S. LIEBER
Professor of Medicine and Pathology,
Mount Sinai School of Medicine (CUNY),
Chief, Section of Liver Disease,
Nutrition and Alcoholism
Bronx Veterans Administration Hospital,
Bronx, New York 10468, U.S.A.

JOHN LINDENBAUM
Professor of Medicine,
Columbia University,
College of Physicians and Surgeons,
Chief, Hematology,
Harlem Hospital Center
New York, New York 10032, U.S.A.

ERNEST P. NOBLE*
Professor of Medicine,
University of California, Irvine,
Department of Psychiatry and Human Behavior,
California College of Medicine,
Irvine, California 92717, U.S.A.

EMANUEL RUBIN
Professor and Chairman,
Department of Pathology,
Mount Sinai School of Medicine (CUNY),
New York, New York 10029, U.S.A.

PAUL D. SAVILLE
Professor of Medicine,
Chairman, Division of Rheumatology,
Department of Medicine,
West Virginia University,
Morgantown, West Virginia 26506, U.S.A.

A. LOUIS SOUTHREN
Professor of Medicine,
Chief, Endocrine Section, Department of Medicine,
New York Medical College,
Flower and Fifth Avenue Hospitals,
New York, New York 10029, U.S.A.

SUJATA TEWARI
Assistant Professor-in-Residence,
University of California, Irvine,
Department of Psychiatry and Human
Behavior, California College of Medicine,
Irvine, California 92717, U.S.A.

HARALD TILLMANNS
Research Fellow,
University of Southern California,
Los Angeles, California 90007, U.S.A.

* Presently Director, National Institute on Alcohol Abuse and Alcoholism, Rockville, Maryland 20852, U.S.A.

Introduction

In the first annual report on Alcohol and Health to Congress (December, 1971), the then HEW Secretary Elliot L. Richardson called alcohol 'the most abused drug in the United States'. The report revealed that nine million Americans are alcohol abusers and that alcoholic individuals represent almost 10 % of the nation's work force. With spreading alcoholism, the incidence of physical damage due to alcohol has greatly increased. A question which is often raised is 'in which way does an alcoholic differ from a non-alcoholic?' Inquiries have focused on psychological make-up, behavioural differences and socioeconomic factors. More recently, however, physical differences have been delineated. Prior to the development of various disease entities, chronic ethanol exposure results in profound biochemical and morphological changes. Consequently an alcoholic does not respond normally to alcohol, or other drugs or even other toxic agents. Some of these persistent biochemical and morphological changes are the consequences of the injurious effects of ethanol, whereas others may represent the possible adaptive responses to the profound changes in intermediary metabolism which are a direct and immediate consequence of the oxidation of ethanol itself. Differentiation between the effects of ethanol directly linked to its oxidation, and the adaptive and injurious effects of ethanol are not simple, and overlap is common. In general, however, metabolic effects are associated with the presence of relatively low ethanol concentrations, whereas injurious effects occur with high ethanol concentrations and/or after prolonged intake. High ethanol concentrations also produce so-called pharmacological effects. The adaptive phase is an intermediate stage which follows repeated administration of moderate to large doses of ethanol. The liver, the main site of ethanol oxidation, displays the broadest spectrum of metabolic response to ethanol. Other tissues however can also be severely affected, including brain, gut, heart, endocrine systems, bone, blood and muscle.

1
Metabolism of Ethanol

C. S. LIEBER

1.1 PATHWAYS OF ETHANOL OXIDATION 1
1.1.1 *The alcohol dehydrogenase pathway (ADH)* 2
1.1.2 *Microsomal ethanol-oxidizing system (MEOS)* 6
1.1.3 *Catalase* 9
1.2 PATHWAYS OF ACETALDEHYDE METABOLISM 10
1.3 ALTERATION IN THE METABOLISM OF ETHANOL AND ACETALDEHYDE AFTER CHRONIC ETHANOL CONSUMPTION 11
1.3.1 *Accelerated ethanol metabolism after chronic ethanol consumption* 11
1.3.1.1 Increase in ethanol metabolism related to the ADH pathway 11
1.3.1.2 Non-ADH-related acceleration of ethanol metabolism 12
1.3.1.3 Energy cost related to stimulated microsomal function 15
1.3.2 *Effect of chronic ethanol consumption on acetaldehyde metabolism* 16
1.3.2.1 Mitochondrial acetaldehyde oxidation 16
1.3.2.2 Clinical implications of deranged acetaldehyde metabolism 17
References 21

1.1 PATHWAYS OF ETHANOL OXIDATION

Ethanol can be synthesized endogenously in trace amounts[1] including bacterial fermentation in the gut[2]; it is however primarily an exogenous compound that is readily absorbed from the gastrointestinal tract. Only 2–10 % of that absorbed is eliminated through the kidneys and lungs; the rest must be oxidized in the body, principally in the liver. The rate of disappearance of ethanol from the blood is indeed remarkably decreased or halted by hepatectomy or procedures damaging the liver[3]. Moreover, the predominant role of the liver for ethanol metabolism was shown directly in individuals with portacaval shunts undergoing hepatic vein catheterization[4]. Extrahepatic metabolism of ethanol, although it occurs, is small[5,6]. This relative organ specificity of ethanol for the liver probably explains why, despite the existence of intracellular mechanisms responsible for redox homeostasis, ethanol oxidation produces striking metabolic imbalances in the liver. These effects are

Table 1.1 Characteristics of ethanol metabolism

1. Large caloric load, sometimes in excess of all other nutrients
2. Almost no renal or pulmonary excretion
3. No storage mechanism in the body
4. Oxidation predominantly in the liver
5. No feedback control of rates of ethanol oxidation

aggravated by the lack of feedback mechanism to adjust the rate of ethanol oxidation to the metabolic state of the hepatocyte, and the inability of ethanol, unlike other major sources of calories, to be stored or metabolized to a marked degree in peripheral tissues (Table 1.1). The hepatocyte contains three main pathways for ethanol metabolism, each located in a different subcellular compartment: the alcohol dehydrogenase pathway of the cytosol or the soluble fraction of the cell, the microsomal ethanol oxidizing system located in the endoplasmic reticulum and catalase located in the peroxisomes.

1.1.1 The alcohol dehydrogenase pathway (ADH)

The main pathway for ethanol disposition involves alcohol dehydrogenase (ADH), an enzyme of the cell sap (cytosol) that catalyses the conversion of ethanol to acetaldehyde. The enzyme has a broad substrate specificity, which includes dehydrogenation of steroids[7] and omega oxidation of fatty acids[8]. These compounds may represent the 'physiological' substrates for ADH,

A.

$$CH_3CH_2OH + NAD^+ \xrightarrow[\text{ADH}]{} CH_3CHO + NADH + H^+$$

B.

$$CH_3CH_2OH + NADPH + H^+ + O_2 \xrightarrow[\text{MEOS}]{} CH_3CHO + NADP^+ + 2H_2O$$

C.

$$NADPH + H^+ + O_2 \xrightarrow[\text{NADPH Oxidase}]{} NADP^+ + H_2O_2$$

$$+$$

$$H_2O_2 + CH_3CH_2OH \xrightarrow[\text{Catalase}]{} 2H_2O + CH_3CHO$$

D.

$$\text{HYPOXANTHINE} + H_2O + O_2 \xrightarrow[\text{Xanthine Oxidase}]{} \text{XANTHINE} + H_2O_2$$

$$+$$

$$H_2O_2 + CH_3CH_2OH \xrightarrow[\text{Catalase}]{} 2H_2O + CH_3CHO$$

Figure 1.1 Ethanol oxidation by A, alcohol dehydrogenase (ADH), nicotinamide adenine dinucleotide (NAD), nicotinamide adenine dinucleotide, reduced form (NADH); B, the hepatic microsomal ethanol-oxidizing system (MEOS), nicotinamide adenine dinucleotide phosphate (NADP); C, a combination of NADPH oxidase and catalase; or D, xanthine oxidase and catalase

Table 1.2 Hepatic metabolite concentrations in rats chronically fed ethanol (E) and in their pair-fed controls (C) 90 min after acute intragastric administration of ethanol (3 g/kg) or during moderate starvation (7 and 4 pairs, respectively). The metabolite concentrations are given as means ± SD and expressed in nmol/g fresh weight (from Domschke *et al.*[133])

	90 min after 3 g/kg ethanol		*16-hour starvation*	
	E	*C*	*E*	*C*
Lactate	1153 ± 303	1369 ± 260	871 ± 192	955 ± 266
Pyruvate	60 ± 9	43 ± 9	54 ± 8	52 ± 13
Malate	1015 ± 77	1066 ± 101	565 ± 66	494 ± 56
β-Hydroxybutyrate	440 ± 93	720 ± 189	1509 ± 409	1403 ± 251
Acetoacetate	46 ± 17	29 ± 10	268 ± 105	217 ± 41
Glutamate	5163 ± 928	4781 ± 1308	2152 ± 771	1636 ± 346
Ammonia	882 ± 181	712 ± 130	812 ± 297	827 ± 131
α-Oxoglutarate	38 ± 8	23 ± 4	33 ± 9	22 ± 3

although the small amount of endogenous ethanol could also play such a role. Hydrogen is transferred from ethanol to the cofactor nicotinamide adenine dinucleotide (NAD), which is converted to its reduced form (NADH) (Figure 1.1A). As a net result, ethanol oxidation generates an excess of reducing equivalents in the liver, primarily as NADH. The altered redox state of the cytosol can be calculated from the measurement of the lactate and pyruvate in control rats given ethanol (Tables 1.2 and 1.3). These results are similar to those obtained by Veech *et al.*[9] The altered redox state in turn is responsible for a variety of metabolic abnormalities, which will be discussed in a subsequent chapter. Some of these, such as hyperlactacidaemia, are linked to the utilization of the excess NADH in the cytosol (Figure 1.2). The H can also be transferred to NADP and the increased NADPH can be utilized for synthetic pathways in the cytosol and microsomal functions, as illustrated in Figure 1.2 and discussed in more detail subsequently.

Some of the excess hydrogen equivalents can also be transferred from the

Table 1.3 Cytoplasmic and mitochondrial ratios of free pyridine nucleotides in rat livers calculated from values given in Table 1.2. The values compiled are the means ± SD of the ratios calculated for each individual animal (from Domschke *et al.*[133])

	90 min after 3 g/kg ethanol		*16-hour starvation*	
	E	*C*	*E*	*C*
Cytoplasm				
(NAD)/(NADH)	485 ± 96	292 ± 70	574 ± 143	537 ± 122
(NADP)/(NADPH)	0.00198 ± 0.00036	0.00138 ± 0.00031	0.00327 ± 0.00078	0.00358 ± 0.00102
Mitochondria				
(NAD)/(NADH)	2.25 ± 0.79	0.82 ± 0.27	3.60 ± 0.79	3.21 ± 0.84
(NADP)/(NADPH)	2.560 ± 0.540	1.490 ± 0.530	5.060 ± 1.720	4.010 ± 1.090

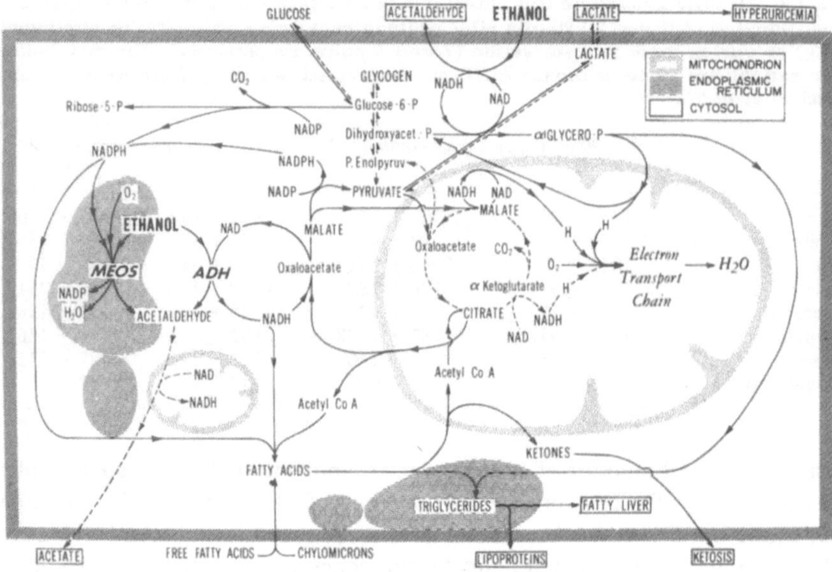

Figure 1.2 Metabolism of ethanol in the hepatocyte. Pathways which are decreased after ethanol abuse are represented by dashed lines. ADH, alcohol dehydrogenase: MEOS, microsomal ethanol-oxidizing system; NAD, nicotinamide adenine dinucleotide; NADH, nicotinamide adenine dinucleotide, reduced form; NADP, nicotinamide adenine dinucleotide phosphate; NADPH, nicotinamide adenine dinucleotide phosphate, reduced form

cytosol into the mitochondria. Since the mitochondrial membrane is normally impermeable to NADH, it is generally believed that the reducing equivalents of NADH are transferred to the mitochondrial respiratory chain via shuttle mechanisms. Thus, NADH reduces the oxidized partner of the shuttle pair (i.e. oxaloacetate) in the presence of the cytoplasmic enzyme, thereby regenerating NAD. The reduced component (i.e. malate) now traverses the mitochondrial membrane where it reacts with the mitochondrial enzyme and NAD (or FAD in the case of α-glycerophosphate) to generate NADH or FADH plus the oxidized partner. FADH and NADH are oxidized by the respiratory chain and the oxidized partner enters the cytoplasm where it is available for another round of the shuttle cycle. The altered redox state of the mitochondria can be calculated from changes of the β-hydroxybutyrate and acetoacetate in control rats given ethanol (Tables 1.2 and 1.3). Several 'shuttle' mechanisms have been proposed, three of which are illustrated in Figure 1.2, namely the malate cycle[10] (quantitatively probably the most important one), the fatty acid elongation cycle[11,12], and the α-glycerophosphate cycle[13]. Whereas the latter shuttle seems to play an important role in some tissues, i.e. insect flight muscle, its significance in the liver has been questioned because the activity of hepatic α-glycerophosphate dehydrogenase is low, except in special situations such as hyperthyroidism[14] or treatment with clofibrate[15]. Normally, fatty acids are oxidized via β-oxidation and the citric acid cycle of the mitochondria, which serves as 'hydrogen' donor for the mitochondrial electron transport chain. When ethanol is oxidized, however, the generated hydrogen equivalents which are 'shuttled' into the mitochondria supplant the citric acid cycle as a source of hydrogen.

As emphasized before[16,17] other metabolic effects of alcohol that can be attributed to the generation of NADH include interference with galactose, serotonin and other amine metabolism. The increased availability of NADH also results in alteration of hepatic steroid metabolism in favour of the reduced compounds[18,19]. It is noteworthy that ADH activity was found in testicles[20] which makes it probable that ethanol ingestion is associated with high testicular concentrations of NADH, which could alter testicular sex steroidogenesis. Specifically, the conversion of pregnenolone to progesterone, a rate-controlling step in testosterone formation, is NAD-dependent and might be inhibited by the excessive accumulation of NADH. Similarly, the 3 and 17 β-OH-steroid reductases are NAD-dependent and important in androgen biosynthesis. Thus, alcohol ingestion may directly decrease testosterone biosynthesis. This, in addition to enhanced testosterone degradation secondary to the 'induced' hepatic microsomal testosterone dehydrogenase[21], may explain decreased plasma testosterone levels. Furthermore, vitamin A, which is essential for spermatogenesis[22], is absorbed and transported in plasma as retinol, but peripheral oxidation to retinal is essential for activation[23]. As in the liver and in the retina[24], testicular retinal formation is dependent on alcohol dehydrogenase. Ethanol competitively inhibits testicular retinal formation *in vitro*. Testicular deficiency of activated vitamin A should result in aspermatogenesis. Indeed, ethanol ingestion was found to induce gonadal atrophy in laboratory animals[25].

Although alcohol dehydrogenase may account for the bulk of ethanol oxidation in the normal state, ethanol metabolism was found to persist even in the presence of pyrazole (a potent ADH inhibitor) both *in vivo*[26] and *in vitro* in isolated perfused liver[27], liver slices[28] and isolated liver cells[29,30,31]. Furthermore, in the presence of pyrazole, glucose labelling from (1R-^{3}H) ethanol was nearly abolished, while H^{3}HO production was inhibited less than 50 %. In view of the stereospecificity of ADH for (1R-^{3}H) ethanol, these findings again suggest 'the presence of a significant pathway not mediated by cytosolic ADH[32]. The rate of this non-ADH-mediated oxidation varied depending on the concentrations of ethanol used, from 20–25 %[26,27,33] to half or more[29,30,31] of the total ethanol metabolism. Additional evidence that this pyrazole insensitive residual ethanol metabolism is not ADH-mediated was derived from the fact that the cytosolic redox state was unaffected[34]. These findings raise the question of the nature of the ADH-independent pathway. Theoretically, two enzyme systems could account for the latter, namely the microsomal ethanol oxidizing system and catalase.

1.1.2 Microsomal ethanol-oxidizing system (MEOS)

The first indication of an interaction of ethanol with the microsomal fraction of the hepatocyte was provided by the morphological observation that in rats ethanol feeding results in a proliferation of the smooth endoplasmic reticulum (SER)[35,36]. This increase in SER resembles that seen after the administration of a wide variety of xenobiotic compounds including known hepatotoxins[37], numerous therapeutic agents[38] and food additives[39]. Most of these substances which induce a proliferation of the SER are metabolized, at least in part, in the microsomal fraction of the hepatocyte which comprises the SER. The observation that ethanol produces proliferation of the SER raised the possibility that, in addition to its oxidation by ADH in the cytosol, ethanol may also be metabolized by the microsomes. A microsomal system capable of methanol oxidation was described[40] but its capacity for ethanol oxidation was extremely low. Subsequently, a microsomal ethanol oxidizing system with a rate of ethanol oxidation 10 times higher than reported by Orme-Johnson and Ziegler[40] was revealed[28,41]. The striking increase in the non-ADH fraction of ethanol metabolism with increasing ethanol concentrations[29,30,31] is consistent with the known K_m for ADH and MEOS: whereas the former has a K_m varying from 0.26–2 mM[42–45], the latter has a value of 8–10 mM[33]. *In vitro*, the K_m of ADH is even lower[45]. The *in vitro* K_m of MEOS agrees well with the corresponding value of the pyrazole-insensitive pathway of 8.8 mM *in vivo*[26], suggesting that MEOS may play a significant role in ethanol metabolism.

Differentiation of MEOS in total microsomes from that of alcohol dehydrogenase was achieved by subcellular localization, pH optimum *in vitro*, cofactor requirements (Figure 1.1B) and effects of inhibitors such as pyrazole[46,47]. Studies with inhibitors have also indicated that a major fraction of the ethanol-oxidizing activity in microsomes is independent from catalase[28,40,46,47]. The concept that hepatic microsomes contain a catalase-independent pathway for ethanol oxidation has been supported by various studies[48,49,50]. Similarly, a clear dissociation of the NADPH-dependent from a H_2O_2-mediated ethanol oxidation in microsomes has been demonstrated by the use of aminotriazole *in vitro*[51]. Aminotriazole is an inhibitor of catalase[27] and also of microsomal enzymes[52] and of ADH[44]: it completely abolished the H_2O_2-dependent peroxidation of ethanol by inactivation of catalase, whereas the NADPH-mediated microsomal ethanol oxidation was only slightly reduced[51]. A similar dissociation was also observed using pyrazole which inactivates catalase *in vivo*[46], and azide which inhibits catalase *in vitro*[28]. This dissociation was also found in preparations with the same control rates of H_2O_2 and NADPH-mediated ethanol metabolism, to obviate the objection that effectiveness of inhibition might differ if the ratio of H_2O_2 generated and amount of catalase varies[47]. Thus, under experimental conditions with complete abolition of the peroxidatic activity of catalase, the NADPH-dependent ethanol oxidation still proceeded at a significant rate; this again dissociates the NADPH-dependent MEOS activity from a process involving catalase-H_2O_2.

Some other groups, however, have attributed all of the ethanol-oxidizing activity in microsomes to NADPH oxidase-dependent H_2O_2 generation (Figure 1.1C) combined either with peroxidatic activity of catalase alone[53], or with catalase and another unidentified enzyme[54], or even with catalase and alcohol dehydrogenase[55]. More recently, however, MEOS was solubilized and isolated

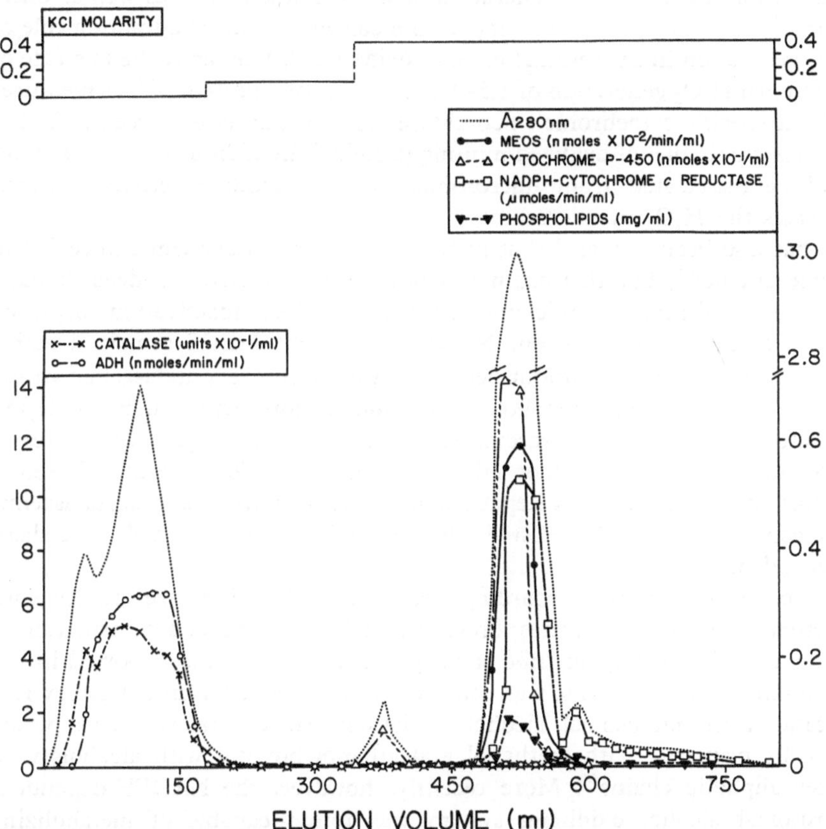

Figure 1.3 Separation of MEOS from ADH and catalase activities by ion exchange column chromatography on DEAE-cellulose. Sonicated microsomes from rats fed laboratory chow were further solubilized by treatment with sodium deoxycholate and put onto a DEAE-cellulose column (2.5 × 45 cm). The separation of the enzyme activities was achieved by a stepwise increase of the salt gradient (from Teschke *et al.*[57])

from alcohol dehydrogenase and catalase activities by DEAE-cellulose column chromatography[50,56,57] (Figure 1.3). Differentiation of MEOS from ADH in the column fractions was shown by the failure of NAD to promote ethanol oxidation at pH 9.6, by cofactor requirements, by the apparent K_m for ethanol (7.2 mM), and by the insensitivity of the microsomal ethanol-oxidizing system to the ADH inhibitor pyrazole. MEOS was also distinguished from a process involving catalase-H_2O_2 by the lack of catalatic activity, by the apparent K_m

for oxygen (8.3 μM), by the insensitivity to the catalase inhibitors azide and cyanide, and by the inability of a H_2O_2 generating system (glucose–glucose oxidase) to sustain ethanol oxidation in the isolated column fraction[57]. Thus, using specific and sensitive methods, MEOS activity could be clearly differentiated from an enzymatic process involving peroxidatic activity of catalase, microsomal H_2O_2 generation or both. These results as well as other reports[48,49,50] therefore fail to support the concept of the rate-limiting role of H_2O_2 generation in microsomal ethanol oxidation[53]. Similarly, the low rate of microsomal H_2O_2 generation of 1.5–1.7 nmol/min/mg protein[53,58], as measured with the specific cytochrome *c* peroxidase method, can hardly account for the rate of 8 nmol ethanol-oxidized/min/mg protein[53]. In addition, MEOS activity could be dissociated from microsomal NADPH oxidase activity[59], which generates the H_2O_2 in microsomes[60].

It has also been reported that microsomes from acatalasaemic mice fail to oxidize ethanol[61], but this claim has now been retracted[62]. Indeed, hepatic microsomes of acatalasaemic mice subjected to heat inactivation displayed decreased catalatic activity but NADPH-dependent MEOS remained active and unaffected[63]. Even without heat inactivation, in the acatalasaemic strain, the NADPH-dependent metabolism was much more active than the H_2O_2-mediated one, whereas microsomes of control mice displayed equal rates of H_2O_2 and NADPH-dependent ethanol oxidation[62]. These results therefore support the conclusion that hepatic microsomes of normal and acatalasaemic mice contain a NADPH-mediated ethanol-oxidizing system which is catalase-independent.

Of particular interest regarding the nature of MEOS are studies with different alcohols as substrates. Previously, a NADPH-dependent oxidation of methanol and ethanol, but not of propanol or butanol was reported in the microsomal fraction[40]. This was considered as evidence for an obligatory role of catalase in microsomal alcohol oxidation[53] since catalase reacts peroxidatically primarily with methanol and ethanol but not with alcohols with longer aliphatic chains[64]. More recently, however, the NADPH-dependent microsomal alcohol oxidizing system was found capable of metabolizing methanol, ethanol, propanol and butanol to their respective aldehydes in whole hepatic microsomes as well as in column fractions which contained the microsomal components cytochrome P-450, NADPH-cytochrome *c* reductase and phospholipids, but no ADH or catalase activity[65,66]. In whole hepatic microsomes, the oxidation rate of ethanol is approximately twice that of butanol in the presence of NADPH. With a H_2O_2-generating system, rates similar to the NADPH-dependent oxidation are achieved with ethanol, whereas butanol is a substrate only for the NADPH-dependent microsomal system but, unlike ethanol, is not a substrate for catalase-H_2O_2. The latter finding is in excellent agreement with previous reports regarding the substrate specificity of catalase[64,67,68]. The system of Orme-Johnson and Ziegler[40] did not oxidize propanol and butanol, which suggests that their low acidity may well have been due to contaminating catalase. Non-enzymatic oxidation of ethanol has been demonstrated in biological extracts with an acid pH optimum[69] which clearly differentiates it from MEOS.

1.1.3 Catalase

The hepatocyte contains catalase primarily in the peroxisomes, the mitochondria and also small amounts in the isolated microsomes. In the latter fraction, catalase is considered to be a contaminant rather than a component of the membrane of the endoplasmic reticulum itself[70].

It has been shown that catalase is capable of oxidizing ethanol *in vitro* in the presence of a H_2O_2-generating system[67] (Figure 1.1C and 1.1D). However, a significant role of catalase in ethanol metabolism has been rejected by many[27,44,71,72]. It is generally accepted that the H_2O_2-mediated ethanol peroxidation by catalase is limited by the rate of H_2O_2 generated rather than the amount of catalase itself. Thus, an indirect answer to the question of the extent of the role catalase plays in ethanol metabolism can be derived from the rate of H_2O_2 generated in the liver. The physiological rate of H_2O_2 production has been estimated to be 3.6 μmol/h/g of liver[58] which represents 2 % of the *in vivo* rate of ethanol oxidation of 178 μmol/h/g of liver[26] assuming 3.5 g of liver per 100 g b.w. Actually, the rate of 2 % of ethanol being oxidized possibly by a catalase–H_2O_2-mediated mechanism is probably an overestimate, since not all of the H_2O_2 generated in the liver can be utilized by the peroxidatic reaction of catalase[73]. Furthermore, the H_2O_2 produced by the microsomes (which comprise the endoplasmic reticulum upon subcellular fractionation) does not contribute to ethanol oxidation in perfused liver[74] although this fraction furnishes almost half of the total hepatic H_2O_2 generation[58]. Similarly, a comparison of the rate of H_2O_2 generation[58] with the pyrazole-insensitive ethanol oxidation of 53 μmol/h/g *in vivo*[26] reveals that catalase–H_2O_2 can account for not more than 5 % of the non-ADH-mediated pathway. Studies with perfused livers have also shown a similar striking discrepancy between the rate of H_2O_2 generation with that of ethanol oxidation. The rate of H_2O_2 production in perfused liver of 3 μmol/h/g of liver[75] accounts for less than 10 % of the ADH-independent pathway estimated to be 40–50 μmol ethanol-oxidized/h/g of perfused liver[76]. Finally, the hepatic oxygen concentration which was estimated to be less than 50 μM may be far too low for significant rates of peroxisomal H_2O_2 generation which has an apparent K_m of 100 μM for oxygen[58]. To evaluate a possible role of catalase in ethanol metabolism, aminotriazole (a catalase inhibitor) has been widely used. However, no significant change of the metabolic rate of ethanol oxidation was observed, both *in vivo*[44,77] and *in vitro* in liver slices[77] and perfused liver[27]. Thus, under physiological conditions, catalase appears to play no major role and cannot account quantitatively for the ADH-independent pathway of ethanol metabolism.

Moreover, the statement that catalase totally accounts for microsomal ethanol oxidation has now been retracted[78].

1.2 PATHWAYS OF ACETALDEHYDE METABOLISM

It is now generally accepted that more than 90 % of the acetaldehyde formed from ethanol is normally oxidized by the liver[79]. Several enzyme systems responsible for acetaldehyde oxidation have been described[80,81] and characterized by their differential affinities for the substrate[82,83]. Observations that acetaldehyde levels in the liver after ethanol administration are only between 100 and 250 μM[84,85], have led to the conclusion that mitochondrial NAD-dependent aldehyde dehydrogenase, characterized by a high affinity for the substrate (an apparent K_m for acetaldehyde of below 10 μM) is the main pathway for the acetaldehyde oxidation in the liver[86]. The nature of this enzyme activity is, however, relatively unknown.

It was found by Hasumura *et al.*[87] that isolated, intact rat liver mitochondria are capable of oxidizing acetaldehyde at the rate of approximately 15 nmol/min/mg protein at 30 °C with 180 μM acetaldehyde as substrate. Concomitantly, the mitochondria consumed oxygen at the same rate. This reaction was markedly affected by several modifiers of the mitochondrial respiratory chain; ADP increased the rate of acetaldehyde oxidation by 88 %. Also significant is the stimulation of the oxidation observed upon addition of 2,4-dinitrophenol, an uncoupler of the mitochondrial respiratory chain. A similar stimulatory effect of dinitrophenol on acetaldehyde oxidation was found in perfused livers[88]. In sharp contrast, rotenone, an inhibitor of mitochondrial respiration at Site 1, virtually abolished the rate of acetaldehyde oxidation. As reported for isolated hepatocytes[86], acetaldehyde oxidation in the isolated mitochondria was also diminished by the addition of substrates for mitochondrial NAD-linked dehydrogenases. These results clearly indicate that the oxidation of acetaldehyde in liver mitochondria is linked to the mitochondrial respiratory chain at the site of NAD-linked dehydrogenases. Since the ADP : O ratio with 180 μM acetaldehyde was 2.6, a ratio similar to that of glutamate as substrate, it is also likely that the oxidation is coupled with oxidative phosphorylation. Indeed, little acetaldehyde is oxidized in mitochondria in which membranes are disrupted by sodium deoxycholate. In the disrupted mitochondria, however, acetaldehyde oxidation is fully restored upon addition of NAD, suggesting that the ability of mitochondria to supply NAD controls the rate of acetaldehyde oxidation in intact mitochondria. Acetaldehyde is a very reactive compound and may be responsible for a variety of toxic effects of ethanol, to be discussed subsequently.

1.3 ALTERATION IN THE METABOLISM OF ETHANOL AND ACETALDEHYDE AFTER CHRONIC ETHANOL CONSUMPTION

1.3.1 Accelerated ethanol metabolism after chronic ethanol consumption

Regular drinkers tolerate large amounts of alcoholic beverages, mainly because of central nervous system adaptation. In addition, alcoholics develop increased rates of blood ethanol clearance, so-called metabolic tolerance[89,90]. Experimental ethanol administration also results in an increased rate of ethanol metabolism[28,91,92]. The mechanism of this acceleration is the subject of debate.

1.3.1.1 Increase of ethanol metabolism related to the ADH pathway

There is a controversy over whether ethanol consumption affects activities of hepatic ADH, with increases[93,94] or no change[28,95–101], or even decreases reported. Some who found a moderate initial increase subsequently observed a return to normal or a decrease after prolonged ethanol feeding[102,103]. In alcoholics, hepatic ADH was found to be lowered even in the absence of liver damage[104]. Extrahepatic ADH, particularly the gastric one, has been reported to increase after alcohol feeding[94] but this has not been confirmed either after acute or chronic ethanol administration[105].

Actually, the question of whether there is a moderate change in hepatic ADH activity may not have direct bearing on the problem of rates of alcohol metabolism since it is generally recognized that ADH activity is usually not the rate-limiting factor in that pathway. There are numerous examples of the lack of correlation between rates of ethanol oxidation and hepatic ADH activity. For instance, the increase in ADH activity after propylthiouracil was associated with a slowing of ethanol metabolism[106]. ADH was found to be heterogeneous, and several isoenzymes have been described in human liver[107–109]. In addition, an atypical ADH has been isolated[110] which, *in vitro*, has a much higher activity at physiological pH than does the normal variety. Although those individuals with 'atypical' ADH have enzyme activities several times higher than normal *in vitro*, this is not accompanied by an acceleration of the metabolism of ethanol *in vivo*[111]. This discrepancy supports the view that in the process of ADH-mediated ethanol oxidation ADH itself is not rate-limiting but that velocities may depend on availability of the cofactor NAD, especially the speed of the reoxidation of the ADH–NADH complex. As an example of an accelerator of ethanol metabolism which may involve the ADH pathway, fructose can be cited[112]. Its action[113,114] may be due to a speeding up of the reoxidation of NADH[115], either directly or indirectly. Indeed, fructose results in rapid production of *d*-glyceraldehyde and pyruvate both of which stimulate the 'malic enzyme shuttle'[116,117] (Figure 1.2). In any event, in view of the moderate nature of the fructose effect and the potential hepatotoxicity of the compound, its use is presently not recommended.

Another mechanism which could contribute to the acceleration of ADH dependent-ethanol metabolism after ethanol consumption (based on increased NADH reoxidation) involves enhanced ATPase activity (susceptible to ouabain inhibition)[118] and the creation of a hypermetabolic state akin to hyperthyroidism[119,120]. Mitochondrial mechanisms which have been postulated include enhanced shuttling of the H equivalent from the cytosol to the mitochondria after chronic ethanol feeding, but this possibility could not be confirmed[121]. After halothane treatment, however, both increased rates of ethanol clearance and malic enzyme activities were described[122] possibly implicating the 'malic shuttle' previously discussed in this chapter. The effect of 2,4-dinitrophenol, an uncoupler of oxidative phosphorylation, is controversial, with increases[88,123] and decreases[124] of ethanol metabolism reported. In general, it must be pointed out that if following chronic ethanol consumption, changes affecting the ADH pathway (such as ATPase activity) were responsible exclusively for the acceleration of ethanol metabolism, the latter should be fully abolished by pyrazole treatment, but this was not the case[26,28] although levels of pyrazole were comparable[125]. This raises the possibility of the involvement of non-ADH pathways, shown to play a significant role in liver tissue[126].

1.3.1.2 Non-ADH-related acceleration of ethanol metabolism

Following chronic ethanol consumption, MEOS significantly increases in activity[33,41]. This is associated with an increase in various constituents of the smooth fraction of the membranes involved in drug metabolism, such as phospholipids, cytochrome P-450 reductase and cytochrome P-450[127,128]. The increase of cytochrome P-450 was particularly striking for cyanide binding form 1, which may be preferentially involved in MEOS activity[59,129,130]. Evidence in favour of an increase of a special species of cytochrome P-450 after ethanol treatment was also derived recently from inhibitor studies[131]. Calculations show that when corrected for microsomal losses during the preparative procedure, the rise in MEOS activity can account for one-half to two-thirds of the increase in blood ethanol clearance[26]. The unaccounted-for difference may actually result from a secondary increase in oxidation via ADH, a pathway limited by the rate of NADH reoxidation. This indeed could be accelerated by an increase in MEOS activity, since the latter is associated with enhanced NADPH utilization, and the NADPH: NADP and NADH: NAD systems are linked[132]. For instance, NADH could reduce oxaloacetate to malate, which could be oxidized to pyruvate with generation of NADPH. Pyruvate could regenerate the oxaloacetate in an ATP requiring reaction. The hypothesis of the link of the oxidation of ethanol with the reduction of oxaloacetate was already proposed in 1968[16] (Figure 1.2). Experimental evidence indirectly supporting this concept has been provided more recently[117]. Consistent with the concept of the interaction of the NAD and NADP systems is the observation that acute administration of ethanol leads to a smaller shift of the reduced state in livers from animals adapted to ethanol than in those from control rats[133] both in cytosolic and mitochondrial redox levels (Tables 1.2 and 1.3). Moreover, evidence is accumulating that NADH may serve as partial electron donor for microsomal drug-detoxifying systems[134]. Interestingly, upon addition of ethanol to microsomes, a modified type 2 binding spectrum appears, the magnitude of which is tripled by ethanol treatment[135]. Increases of MEOS activity in alcoholics or after chronic alcohol feeding were also found in man[136,137] which decreased after discontinuation of alcohol; there was no strict parallelism between the increases in blood ethanol clearances and enzyme activity conceivably related to changes in blood flow and/or liver mass, which were not assessed. It should also be pointed out that the method for MEOS measurement in liver biopsy has not been validated (Lieber and DeCarli, unpublished observation).

Indirect evidence that MEOS activity may play a role *in vivo* can be derived from the fact that other drugs (such as barbiturates) which increase total hepatic MEOS activity[28] were also found to enhance rates of blood ethanol clearance[26,138–140]. Some other studies failed to verify this effect[141,142]. In the latter investigations, however, long-acting barbiturates were used and ethanol clearance was tested in close association with barbiturate administration, at a time when blood barbiturate levels were probably elevated. Under these conditions, it was found that barbiturates interfere with blood ethanol clearance[26]. Interestingly, asthmatics were found to exhibit an accelerated clearance of ethanol from the blood, possibly as a result of longstanding drug consumption[143]. Similarly, diabetics were reported to display accelerated ethanol metabolism in association with tolbutamide treatment[100]. Prolonged diphenylhydantoin administration to rats also increased MEOS activity[144]. The converse effect, namely increased drug metabolism and activity of microsomal drug metabolizing enzymes after chronic ethanol consumption (and their inhibition in the presence of ethanol), will be discussed in detail in another chapter.

There is also some debate over whether, in rats, ethanol feeding enhances catalase activity. Both an increase[145] and no change[28,93,96] have been reported. In man there was no increase[90]. This question however may not be fully relevant to the rate of ethanol metabolism since, as discussed before, peroxidative metabolism of ethanol in the liver is probably limited by the rate of hydrogen peroxide formation rather than by the amount of available catalase[58]. Ethanol consumption does, however, enhance the activity of hepatic NADPH oxidase[28,74,145] which as illustrated in Figure 1.1C, can participate in H_2O_2 generation. It is conceivable that this mechanism contributes to ethanol metabolism *in vivo* (and to its increase after chronic ethanol consumption) by furnishing the H_2O_2 needed for peroxidative oxidation of ethanol. As discussed before, however, the amount of H_2O_2 generated by the liver is small[58,73] and

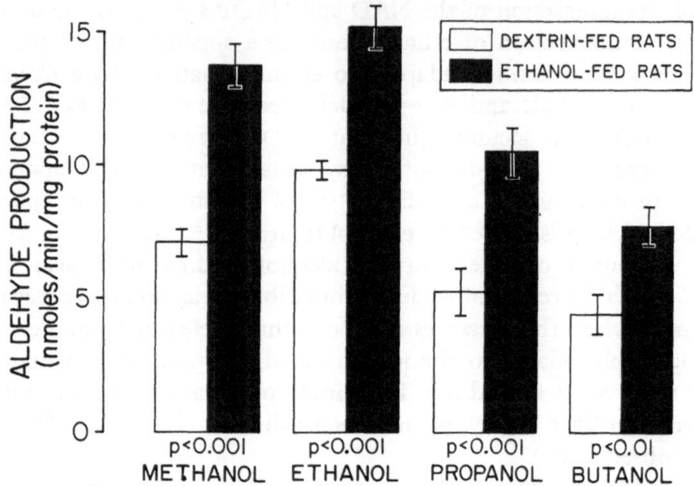

Figure 1.4 Effect of chronic ethanol consumption (6–8 weeks) on the activity of MEOS. Female rats were pair-fed nutritionally adequate liquid diets containing either ethanol or dextrin as controls. The values represent means (± SEM). The experimental conditions were as described by Teschke *et al.*[57]

even when increased by ethanol consumption could not account for the rate of ethanol clearance observed[146,147]. Moreover, acute ethanol administration was found recently to inhibit NADPH oxidase activity[59]. Catalase appears to participate primarily in the oxidation of methanol, at least in the rat, whereas in the monkey alcohol dehydrogenase may play a greater role in that respect[148]. In addition to the enhancement of MEOS activity, chronic ethanol feeding resulted in a striking increase of microsomal NADPH-dependent oxidations of methanol, ethanol, propanol and butanol (Figure 1.4). These experiments therefore show that the adaptive response observed after chronic ethanol consumption can be ascribed predominantly to a catalase–H_2O_2 independent mechanism since it was also demonstrated with propanol and butanol as substrates which virtually fail to react peroxidatically with catalase–H_2O_2. Furthermore, in liver slices, the pyrazole-insensitive pathway is also unaffected by the catalase inhibitor azide at concentrations which abolish H_2O_2-mediated ethanol oxidation, with D-amino acids as H_2O_2 source (Teschke, Hasumura and Lieber, unpublished observation). Moreover, evidence for the activity of MEOS was derived from the concentration dependency of ethanol oxidation. When the rates of ethanol oxidation by liver slices of rats fed ethanol chronically and of their pair-fed controls were compared at different ethanol concentrations there was no significant difference of ethanol oxidation rates between the two groups at low ethanol concentration whereas at 30 mM and above significant increases were observed in ethanol-fed rats compared to the rates of increase in the controls and those at low concentration. Significant differences of ethanol oxidation rates between the two groups were maintained

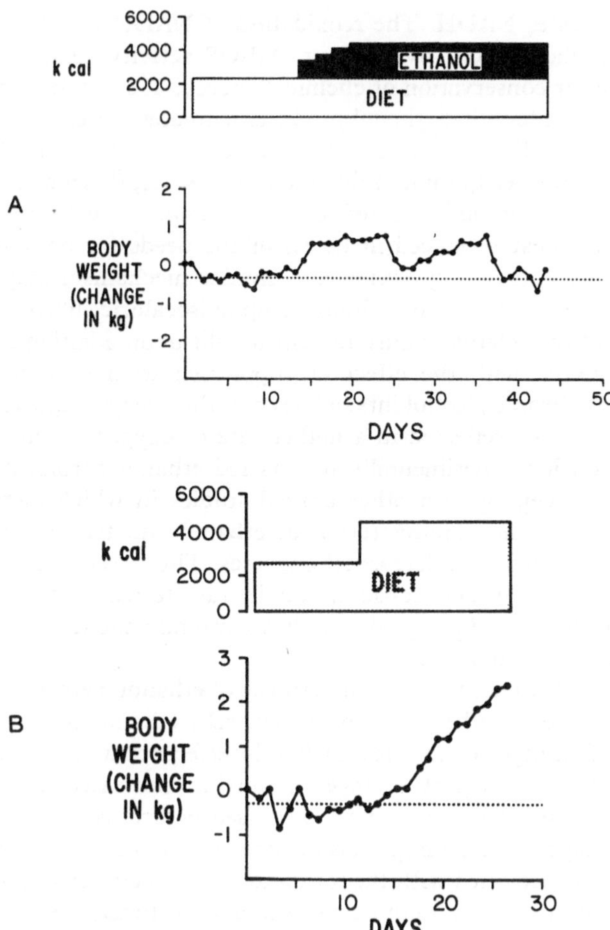

Figure 1.5 Effect on body weight of the addition of 2000 kcal daily as ethanol (A) or chocolate (B) to the diet of the same subject. The dotted line represents the mean change during the control period (from Pirola and Lieber[152])

even after the inhibition of ADH by 2 mM pyrazole and catalase by 1 mM azide[31]. Because of this insensitivity to the inhibitors and because the activating effect of high ethanol concentrations is consistent with the saturation of MEOS (K_m = 8–9 mM for ethanol), the adaptive increase of ethanol oxidation in the liver after chronic ethanol feeding most likely involves the activity of MEOS.

1.3.1.3 Energy cost related to stimulated microsomal function

Oxidation of foreign compounds by the microsomes requires NADPH and O_2; as discussed before, this is also the case for the microsomal ethanol-oxidizing system (Figure 1.1B), whereas ethanol oxidation by the ADH pathway requires

NAD and generates NADH. The reoxidation of NADH can be coupled with oxidative phosphorylation. By contrast, MEOS activity generates only heat without apparent conservation of chemical energy. This could conceivably be responsible for the fact that ethanol produces a greater increase in oxygen consumption in alcoholics than in normal individuals[149], since MEOS might be 'induced' in the former but not in the latter. Moreover, this may also cause the lesser growth[150,151] in animals fed ethanol compared with isocaloric carbohydrate since heat produced in excess of the needs for body temperature regulation represents energy wastage. A similar mechanism may explain, at least in part, the weight loss of volunteers upon isocaloric substitution of food by ethanol and the relative failure to gain weight upon addition of ethanol to the diet compared with the effect of supplementation of other calories[152] (Figure 1.5). If chronic alcohol intake increases the energy requirements of the body, this should be reflected in a higher rate of oxygen consumption. This was indeed verified experimentally in rats fed ethanol chronically[153]. These findings are in keeping with other animal studies in which metabolic rates were increased by the administration of ethanol and barbiturates in doses known to induce hepatic microsomal enzymes. Thus pretreatment with barbiturates enhanced oxygen consumption in rats tested under various conditions: in the absence of drugs, during hexobarbital anaesthesia and after the administration of aminopyrine[153].

In addition to the energy-wasteful pathway of ethanol metabolism, there are of course a number of other mechanisms whereby ethanol might affect the efficient disposal of ingested calories, such as interference with digestion and absorption, and physiological changes requiring increased expenditure of energy[152]. Increased ATPase activity, discussed before, could also contribute to energy wastage. Ethanol might also enhance other catabolic pathways that are not effectively coupled with the formation of high energy phosphate bonds such as the initial steps in amino acid degradation. Indeed, it is possible that ethanol could increase protein catabolism as suggested by changes in urinary nitrogen[154]. In any event, ethanol calories do not fully 'count', at least at a relatively high ethanol intake. This applies especially to alcoholics in whom ethanol represents a large fraction of the total calories, and is metabolized, in part, by the MEOS which, as discussed before, is 'induced' by chronic ethanol consumption.

1.3.2 Effect of chronic ethanol consumption on acetaldehyde metabolism

1.3.2.1 Mitochondrial acetaldehyde oxidation

Chronic ethanol consumption results in a significant reduction of the capacity of rat liver mitochondria to oxidize acetaldehyde, regardless of the presence of substrates for NAD-linked dehydrogenase. Since prolonged intake of ethanol depresses the oxidation of some NAD-dependent substrates[155], the observed reduction of acetaldehyde metabolism can be ascribed, at least in part, to the decreased ability of NADH reoxidation in mitochondria of ethanol-fed animals[87]. It was reported, however, that chronic ethanol consumption did not change[95,156,157] or even increased[102,158] the activity of hepatic NAD-dependent aldehyde dehydrogenase. In all of these reports, the enzyme activity was assayed in a system in which very high concentrations of acetaldehyde between 3 and 12 mM was used as substrate. These levels are one order of magnitude higher than the acetaldehyde concentrations observed in liver after ethanol administration[84,85]. In a more recent study, it was found that the activity of the NAD-dependent aldehyde dehydrogenase, characterized by high affinity for acetaldehyde, remained unchanged following chronic ethanol consumption in disrupted mitochondria supplied with NAD. The discrepancy between the decreased rate of acetaldehyde oxidation in intact mitochondria and the unaffected enzyme activity in disrupted organelles suggests that the rate-limiting step of acetaldehyde oxidation in hepatic mitochondria is the mitochondrial capacity to reoxidize NADH rather than the aldehyde dehydrogenase activity itself[87]. In any event, the decreased capacity of mitochondria of alcohol-fed animals to oxidize acetaldehyde, associated with unaltered or even enhanced rates of ethanol oxidation (and therefore acetaldehyde generation) may result in an imbalance between production and disposition of acetaldehyde. Such a mechanism may result in the elevated acetaldehyde levels observed after chronic ethanol consumption, as described in the following section.

1.3.2.2 Clinical implications of deranged acetaldehyde metabolism

The metabolic effects of acetaldehyde have long remained unclear, even though it had been speculated that this compound may contribute to the complications of alcohol[159]. In recent years Truitt[160] studied acetaldehyde levels after oral administration of ethanol to alcoholics and non-alcoholics but no statistically significant differences were found. Freund and O'Hollaren[161] found a plateau of acetaldehyde concentration in human alveolar air after ethanol administration, but the relation to ethanol metabolism was not clarified. Majchrowicz and Mendelson[162] also found elevated levels in alcoholics, but they related this to the amount of acetaldehyde contained as a congener in alcoholic beverage because of the lack of relationship between blood ethanol and acetaldehyde concentrations in their clinical study. A similar conclusion was reached by Magrinat *et al.*[163]

More recently, Korsten *et al.*[164] found a relationship between blood acetaldehyde and ethanol levels in humans after intravenous administration of ethanol yielding concentrations high enough to saturate intrahepatic ethanol oxidizing systems including ADH, MEOS and catalase. This study revealed that the acetaldehyde level remained relatively constant despite wide variations in blood ethanol above 150 mg/100 ml, but the acetaldehyde plateau abruptly terminated when ethanol concentration reached a mean level of 20–25 mM, a concentration which corresponds to MEOS desaturation (Figure 1.6). Moreover, the plateau level of acetaldehyde was significantly higher in alcoholics (42.7 ± 1.2 μM) than in non-alcoholics (26.5 ± 1.5) (Figure 1.7).

The finding that at high blood ethanol concentrations blood acetaldehyde is maintained at a relatively constant level implies that, under these conditions,

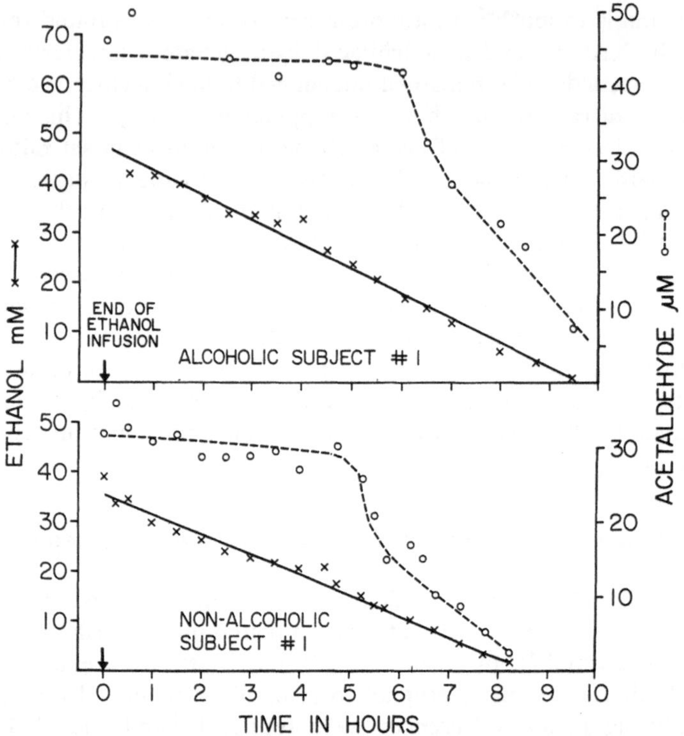

Figure 1.6 Blood acetaldehyde and ethanol levels after intravenous alcohol infusion in an alcoholic and a non-alcoholic subject. The plateau acetaldehyde level of the former fluctuated around a higher mean than that of the latter. In both, however, acetaldehyde sharply declined at an ethanol concentration of about 20 mM (from Korsten *et al.*[164])

release of acetaldehyde from the liver and disappearance of acetaldehyde from the blood must be equal. Since the concentrations of acetaldehyde observed during this plateau were far above those needed to saturate the major pathway for acetaldehyde dehydrogenation[83,165], acetaldehyde metabolism must be constant, and it follows that acetaldehyde production must also be constant. If the latter is true, it implies that the enzyme system involved in ethanol oxidation is saturated and maintains a constant reaction velocity independent of substrate levels. However, this study revealed that at a mean ethanol level of

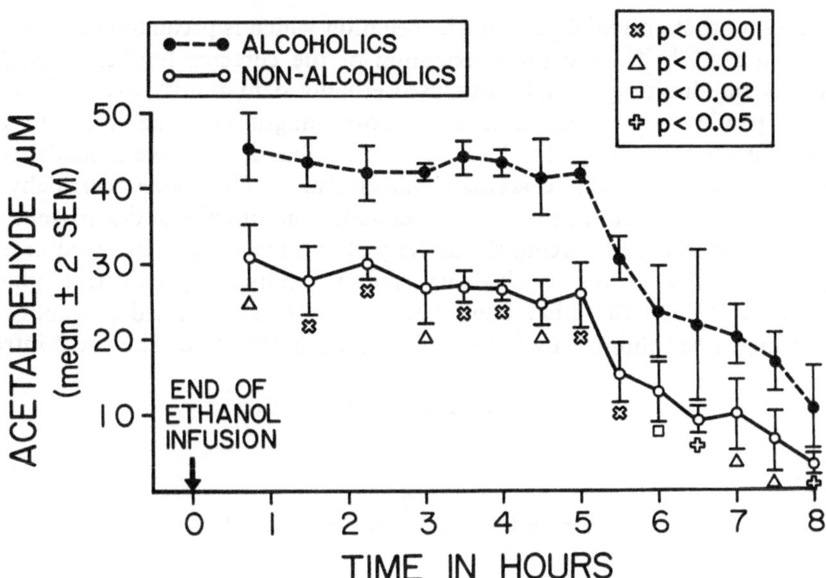

Figure 1.7 Comparison of blood acetaldehyde levels of alcoholic and non-alcoholic subjects after intravenous alcohol infusion. The significance level of the difference of the means is noted (from Korsten *et al.*[164])

110 mg/100 ml, acetaldehyde levels abruptly decreased. Acetaldehyde disappearance should still be constant, since the acetaldehyde concentrations were still far above those needed to saturate acetaldehyde dehydrogenation. Furthermore, the latter has not been shown to be inhibited by that ethanol level. Since the acetaldehyde levels drop at this point, it follows that production of acetaldehyde decreased. The main pathway for hepatic ethanol oxidation to acetaldehyde proceeds via ADH. However, given the K_m of alcohol dehydrogenase (0.5–2 mM)[42,43], it is obvious that at an ethanol concentration of 110 mg/100 ml (24 mM), ADH is still fully saturated. By contrast, MEOS has a K_m of about 8 mM for ethanol in microsomes and 8.8 mM *in vivo*[26,28]. The activity of such a system can be expected to decrease at blood ethanol levels associated with the drop in blood acetaldehyde. Catalase represents a second possible non-ADH pathway for ethanol oxidation but its capacity is limited as discussed before.

Thus, the observed abrupt fall in blood acetaldehyde concentration at blood ethanol levels which are fully saturating for ADH suggests the *in vivo* operation of a non-ADH pathway of alcohol metabolism.

The microsomal ethanol-oxidizing system has been shown to increase in activity after chronic alcohol feeding. This induction may explain, at least in part, the higher plateau levels in alcoholics. On the other hand, the decreased capacity of the mitochondria to oxidize acetaldehyde in the liver (described before) could also explain this higher level of acetaldehyde in alcoholics[87].

It follows that acetaldehyde dehydrogenation which is predominantly intramitochondrial[30,83,165], and the reoxidation of the cofactor NADH to NAD, which is rate-limiting in ADH-catalysed ethanol oxidation[166] and is also, in part, dependent on mitochondrial integrity, might both be impaired by chronic alcohol consumption. Thus, on the one hand, defective acetaldehyde dehydrogenation may retard acetaldehyde clearance. The higher acetaldehyde concentrations that result may in turn enhance the functional disturbance of the mitochondria (by reducing the activity of various shuttles involved in the disposition of reducing equivalents and by inhibiting oxidative phosphorylation)[167]. On the other hand, the rate of ADH-catalysed ethanol oxidation might be inhibited by failure of reoxidized NADH by the usual intra-

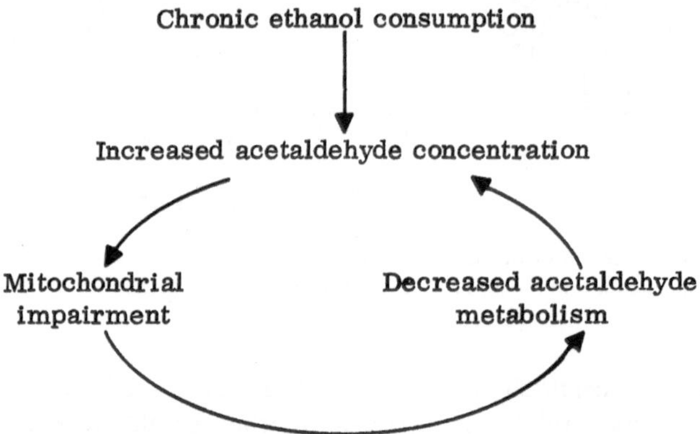

Figure 1.8 Possible relation between ethanol consumption, altered acetaldehyde levels, and mitochondrial impairment (from Hasumura *et al.*[87])

mitochondrial routes. In this respect induction of non-ADH pathways would be considered compensatory. Indeed, such induction may explain why in other human studies[89,136] the rate of ethanol clearance of alcoholics was either equal to or faster than that of non-alcoholics. This 'induction' may be the source of greater production of the toxic metabolite (acetaldehyde) resulting in a 'vicious cycle' (Figure 1.8): acetaldehyde causes mitochondrial dysfunction which in turn promotes higher acetaldehyde levels; this circular process could result in progressive elevation of acetaldehyde and liver damage, which will be discussed in a subsequent chapter.

These findings increase our understanding not only of ethanol metabolism but possibly of the pathogenesis of some of its complications. Numerous toxic effects have been attributed to acetaldehyde[168]. It was alluded to before that the metabolism of some amines (such as serotonin and norepinephrine) shifts from that conversion to the acid to the production of the reduced (alcoholic) compound, in part because of the increased NADH/NAD ratio. In addition, the major reason for this change appears to be the competitive inhibition of the corresponding aldehyde dehydrogenase by acetaldehyde. Acetaldehyde also stimulates the release of catecholamines[169]; moreover it has been shown to participate in and to favour the condensation reactions of biogenic amines[170,171]. The products of these interactions could have addictive properties if sufficient amounts were generated *in vivo*. Furthermore, acetaldehyde appears to displace pyridoxal phosphate from its protein binding, thereby promoting degradation of the vitamin. This may contribute to the low plasma levels of this vitamin in alcoholics[172]. Finally, myocardial protein synthesis was impaired by acetaldehyde[173,174] at concentrations comparable to those found in the blood (Figure 1.7); this effect might contribute to the development of alcoholic cardiomyopathy. With regard to the brain, alterations of CNS amine levels were reported in experimental animals with concentrations of acetaldehyde comparable to those we found after intravenous alcohol administration. Moreover, withdrawal symptoms were observed when acetaldehyde administration was discontinued. These symptoms were similar to those during alcohol withdrawal syndromes[175]. Thus, the high levels of blood acetaldehyde found at high alcohol concentrations may have fundamental pathogenetic consequences in the alcoholic since he has significantly higher blood acetaldehyde levels than the non-alcoholic. The detailed effects of acetaldehyde on various tissues, especially the liver, will be discussed in subsequent chapters.

The exact fate of acetaldehyde is still the subject of debate. That acetylCoA is formed from ethanol is indicated by the observation that ethanol[C^{14}] can be traced to a variety of metabolites of which acetylCoA is a precursor, such as fatty acids, cholesterol, glycerol, glycogen, amino acids, and protein[5,17,176–180]. It is noteworthy that a large fraction of the carbon skeleton of ethanol is incorporated in hepatic lipids after ethanol administration[181,182]. The acetaldehyde which results from the oxidation of ethanol could be converted to acetylCoA via acetate. The reverse possibility, namely that ethanol is converted directly to acetylCoA which in turn could be either incorporated into various metabolites or yield acetate, has not been ruled out. In any event, acetate has been found to increase in the blood markedly after ethanol administration[81,183].

Although *in vitro* the liver can readily utilize acetate, *in vivo* most of the acetate is metabolized in peripheral tissues[4,184]. The effects of a rise of circulating acetate on intermediary metabolism in various tissues have not been defined, except for adipose tissue where it was found to be responsible, at least in part, for the decreased release of free fatty acids (FFA) and the fall of circulating FFA[183].

References

1. McManus, I. R., Contag, A. O. and Olson, R. E. (1966). Studies on the identification and origin of ethanol in mammalian tissues. *J. Biol. Chem.*, **241**, 349
2. Krebs, H. A. and Perkins, J. R. (1970). The physiological role of liver alcohol dehydrogenase. *Biochem. J.*, **118**, 635
3. Thompson, G. N. (1956). *Alcoholism*. Springfield, Ill.: C. C. Thomas

4. Winkler, K., Lundquist, F. and Tygstrup, N. (1969). The hepatic metabolism of ethanol in patients with cirrhosis of the liver. *Scand. J. Clin. Lab. Invest.*, **23**, 59
5. Forsander, O. A. and Raiha Niels, C. R. (1960). Metabolites produced in the liver during alcohol oxidation. *J. Biol. Chem.*, **235**, 34
6. Larsen, J. A. (1959). Extrahepatic metabolism of ethanol in man. *Nature (London)*, **184**, 1236
7. Okuda, K. and Takigawa, N. (1970). Rat liver 5β-cholestane-3α,7α,12α,26-tetrol dehydrogenase as a liver alcohol dehydrogenase. *Biochem. Biophys. Acta*, **220**, 141
8. Björkhem, I. (1972). On the role of alcohol dehydrogenase in Ω-oxidation of fatty acids. *Eur. J. Biochem.*, **30**, 441
9. Veech, R. L., Guynn, R. and Veloso, D. (1972). The time-course of the effects of ethanol on the redox and phosphorylation states of rat liver. *Biochem. J.*, **127**, 387
10. Chappell, J. B. (1968). Systems used for the transport of substrates into mitochondria. *Br. Med. Bull.*, **24**, 150
11. Whereat, A. F., Orishimo, M. W. and Nelson, J. (1969). The location of different synthetic systems for fatty acids in inner and outer mitochondrial membranes from rabbit heart. *J. Biol. Chem.*, **244**, 6498
12. Grunnet, N. (1970). Oxidation of extramitochondria NADH by rat liver mitochondria: possible role of acyl-CoA elongation enzymes. *Biochem. Biophys. Res. Commun.*, **41**, 909
13. Bücher, T. and Klingenberg, M. (1958). Wege des Wasserstoffs in der lebendigen Organisation. *Angewandte Chem.*, **70**, 552
14. Hassinen, I. (1967). Hydrogen transfer into mitochondria in the metabolism of ethanol. *Ann. Med. Exp. Biol. Fenn.*, **45**, 35
15. Kähönen, M. T., Ylikahri, R. H. and Hassinen, I. (1971). Ethanol metabolism in rats treated with ethyl-α-p-chlorophenoxyisobutyrate (clofibrate). *Life Sci. (Part II)*, **10**, 661
16. Lieber, C. S. (1968). Metabolic effects produced by alcohol in the liver and other tissues. *Adv. Intern. Med.*, **14**, 151
17. Lieber, C. S. and Davidson, C. S. (1962). Some metabolic effects of ethyl alcohol. *Am. J. Med.*, **33**, 319
18. Cronholm, T. and Sjovall, J. (1970). Effect of ethanol metabolism on redox state of steroid sulphates in man. *Eur. J. Biochem.*, **13**, 124
19. Admirand, W. H., Cronholm, T. and Sjovall, J. (1970). Reduction of dehydroepiandrosterone sulfate in the liver during ethanol metabolism. *Biochim. Biophys. Acta*, **202**, 343
20. Van Thiel, D. H., Gavaler, J. and Lester, R. (1974). Ethanol inhibition of vitamin A metabolism in the testes: possible mechanism for sterility in alcoholics. *Science*, **186**, 941
21. Rubin, E., Lieber, C. S., Altman, K., Gordon, G. G. and Southren, A. L. (1976). Prolonged ethanol consumption increases testosterone metabolism in the liver. *Science*, **191**, 563
22. McHowell, J., Thompson, J. N. and Pitt, G. A. J. (1967). Changes in the tissues of guinea-pigs fed on a diet free from vitamin A but containing methyl retinoate. *Br. J. Nutr.*, **21**, 37
23. Olson, J. A. (1967). The metabolism of vitamin A. *Pharmacol. Rev.*, **19**, 559
24. Mezey, E. and Holt, P. R. (1971). The inhibitory effect of ethanol on retinol oxidation by human liver and cattle retina. *Exp. Molec. Pathol.*, **15**, 148
25. Van Thiel, D. H., Gavaler, J. S., Lester, R. and Goodman, M. D. (1975). Alcohol-induced testicular atrophy. An experimental model for hypogonadism occurring in chronic alcoholic men. *Gastroenterology*, **69**, 326
26. Lieber, C. S. and DeCarli, L. M. (1972). The role of the hepatic microsomal ethanol oxidizing system (MEOS) for ethanol metabolism *in vivo*. *J. Pharmacol. Exp. Ther.*, **181**, 279
27. Papenberg, J., von Wartburg, J. P. and Aebi, H. (1970). Metabolism of ethanol and fructose in the perfused rat liver. *Enzym. Biol. Clin.*, **11**, 237
28. Lieber, C. S. and DeCarli, L. M. (1970). Reduced nicotinamide-adenine dinucleotide phosphate oxidase: activity enhanced by ethanol consumption. *Science*, **170**, 78

29. Thieden, H. I. D. (1971). The effect of ethanol concentration on ethanol oxidation rate in rat liver slices. *Acta Chem. Scand.*, **25**, 3421
30. Grunnet, N., Quistorff, B. and Thieden, H. I. D. (1973). Rate-limiting factors in ethanol oxidation by isolated rat liver parenchymal cells. *Eur. J. Biochem.*, **40**, 275
31. Matsuzaki, S. and Lieber, C. S. (1975). ADH-independent ethanol oxidation in the liver and its increase by chronic ethanol consumption. *Gastroenterology*, **69**, 845
32. Rognstad, R. and Clark, D. G. (1974). Tritium as a tracer for reducing equivalents in isolated liver cells. *Eur. J. Biochem.*, **42**, 51
33. Lieber, C. S. and DeCarli, L. M. (1970). Effect of drug administration on the activity of the hepatic microsomal ethanol oxidizing system. *Life Sci.*, **9**, 267
34. Grunnet, N. and Thieden, H. I. D. (1972). The effect of ethanol concentration upon *in vivo* metabolite levels of rat liver. *Life Sci. (Part II)*, **11**, 983
35. Iseri, O. A., Gottlieb, L. S. and Lieber, C. S. (1964). The ultrastructure of ethanol-induced fatty liver. *Fed. Proc.*, **23**, 579
36. Iseri, O. A., Lieber, C. S. and Gottlieb, L. S. (1966). The ultrastructure of fatty liver induced by prolonged ethanol ingestion. *Am. J. Pathol.*, **48**, 535
37. Meldolesi, J. (1967). On the significance of the hypertrophy of the smooth endoplasmic reticulum in liver cells after administration of drugs. *Biochem. Pharmacol.*, **16**, 125
38. Conney, A. H. (1967). Pharmacological implications of microsomal enzyme induction. *Pharmacol. Rev.*, **19**, 317
39. Lane, B. P. and Lieber, C. S. (1967). Effects of butylated hydroxytoluene on the ultrastructure of rat hepatocytes. *Lab. Invest.*, **16**, 341
40. Orme-Johnson, W. H. and Ziegler, D. M. (1965). Alcohol mixed function oxidase activity of mammalian liver microsomes. *Biochem. Biophys. Res. Commun.*, **21**, 78
41. Lieber, C. S. and DeCarli, L. M. (1968). Ethanol oxidation by hepatic microsomes: adaptive increase after ethanol feeding. *Science*, **162**, 917
42. Reynier, M. (1969). Pyrazole inhibition and kinetic studies of ethanol and retinol oxidation catalyzed by rat liver alcohol dehydrogenase. *Acta Scand.*, **23**, 1119
43. Makar, A. B. and Mannering, G. J. (1970). Kinetics of ethanol metabolism in the intact rat and monkey. *Biochem. Pharmacol.*, **19**, 2017
44. Feytmans, E. and Leighton, F. (1973). Effects of pyrazole and 3-amino-1,2,4-triazole on methanol and ethanol metabolism by the rat. *Biochem. Pharmacol.*, **22**, 349
45. Lindros, K. O., Oshino, N., Parrilla, R. and Williamson, J. R. (1974). Characteristics of ethanol and acetaldehyde oxidation on flavin and pyridine nucleotide fluorescence changes in perfused rat liver. *J. Biol. Chem.*, **249**, 7956
46. Lieber, C. S., Rubin, E. and DeCarli, L. M. (1970). Hepatic microsomal ethanol-oxidizing system (MEOS): differentiation from alcohol dehydrogenase and NADPH oxidase. *Biochem. Biophys. Res. Commun.*, **40**, 858
47. Lieber, C. S. and DeCarli, L. M. (1973). The significance and characterization of hepatic microsomal ethanol oxidation in the liver. *Drug Metab. Dispos.*, **1**, 428
48. Hildebrandt, A. G. and Speck, M. (1973). Investigations on metabolism of ethanol in rat liver microsomes. *Arch. Pharmacol. Suppl.*, **277**, 165
49. Hildebrandt, A. G., Speck, M. and Roots, I. (1974). The effects of substrates of mixed function oxidase on ethanol oxidation in rat liver microsomes. *Naunyn-Schmiedeberg's Arch. Pharmacol.*, **281**, 371
50. Mezey, E., Potter, J. J. and Reed, W. D. (1973). Ethanol oxidation by a component of liver microsomes rich in cytochrome P-450. *J. Biol. Chem.*, **248**, 1183
51. Khanna, J. M., Kalant, H. and Lin, G. (1970). Metabolism of ethanol by rat liver microsomal enzymes. *Biochem. Pharmacol.*, **19**, 2493
52. Kato, R. (1967). Effect of administration of 3-aminotriazole on the activity of microsomal drug metabolizing enzyme systems of rat liver. *Jap. J. Pharmacol.*, **17**, 56
53. Thurman, R. G., Ley, H. G. and Scholz, R. (1972). Hepatic microsomal ethanol oxidation. Hydrogen peroxide formation and the role of catalase. *Eur. J. Biochem.*, **25**, 420

54. Roach, M. K., Reese, W. N. and Creaven, P. J. (1969). Ethanol oxidation in the microsomal fraction of rat liver. *Biochem. Biophys. Res. Commun.*, **36,** 596
55. Isselbacher, K. J. and Carter, E. A. (1970). Ethanol oxidation by liver microsomes: evidence against a separate and distinct enzyme system. *Biochem. Biophys. Res. Commun.*, **39,** 530
56. Teschke, R., Hasumura, Y., Joly, J.-G., Ishii, H. and Lieber, C. S. (1972). Microsomal ethanol-oxidizing system (MEOS): purification and properties of a rat liver system free of catalase and alcohol dehydrogenase. *Biochem. Biophys. Res. Commun.* **49,** 1187
57. Teschke, R., Hasumura, Y. and Lieber, C. S. (1974). Hepatic microsomal ethanol oxidizing system: solubilization, isolation and characterization. *Arch. Biochem. Biophys.*, **163,** 404
58. Boveris, A., Oshino, N. and Chance, B. (1972). The cellular production of hydrogen peroxide. *Biochem. J.*, **128,** 617
59. Hasumura, Y., Teschke, R. and Lieber, C. S. (1975). Hepatic microsomal ethanol oxidizing system (MEOS): dissociation from reduced nicotinamide adenine dinucleotide phosphate-oxidase and possible role of form 1 of cytochrome P-450. *J. Pharmacol. Exp. Ther.*, **194,** 469
60. Gillette, J. R., Brodie, B. B. and La Du, B. N. (1957). The oxidation of drugs by liver microsomes: on the role of TPNH and oxygen. *J. Pharmacol. Exp. Ther.*, **119,** 532
61. Vatsis, K. P. and Schulman, M. P. (1973). Absence of ethanol metabolism in 'acatalatic' hepatic microsomes that oxidize drugs. *Biochem. Biophys. Res. Commun.*, **52,** 588
62. Vatsis, K. P. and Schulman, M. P. (1974). An unidentified constituent of ethanol oxidation in hepatic microsomes. *Fed. Proc.*, **33,** 554
63. Lieber, C. S. and DeCarli, L. M. (1974). Oxidation of ethanol by hepatic microsomes of acatalasemic mice. *Biochem. Biophys. Res. Commun.*, **60,** 1187
64. Chance, B. (1947). An intermediate compound in the catalase–hydrogen reaction. *Acta Chem. Scand.*, **1,** 236
65. Teschke, R., Hasumura, Y. and Lieber, C. S. (1974). NADPH-dependent oxidation of methanol, ethanol, propanol and butanol by hepatic microsomes. *Biochem. Biophys. Res. Commun.*, **60,** 851
66. Teschke, R., Hasumura, Y. and Lieber, C. S. (1975). Hepatic microsomal alcohol oxidizing system: affinity for methanol, ethanol, propanol and butanol. *J. Biol. Chem.*, **250,** 7397
67. Keilin, D. and Hartree, E. F. (1945). Properties of catalase. Catalysis of coupled oxidation of alcohols. *Biochem. J.*, **39,** 293
68. Chance, B. and Oshino, N. (1971). Kinetics and mechanisms of catalase in peroxisomes of the mitochondrial fraction. *Biochem. J.*, **122,** 225
69. Sippel, H. W. (1973). Non-enzymatic ethanol oxidation in biological extracts. *Acta Chem. Scand.*, **27,** 541
70. Redman, C. M., Grab, D. J. and Irukulla, R. (1972). The intracellular pathway of newly formed rat liver catalase. *Arch. Biochem. Biophys.*, **152,** 496
71. Bartlett, G. R. (1952). Does catalase participate in the physiological oxidation of alcohols? *Q. J. Stud. Alc.*, **13,** 583
72. Lester, D. and Benson, G. D. (1970). Alcohol oxidation in rats inhibited by pyrazole, oximes and amides. *Science*, **169,** 282
73. Oshino, N., Chance, B., Sies, H. and Bücher, T. (1973). The role of H_2O_2 generation in perfused rat liver and the reaction of catalase compound I and hydrogen donors. *Arch. Biochem. Biophys.*, **154,** 117
74. Thurman, R. G. (1973). Induction of hepatic microsomal reduced nicotinamide adenine dinucleotide phosphate-dependent production of hydrogen peroxide by chronic prior treatment with ethanol. *Molec. Pharmacol.*, **9,** 670
75. Oshino, N., Oshino, R. and Chance, B. (1973). The characteristics of the 'peroxidatic' reaction of catalase in ethanol oxidation. *Biochem. J.*, **131,** 555
76. McKenna, W. R. and Thurman, R. G. (1974). Activation of ethanol utilization by D-amino acids in perfused rat liver. *Fed. Proc.*, **33,** 554

77. Smith, M. E. (1961). Interrelations in ethanol and methanol metabolism. *J. Pharmacol.*, **134**, 233

78. Thurman, R. G. and Brentzel, H. J. (1977). The role of alcohol dehydrogenase in microsomal ethanol oxidation and the adaptive increase in ethanol metabolism due to chronic treatment with ethanol. *Alcoholism: Clin. Exp. Stud.* (In press)

79. Lindros, K. O. (1974). Acetaldehyde oxidation and its role in the overall metabolic effects of ethanol in the liver; in regulation of hepatic metabolism. In F. Lundquist and N. Tygstrup, eds., *Proceedings of the Alfred Benzon Symposium VI, Copenhagen 1973*, p. 417. Copenhagen: Munksgaard

80. Racker, E. (1949). Aldehyde dehydrogenase, a diphosphopyridine nucleotide-linked enzyme. *J. Biol. Chem.*, **177**, 883

81. Lundquist, F., Tygstrup, N., Winkler, K., Mellemgaard, K. and Munck-Petersen, S. (1962). Ethanol metabolism and production of free acetate in the human liver. *J. Clin. Invest.*, **41**, 955

82. Grunnet, N. (1973). Oxidation of acetaldehyde by rat liver mitochondria in relation to ethanol oxidation and the transport of reducing equivalents across the mitochondrial membrane. *Eur. J. Biochem.*, **35**, 236

83. Tottmar, S. O. C., Pettersson, H. and Kiessling, K.-H. (1973). The subcellular distribution and properties of aldehyde dehydrogenases in rat liver. *Biochem. J.*, **135**, 577

84. Eriksson, C. J. P. (1973). Ethanol and acetaldehyde metabolism in rat strains genetically selected for their ethanol preference. *Biochem. Pharmacol.*, **22**, 2283

85. Kesaniemi, Y. A. (1974). Metabolism of ethanol and acetaldehyde in intact rats during pregnancy. *Biochem. Pharmacol.*, **23**, 1157

86. Parrilla, R., Ohkawa, K., Lindros, K. O., Zimmerman, U.-J. P., Kobayashi, K. and Williamson, J. R. (1974). Functional compartmentation of acetaldehyde oxidation in rat liver. *J. Biol. Chem.*, **249**, 4926

87. Hasumura, Y., Teschke, R. and Liber, C. S. (1975). Acetaldehyde oxidation by hepatic mitochondria: decrease after chronic ethanol consumption. *Science*, **189**, 727

88. Eriksson, C. J. P., Lindros, K. O. and Forsander, O. A. (1974). 2,4-dinitrophenol-induced increase in ethanol and acetaldehyde oxidation in the perfused rat liver. *Biochem. Pharmacol.*, **23**, 2193

89. Kater, R. M. H., Carulli, N. and Iber, F. L. (1969). Differences in the rate of ethanol metabolism in recently drinking alcoholic and nondrinking subjects. *Am. J. Clin. Nutr.*, **22**, 1608

90. Ugarte, G., Pereda, T., Pino, M. E. and Iturriaga, H. (1972). Influence of alcohol intake, length of abstinence and meprobamate on the rate of ethanol metabolism in man. *Q. J. Stud. Alc.*, **33**, 698

91. Tobon, F. and Mezey, E. (1971). Effect of ethanol administration on hepatic ethanol and drug-metabolizing enzymes and on rates of ethanol degradation. *J. Lab. Clin. Med.*, **77**, 110

92. Misra, P. S., Lefevere, A., Ishii, H., Rubin, E. and Lieber, C. S. (1971). Increase of ethanol, meprobamate and pentobarbital metabolism after chronic ethanol administration in man and in rats. *Am. J. Med.*, **51**, 346

93. Hawkins, R. D., Kalant, H. and Khanna, J. M. (1966). Effects of chronic intake of ethanol on rate of ethanol metabolism. *Can. J. Physiol. Pharmacol.*, **44**, 241

94. Mistilis, S. P. and Garske, A. (1969). Induction of alcohol dehydrogenase in liver and gastrointestinal tract. *Aust. Ann. Med.*, **18**, 227

95. Raskin, N. H. and Sokoloff, L. (1972). Ethanol-induced adaptation of alcohol dehydrogenase activity in rat brain. *Nature (London)*, **236**, 138

96. Wartburg, von J.-P., Rothlisberger, M. and Eppenberger, H. M. (1961). Hemmung der Athylalkoholoxydation durch Fusselole. *Helv. Med. Acta*, **28**, 696

97. Greenberger, N. J., Cohen, R. B. and Isselbacher, K. J. (1965). The effect of chronic ethanol administration on liver alcohol dehydrogenase activity in the rat. *Lab. Invest.*, **14**, 264

98. Morrison, G. R. and Brock, F. E. (1967). Quantitative measurement of alcohol dehydrogenase activity within the liver lobule of rats after prolonged ethanol ingestion. *J. Nutr.*, **92,** 286
99. Videla, L. and Israel, Y. (1970). Factors that modify the metabolism of ethanol in rat liver and adaptive changes produced by its chronic administration. *Biochem. J.*, **118,** 275
100. Carulli, N., Manenti, F., Gallo, M. and Salvioli, G. F. (1971). Alcohol–drugs interaction in man: alcohol and tolbutamide. *Eur. J. Clin. Invest.*, **1,** 421
101. Singlevich, T. E. and Barboriak, J. J. (1971). Ethanol and induction of microsomal drug-metabolizing enzymes in the rat. *Toxicol. Appl. Pharmacol.*, **20,** 284
102. Dajani, R. M., Danielski, J. and Orten, J. M. (1963). The utilization of ethanol. II. The alcohol–acetaldehyde dehydrogenase systems in the livers of alcohol-treated rats. *J. Nutr.*, **80,** 196
103. Figueroa, R. B. and Klotz, A. P. (1962). Alterations of liver alcohol dehydrogenase and other hepatic enzymes in alcoholic cirrhosis. *Gastroenterology*, **43,** 10
104. Ugarte, G., Pino, M. E. and Insunza, I. (1967). Hepatic alcohol dehydrogenase in alcoholic addicts with and without hepatic damage. *Am. J. Dig. Dis.*, **12,** 589
105. de Saint-Blanquat, G., Fritsch, P. and Derache, R. (1972). Activité alcool–deshydrogenasique de la muqueuse gastrique sous l'effet de differents traitements ethanoliques chez le rat. *Path. Biol.*, **20,** 249
106. Hillbom, M. E. (1971). Regulation of hepatic elimination of ethanol *in vivo*. *FEBS Lett.*, **17,** 303
107. Schenker, T. M., Teeple, L. J. and von Wartburg, J. P. (1971). Heterogeneity and polymorphism of human liver alcohol dehydrogenase. *Eur. J. Biochem.*, **24,** 271
108. Pietruszko, R., Theorell, H. and de Zalenski, C. (1972). Heterogeneity of alcohol dehydrogenase from human liver. *Arch. Biochem. Biophys.*, **153,** 279
109. Li, T.-K. and Magnes, L. J. (1975). Identification of a distinctive molecular form of alcohol dehydrogenase in human livers with high activity. *Biochem. Biophys. Res. Commun.*, **63,** 202
110. von Wartburg, J.-P., Papenberg, J. and Aebi, H. (1965). An atypical human alcohol dehydrogenase. *Can. J. Biochem.*, **43,** 889
111. Edwards, J. A. and Price Evans, D. A. (1972). Ethanol metabolism in subjects possessing typical and atypical liver alcohol dehydrogenase. *Clin. Pharmacol. Ther.*, **8,** 824
112. Lundquist, F. and Wolthers, H. (1958). The influence of fructose on the kinetics of alcohol elimination in man. *Acta Pharmacol.* **14,** 290
113. Thieden, H. I. D. and Lundquist, F. (1967). The influence of fructose and its metabolites on ethanol metabolism *in vitro*. *Biochem. J.*, **102,** 177
114. Lowenstein, L. M., Simone, R., Boulter, P. and Nathan, P. (1970). Effect of fructose on alcohol concentrations in the blood in man. *J. Am. Med. Ass.*, **213.** 1899
115. Holzer, H. and Schneider, S. (1955). Zum Mechanismus der Beeinflussung der Alkoholoxydation in der Leber Durch Fructose. *Klin. Wochenschr.*, **33,** 1006
116. Thieden, H. I. D., Grunnet, N., Damgaard, S. E. and Sestoft, L. (1972). Effect of fructose and glyceraldehyde on ethanol metabolism in human liver and in rat liver. *Eur. J. Biochem.*, **30,** 250
117. Damgaard, S. E., Sestoft, L., Lundquist, F. and Tygstrup, N. (1972). The interrelationship between fructose and ethanol metabolism in the isolated perfused pig liver. *Acta Med. Scand. Suppl.*, **542,** 131
118. Bernstein, J., Videla, L. and Israel, Y. (1973). Metabolic alterations produced in the liver by chronic ethanol administration. II. Changes related to energetic parameters of the cell. *Biochem. J.*, **134,** 515
119. Israel, Y., Videla, L., Fernandes-Videla, V. and Bernstein, J. (1975). Effects of chronic ethanol treatment and thyroxine administration on ethanol metabolism and liver oxidative capacity. *J. Pharmacol. Exp. Ther.*, **192,** 565
120. Bernstein, J., Videla, L. and Israel, Y. (1975). Hormonal influences in the development of

the hypermetabolic state of the liver produced by chronic administration of ethanol. *J. Pharmacol. Exp. Ther.*, **192,** 583

121. Cederbaum, A. I., Lieber, C. S., Toth, A., Beattie, D. S. and Rubin, E. (1973). Effects of ethanol and fat on the transport of reducing equivalents into rat liver mitochondria. *J. Biol. Chem.*, **248,** 4977
122. Ugarte, G., Pino, M. E., Pereda, T. and Iturriaga, H. (1973). Increased blood ethanol elimination in rats treated with halothane. *Pharmacology,* **9,** 275
123. Seiden, H., Israel, Y. and Kalant, H. (1974). Activation of ethanol metabolism by 2,4-dinitrophenol in the isolated perfused rat liver. *Biochem. Pharmacol.*, **23,** 2334
124. Krarup, N. and Olsen, C. (1974). Energy requirement of the transport of reducing equivalents from cytosol to mitochondria in perfused rat liver. *Life Sci.*, **15,** 65
125. Koes, M., Ward, T. and Pennington, S. (1974). Lipid peroxidation in chronic ethanol-treated rats: *in vitro* uncoupling of peroxidation from reduced nicotine adenosine dinucleotide phosphate oxidation. *Lipids,* **9,** 899
126. Teschke, R., Hasumura, Y. and Lieber, C. S. (1976). Hepatic ethanol metabolism: Respective roles of alcohol dehydrogenase, the microsomal ethanol oxidizing system and catalase. *Arch. Biochem. Biophys.* **175,** 635
127. Ishii, H., Joly, J.-G. and Lieber, C. S. (1973). Effect of ethanol on the amount and enzyme activities of hepatic rough and smooth microsomal membranes. *Biochim. Biophys. Acta,* **291,** 411
128. Joly, J.-G., Ishii, H., Teschke, R., Hasumura, Y. and Lieber, C. S. (1973). Effect of chronic ethanol feeding on the activities and submicrosomal distribution of reduced nicotinamide adenine dinucleotide phosphate (NADPH)–cytochrome P-450 reductase and the demethylases for aminopyrine and ethylmorphine. *Biochem. Pharmacol.*, **22,** 1532
129. Joly, J.-G., Ishii, H. and Lieber, C. S. (1972). Microsomal cyanide binding cytochrome: its role in hepatic ethanol oxidation. *Gastroenterology,* **62,** 174
130. Comai, K. and Gaylor, J. L. (1973). Existence and separation of three forms of cytochrome P-450 from rat liver microsomes. *J. Biol. Chem.*, **248,** 4947
131. Ullrich, V., Weber, P. and Wollenberg, P. (1975). Tetrahydrofurane – an inhibitor for ethanol-induced liver microsomal cytochrome P-450. *Biochem. Biophys. Res. Commun.*, **64,** 808
132. Veech, R. L., Eggleston, L. V. and Krebs, H. A. (1969). The redox state of free nicotinamide-adenine dinucleotide phosphate in the cytoplasm of rat liver. *Biochem. J.*, **115,** 609
133. Domschke, S., Domschke, W. and Lieber, C. S. (1974). Hepatic redox state: attenuation of the acute effects of ethanol induced by chronic ethanol consumption. *Life Sci.*, **15,** 1327
134. Cohen, B. S. and Estabrook, R. W. (1971). Microsomal electron transport reactions. III. Cooperative interactions between reduced diphosphopyridine nucleotide and reduced triphosphopyridine nucleotide-linked reaction. *Arch. Biochem. Biophys.*, **143,** 54
135. Rubin, E., Lieber, C. S., Alvares, A. P., Levin, W. and Kuntzman, R. (1971). Ethanol binding to hepatic microsomes: its increase by ethanol consumption. *Biochem. Pharmacol.*, **20,** 229
136. Mezey, E. and Tobon, F. (1971). Rates of ethanol clearance and activities of the ethanol-oxidizing enzymes in chronic alcoholic patients. *Gastroenterology,* **61,** 707
137. Kostelnik, M. E. and Iber, F. L. (1973). Correlation of alcohol and tolbutamide blood clearance rates with microsomal alcohol-metabolizing enzyme activity. *Am. J. Clin. Nutr.*, **26,** 161
138. Fischer, H.-D. (1962). Der Einfluss von Barbituraten auf die Entgiftungsgeschwindigkeit des Athanols. (The influence of barbiturates on the rate of detoxication of ethyl alcohol.) *Biochem. Pharmacol.*, **11,** 307
139. Mezey, E. and Robles, E. A. (1974). Effects of phenobarbital administration on rates of ethanol clearance and on ethanol-oxidizing enzymes in man. *Gastroenterology,* **66,** 248
140. Ruebner, B. H., Krieger, R. I., Miller, J. L., Tsao, M. and Rorvik, M. (1975). Hepatic and

metabolic effects of ethanol on rhesus monkeys. In M. M. Gross, ed., *Advances in Experimental Medicine and Biology. Alcohol Intoxication and Withdrawal II*, Vol. 59, p. 395

141. Tephly, T. R., Tinelli, F. and Watkins, W. D. (1969). Alcohol metabolism: role of microsomal oxidation *in vivo*. *Science*, **166**, 627
142. Klaassen, C. S. (1969). Ethanol metabolism in rats after microsomal metabolizing enzyme induction. *Proc. Soc. Exp. Biol. Med.*, **132**, 1099
143. Sotaniemi, E., Isoaho, R., Huhti, E., Huikko, M. and Koivisto, O. (1972). Increased clearance of ethanol from the blood of asthmatic patients. *Ann. Allerg.*, **30**, 254
144. Andreasen, P. B. and Bremmelgaard, A. (1974). Effect of diphenylhydantoin on the hepatic microsomal ethanol oxidizing system in the rat. *Pharmacol.*, **12**, 237
145. Carter, E. A. and Isselbacher, K. J. (1971). The role of microsomes in the hepatic metabolism of ethanol. *Ann. N.Y. Acad. Sci.*, **179**, 282
146. Lieber, C. S. (1973). Hepatic and metabolic effects of alcohol (1966–1973). *Gastroenterology*, **65**, 821
147. Videla, L., Bernstein, J. and Israel, Y. (1973). Metabolic alterations produced in the liver by chronic ethanol administration. Increased oxidative capacity. *Biochem. J.*, **134**, 507
148. Makar, A. B., Tephly, T. R. and Mannering, G. J. (1968). Methanol metabolism in the monkey. *Molec. Pharmacol.*, **4**, 471
149. Tremolières, J. and Carré, L. (1961). Études sur les modalités d'oxydation de l'alcool chez l'homme normal et alcoolique. *Rev. de l'Alcoolisme*, **7**, 202
150. Lieber, C. S., Jones, D. P. and DeCarli, L. M. (1965). Effects of prolonged ethanol intake: production of fatty liver despite adequate diets. *J. Clin. Invest.*, **44**, 1009
151. Saville, P. D. and Lieber, C. S. (1965). Effect of alcohol on growth, bone density and muscle magnesium in the rat. *J. Nutr.*, **87**, 477
152. Pirola, R. C. and Lieber, C. S. (1972). The energy cost of the metabolism in drugs, including ethanol. *Pharmacology*, **7**, 185
153. Pirola, R. C. and Lieber, C. S. (1976). Energy wastage in rats given drugs that induce microsomal enzymes. *J. Nutr.* (In press)
154. Rodrigo, C., Antezana, C. and Baraona, E. (1971). Fat and nitrogen balances in rats with alcohol-induced fatty liver. *J. Nutr.*, **101**, 1307
155. Cederbaum, A. I., Lieber, C. S. and Rubin, E. (1974). The effect of acetaldehyde on mitochondrial function. *Arch. Biochem. Biophys.*, **161**, 26
156. Redmond, G. and Cohen, G. (1971). Induction of liver acetaldehyde dehydrogenase: possible role in ethanol tolerance after exposure to barbiturates. *Science*, **171**, 387
157. Tottmar, S. O. C., Kiessling, K.-H. and Forsling, M. (1974). Effects of phenobarbital and ethanol on rat liver aldehyde dehydrogenases. *Acta Pharmacol. Toxicol.*, **35**, 270
158. Horton, A. A. (1971). Induction of aldehyde dehydrogenase in a mitochondrial fraction. *Biochim. Biophys. Acta*, **253**, 514
159. Truitt, E. B. and Duritz, G. (1966). The role of acetaldehyde in the actions of ethanol. In R. P. Maickel, ed. *Biochemical Factors in Alcoholism*, p. 61. New York: Pergamon Press
160. Truitt, E. B. (1971). Blood acetaldehyde levels after alcohol consumption by alcoholics and nonalcoholic subjects. In M. K. Roach, W. M. McIsaac and P. J. Creaven, eds. *Biological Aspects of Alcohol*, p. 212. Austin and London: University of Texas Press
161. Freund, G. and O'Hollaren, P. (1965). Acetaldehyde concentrations in alveolar air following a standard dose of ethanol in man. *Lipid Res.*, **6**, 471
162. Majchrowicz, E. and Mendelson, J. H. (1970). Blood concentration of acetaldehyde and ethanol in chronic alcoholics. *Science*, **168**, 1100
163. Magrinat, G., Dolan, J. P., Biddy, R. L., Miller, L. D. and Korol, B. (1973). Ethanol and methanol metabolites in alcohol withdrawal. *Nature (London)*, **244**, 234
164. Korsten, M. A., Matsuzaki, S., Feinman, L. and Lieber, C. S. (1975). High blood acetaldehyde levels after ethanol administration in alcoholics. *N. Engl. J. Med.*, **292**, 386

165. Marjanen, L. (1972). Intracellular localization of aldehyde dehydrogenase in rat liver. *Biochem. J.*, **127,** 633
166. Theorell, H. and Bonnichsen, R. (1951). Studies on liver alcohol dehydrogenase. *Acta Chem. Scand.*, **5,** 1105
167. Cederbaum, A. I., Lieber, C. S. and Rubin, E. (1974). Effects of chronic ethanol treatment on mitochondrial functions. *Arch. Biochem. Biophys.*, **165,** 560
168. Walsh, M. J. (1971). Role of acetaldehyde in the interactions of ethanol with neuroamines. In M. K. Roach, W. M. McIsaac and P. J. Creaven, eds. *Biological Aspects of Alcohol*, p. 233. Austin and London: University of Texas Press
169. Eade, N. R. (1959). Mechanism of sympathomimetic action of aldehydes. *J. Pharmacol. Exp. Ther.*, **127,** 29
170. Davis, V. E. and Walsh, M. J. (1970). Alcohol, amines and alkaloids: possible biochemical basis for alcohol addiction. *Science*, **167,** 1005
171. Cohen, G. and Collins, M. (1970). Alkaloids from catecholamines in adrenal tissue: possible role in alcoholism. *Science*, **167,** 1749
172. Veitch, R. L., Lumeng, L. and Li, T.-K. (1975). Vitamin B_6 metabolism in chronic alcohol abuse: the effect of ethanol oxidation on hepatic pyridoxal 5-phosphate metabolism. *J. Clin. Invest.*, **55,** 1026
173. Schreiber, S. S., Briden, K., Oratz, M. and Rothschild, M. A. (1972). Ethanol, acetaldehyde and myocardial protein synthesis. *J. Clin. Invest.*, **51,** 2808
174. Schreiber, S. S., Oratz, M., Rothschild, M. A., Reff, F. and Evans, C. (1974). Alcoholic cardiomyopathy. II. The inhibition of cardiac microsomal protein synthesis by acetaldehyde. *J. Molec. Cell. Cardiol.*, **6,** 207
175. Ortiz, A., Griffiths, P. J. and Littleton, J. M. (1974). A comparison of the effects of chronic administration of ethanol and acetaldehyde to mice: evidence for a role of acetaldehyde in ethanol dependence. *J. Pharm. Pharmacol.*, **26,** 249
176. Schulman, M. P., Zurek, R. and Westerfeld, W. W. (1957). The pathway of alcohol metabolism. In *Alcoholism*, Pub. 47, p. 29. Washington, D.C.: Am. Ass. Adv. Sci.
177. Curran, G. L. and Rittenberg, D. (1951). The role of ethyl alcohol in the biological synthesis of cholesterol. *J. Biol. Chem.*, **190,** 17
178. Smith, M. E. and Newman, H. W. (1960). Ethanol-1-C^{14} and acetate-1-C^{14} incorporation into lipid fractions in the mouse. *Proc. Soc. Exp. Biol. Med.*, **104,** 282
179. Russell, P. T. and van Bruggen, V. J. T. (1964). Ethanol metabolism in the intact rat. *J. Biol. Chem.*, **239,** 719
180. Schiller, D., Burbridge, T. N., Sutherland, V. C. and Simon, A. (1959). The conversion of labeled ethanol to glycerol and glycogen. *Q. J. Stud. Alc.*, **20,** 432
181. Scheig, R. (1971). Lipid synthesis from ethanol in liver. *Gastroenterology*, **60,** 751
182. Brunengraber, H., Boutry, M., Lowenstein, L. and Lowenstein, J. M. (1974). In R. G. Thurman, T. Yonetani, J. R. Williamson and B. Chance, eds. *Alcohol and Aldehyde Metabolizing Systems*, p. 329. New York: Academic Press
183. Crouse, J. R., Gerson, C. D., DeCarli, L. M. and Lieber, C. S. (1968). Role of acetate in the reduction of plasma free fatty acids produced by ethanol in man. *J. Lipid Res.*, **9,** 509
184. Katz, J. and Chaikoff, I. L. (1955). Synthesis via the Kreb's cycle in the utilization of acetate by rat liver slices. *Biochim. Biophys. Acta*, **18,** 87

2
Metabolic Effects of Alcohol on the Liver

C. S. LIEBER and L. M. DeCARLI

2.1 INTRODUCTION 32
2.2 METABOLIC DERANGEMENT DIRECTLY ASSOCIATED WITH THE OXIDATION OF ETHANOL 32
2.2.1 *Effect of excessive hepatic NADH generation by the alcohol dehydrogenase pathway* 32
2.2.1.1 Hyperlactacidaemia, hyperuricaemia, acidosis 33
2.2.1.2 Enhanced lipogenesis and depressed lipid oxidation 33
2.2.2 *Interaction of ethanol with microsomal functions* 36
2.2.3 *Effects of the metabolites of ethanol: acetaldehyde and acetate* 37
2.3 ADAPTIVE METABOLIC CHANGES FOLLOWING CHRONIC ETHANOL INTAKE 37
2.3.1 *Accelerated ethanol metabolism after chronic ethanol consumption* 38
2.3.2 *Stimulation of the microsomal drug metabolizing enzymes* 38
2.3.2.1 Enhanced drug metabolism (drug tolerance) 38
2.3.2.2 Increased CCl_4 toxicity in alcoholics 39
2.3.3 *Increase in microsomal functions related to lipid metabolism* 40
2.3.3.1 Lipid peroxidation 40
2.3.3.2 Cholesterol metabolism 40
2.3.3.3 Alcoholic hyperlipidaemia 41
2.3.4 *Miscellaneous changes in microsomal functions* 44
2.4 INJURIOUS MANIFESTATIONS OF THE ALTERATIONS OF LIVER METABOLISM ASSOCIATED WITH ALCOHOLISM 45
2.4.1 *Alcoholic fatty liver* 46
2.4.1.1 Origin and mechanisms of fat deposition in the liver 46
2.4.1.2 Alcohol as a direct cause of the fatty liver 48
2.4.1.3 The influence of dietary fat 50
2.4.2 *Transitional lesions from alcoholic fatty liver to hepatitis* 53
2.4.2.1 Accumulation of proteins in the alcoholic fatty liver and impairment of lipoprotein and protein export 53
2.4.2.2 Alterations in protein synthesis 54
2.4.2.3 Development of mitochondrial injury 55
2.4.2.4 Various effects of alcohol upon liver and serum enzymes 57
2.4.2.5 Alterations of the immune system in alcoholic liver injury 58
2.4.3 *Alcoholic hepatitis and cirrhosis* 59

2.5 PREVENTION AND TREATMENT OF ALCOHOLIC LIVER INJURY, PRIMARILY THE FATTY LIVER 64
References 65

2.1 INTRODUCTION

Ethanol exerts different effects on hepatic cellular metabolism depending mainly on the dose and duration of intake. Following the ingestion of a substantial amount of ethanol, its presence alters a number of hepatic functions either because of the change in the hepatic redox state — NADH/NAD ratio — (resulting for instance in reduction of lipid oxidation), or because ethanol when present at high concentrations will inhibit a variety of microsomal functions involving particularly drug metabolism. These effects are not observed at low ethanol concentrations. Furthermore chronic ethanol consumption, at least in its early stages, produces adaptive metabolic changes in the endoplasmic reticulum which result primarily in increased metabolism of drugs and accelerated lipoprotein production. More extended periods of ethanol intake result in damage to cell organelles in what can be considered a third stage of the alcohol effect, namely that of injury (primarily to the mitochondria) possibly involving the effects of acetaldehyde, the first product of ethanol metabolism. Prolongation of ethanol-induced injury eventually culminates in hepatic lesions such as alcoholic hepatitis and cirrhosis. The purpose of this chapter is to describe the metabolic abnormalities which characterize each of these stages of alcohol-induced changes in the liver.

2.2 METABOLIC DERANGEMENT DIRECTLY ASSOCIATED WITH THE OXIDATION OF ETHANOL

2.2.1 Effect of excessive hepatic NADH generation by the alcohol dehydrogenase pathway

As shown in Figure 2.1, the oxidation of ethanol results in the transfer of hydrogen to NAD. The resulting enhanced NADH/NAD ratio, in turn, produces a change in the ratio of those metabolites that are dependent for reduction on the NADH–NAD couple. It was therefore proposed that the altered NADH/NAD ratio is responsible for a number of metabolic abnormalities associated with alcohol abuse[1]. These include reduced gluconeogenesis and hypoglycaemia, discussed in the chapter related to endocrine abnormalities (Chapter 9).

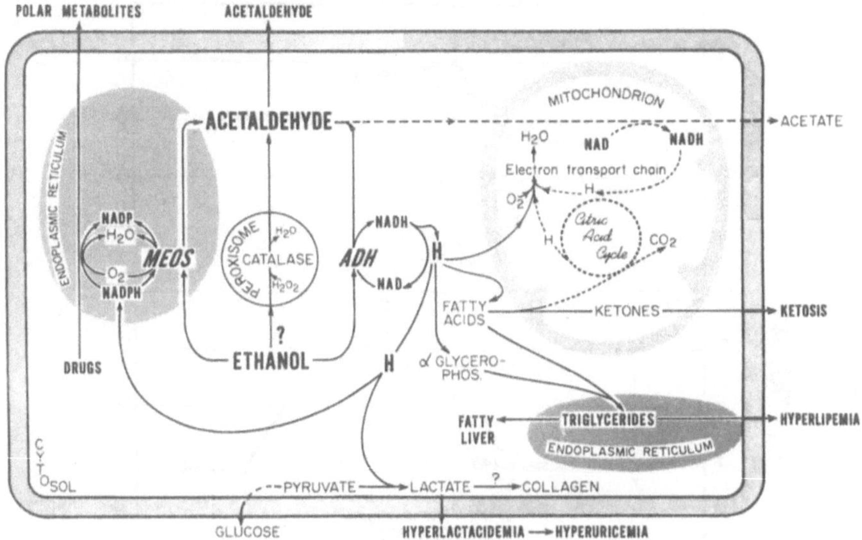

Figure 2.1 Metabolism of ethanol in the hepatocyte and schematic representation of its link to fatty liver, hyperlipaemia, hyperuricaemia, hyperlactacidaemia, ketosis, and hypoglycaemia. ADH — alcohol dehydrogenase; MEOS — microsomal ethanol-oxidizing system; NAD — nicotinamide adenine dinucleotide; NADH — nicotinamide adenine dinucleotide, reduced form; NADP — nicotinamide adenine dinucleotide phosphate; NADPH — nicotinamide adenine dinucleotide phosphate, reduced form. Pathways decreased by ethanol are represented by dashed lines

2.2.1.1 Hyperlactacidaemia, hyperuricaemia, acidosis

The enhanced NADH/NAD ratio reflects itself in an increased lactate/pyruvate ratio that results in hyperlactacidaemia[2,3] because of both decreased utilization and enhanced production of lactate by the liver. The hyperlactacidaemia contributes to acidosis and also reduces the capacity of the kidney to excrete uric acid, leading to secondary hyperuricaemia[3] (Figure 2.2), an observation which has been confirmed more recently[4]. Alcohol-induced ketosis may also promote the hyperuricaemia. The latter may be related to the common clinical observation that excessive consumption of alcoholic beverages frequently aggravates or precipitates gouty attacks[5]. Alcoholic hyperuricaemia can be readily distinguished from the primary variety by its reversibility upon discontinuation of ethanol abuse[3]. A fascinating but as yet hypothetical consequence of the increased availability of lactate may be the stimulation of collagen production and increased hepatic collagen proline hydroxylase activity which may conceivably play a role in collagen accumulation[6].

2.2.1.2 Enhanced lipogenesis and depressed lipid oxidation

The increased NADH/NAD ratio also raises the concentration of α-glycerophosphate[7] that favours hepatic triglyceride accumulation by trapping

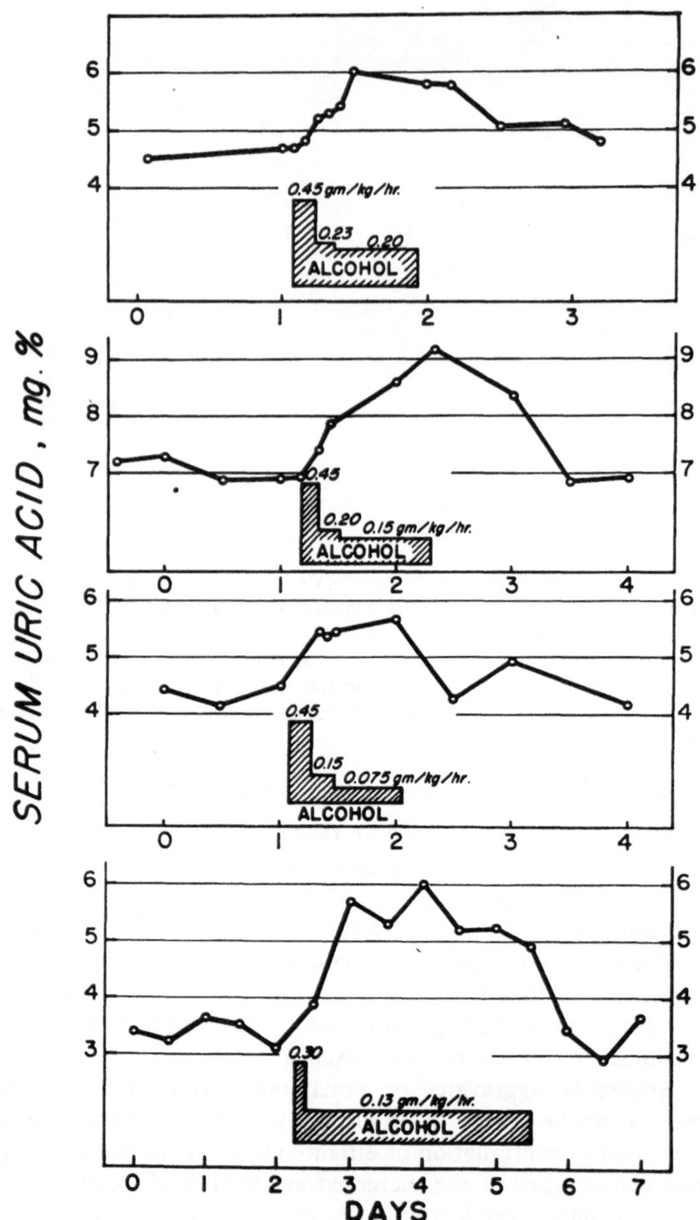

Figure 2.2 Effect of oral ethanol on serum uric acid concentration in four subjects[3]

fatty acids[8]. In addition, excess NADH promotes fatty acid synthesis[9,10] possibly by the elongation pathway or transhydrogenation to nicotinamide adenine dinucleotide phosphate (NADP). Theoretically, enhanced lipogenesis can be considered a means for disposing of the excess hydrogen. *In vivo,* acute administration of a high dose of ethanol did not enhance fatty acid synthesis[11]. Chronic ethanol administration however resulted in enhanced lipogenesis and increased activities of enzymes involved in lipogenesis[12]. Some hydrogen equivalents can be transferred into the mitochondria by the various 'shuttle' mechanisms discussed in the first chapter. The activity of the citric acid cycle

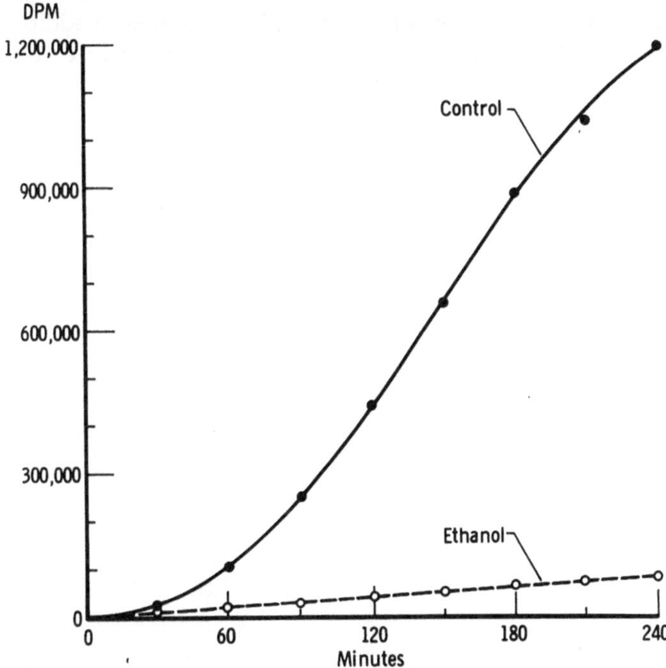

Figure 2.3 Effect of ethanol on total $^{14}CO_2$ production from [^{14}C]labelled chylomicrons in isolated perfused rat livers[14]

is depressed[13,14], partly because of a slowing of the reactions of the cycle that require NAD. Indeed, a major site of interaction of ethanol on the citric acid cycle was found to be on α-ketoglutarate oxidation[15]. Moreover, the redox change associated with ethanol oxidation decreases hepatic concentration of oxaloacetate[16], the availability of which controls the activity of citrate synthetase. The mitochondria will therefore use the hydrogen equivalents originating from ethanol, rather than from the oxidation through the citric acid cycle of two carbon fragments derived from fatty acids. Thus, fatty acids that normally serve as the main energy source for the liver[17] are supplanted by ethanol. Decreased fatty acid oxidation by ethanol has been demonstrated in liver slices[9,18], perfused liver[14] (Figure 2.3), isolated hepatocytes[15], human liver biopsy tissue[19] and *in vivo*[20]. This results in the deposition in the liver of dietary fat, when available, or fatty acids derived from endogenesis synthesis in the absence of dietary fat[21–24] and can be considered a major cause for the development of alcoholic fatty liver.

2.2.2 Interaction of ethanol with microsomal functions

Interactions of the effects of ethanol and various drugs have been widely recognized[25]. Intoxicated individuals are more susceptible to several medications[26]. These various effects are usually attributed to additive or synergistic effects of alcohol and various drugs on the central nervous system.

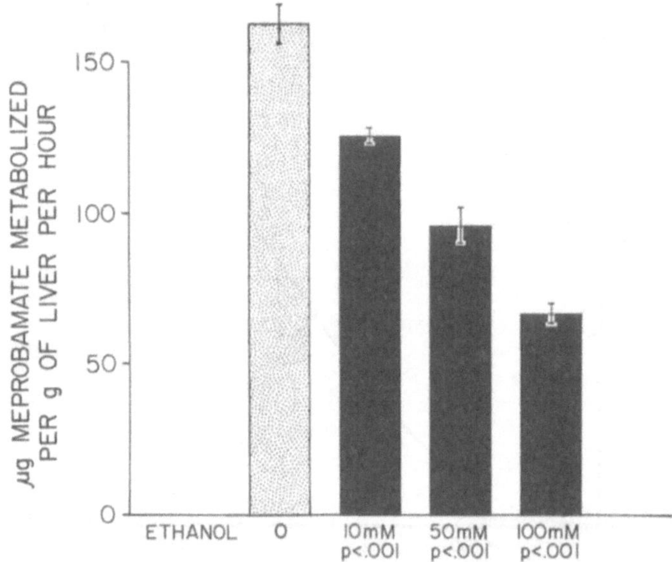

Figure 2.4 Effect of ethanol on metabolism of meprobamate by rat liver slices. Each flask contained 500 mg liver and was incubated for 120 min. Meprobamate concentration was 0.3 mM, including 1 μc [^{14}C]meprobamate[30]

However, the existence of an at least partially common microsomal system for ethanol and drug metabolism (see Chapter 1) sheds new light on the interaction of ethanol and drugs. The increased susceptibility of the inebriated individual could be explained, at least in part, by the effect of ethanol on microsomal drug-detoxifying enzymes. It has indeed been found that ethanol inhibits the metabolism of a variety of drugs *in vitro*[27–29] (Figure 2.4). With some systems, such as aniline hydroxylase, this inhibition is of a competitive nature[30,31]. For some drug metabolizing systems (such as aniline hydroxylase) the inhibitory effect is observed already at low ethanol concentrations whereas for others (such as aminopyrine demethylase) high ethanol concentrations are required[30]. In the latter case, low ethanol concentrations were even stimulatory[32], possibly because of enhanced NADH and the likelihood that NADH may serve as partial electron donor for microsomal drug-detoxifying systems[33]. The inhibitory effects may explain the observation that *in vivo*, simultaneous administration of ethanol and drugs slows the rate of drug metabolism[30,34]. Conversely, drugs also inhibit ethanol oxidation by microsomes *in vitro* in a way which has been considered as strong evidence for a catalase-independent fraction of ethanol metabolism in hepatic microsomes[35]. At a low ethanol concentration, however, its metabolism was stimulated by drugs[36] possibly because of increased reoxidation of NADH again through microsomal utilization. In addition, some drugs inhibit alcohol dehydrogenase[37]. The interaction of ethanol with drug metabolism may have some important practical consequences. Indeed, in the United States more than 50 % of all lethal road accidents are associated with an elevated blood alcohol level[38]. One may wonder to what extent the loss of control on the road may be due not only to ethanol itself, but also to an ethanol–drug interaction, considering that a large segment of the population is given sedatives and tranquillizers.

2.2.3 Effects of the metabolites of ethanol: acetaldehyde and acetate

Acetaldehyde is the first major 'specific' oxidation product of ethanol, whether the latter is oxidized by the classic alcohol dehydrogenase of the cytosol or by the more recently described microsomal system. Except after Antabuse® administration, acetaldehyde concentrations after alcohol ingestion are low, but it has long been speculated that they may contribute to the complication of alcoholism[39]. Some of the effects of acetaldehyde have been discussed in the first chapter of this book; others will be reviewed here in connection with the pathogenesis of liver injury. Although the exact pathway of its metabolism is still the subject of debate, it is generally accepted that aldehyde oxidation proceeds via aldehyde dehydrogenase of which 80 % of the activity is located in the mitochondria[40,41]. Since metabolism of acetaldehyde via aldehyde dehydrogenase results in the generation of NADH, some of the acetaldehyde effects could be attributed to the NADH generation, as discussed before in the case of ethanol. Acetaldehyde however is a very reactive compound which may exert some toxic effects of its own, as reviewed elsewhere in this book. The effects of a rise of circulating acetate on intermediary metabolism of the liver have not been defined.

2.3 ADAPTIVE METABOLIC CHANGES FOLLOWING CHRONIC ETHANOL INTAKE

It is common knowledge that chronic alcohol consumption produces increased tolerance to ethanol. This is generally attributed to central nervous system adaptation. In addition, recent studies have shown the development of metabolic adaptation, that is an accelerated clearance of alcohol from the blood. Furthermore, there is an associated increased capacity to metabolize other drugs as well. Moreover, the liver acquires an enhanced capacity to rid itself of lipids through lipoprotein secretion into the bloodstream. It is noteworthy that these functions which adaptively increase after chronic ethanol feeding involve to a large extent the activity of the hepatic smooth endoplasmic reticulum, which undergoes significant change after chronic alcohol consumption. It was indeed observed more than a decade ago that ethanol feeding results in a proliferation of the smooth membranes of the hepatic endoplasmic reticulum[42,43]. This ultramicroscopic finding was subsequently confirmed[44–46] and established on a biochemical basis by the demonstration of an increase in both phospholipids and total protein content of the smooth membranes[47]. Its functional counterparts include accelerated metabolism of drugs (including ethanol) and lipoprotein production.

2.3.1 Accelerated ethanol metabolism after chronic ethanol consumption

Regular drinkers tolerate large amounts of alcoholic beverages, mainly because of central nervous system adaptation. In addition, alcoholics develop increased rates of blood ethanol clearance, so-called metabolic tolerance[48,49]. Experimental ethanol administration also results in an increased rate of ethanol metabolism[50–52]. The mechanism of this acceleration has been discussed in detail in the first chapter, underlining the role of increased microsomal function.

2.3.2 Stimulation of the microsomal drug metabolizing enzymes

2.3.2.1 Enhanced drug metabolism (drug tolerance)

Repeated ethanol administration results in increased activities of a variety of microsomal drug-detoxifying enzymes[27,28,44,51,53]. Some effects are already observed after a single ethanol dose[54]. Ethanol consumption also increases the content of microsomal cytochrome P-450 and the activity of NADPH-cytochrome P-450 reductase[46,53,55]. These increases occur in the smooth membranes[47,53]. Moreover, it has been shown that microsomal cytochrome P-450, a reductase, and phospholipids play a key role in the microsomal hydroxylation of various drugs[56]. Therefore, the increase in the activity of hepatic microsomal drug-detoxifying enzymes and in the content of cytochrome P-450 induced by ethanol ingestion offers a likely explanation for the recent observation that ethanol consumption enhances the rate of drug clearance *in vivo*. The tolerance of the alcoholic to various drugs has been generally attributed to central nervous system adaptation[57]. However, there is sometimes a dissociation in the time-course of the decreased drug sensitivity of the animals and the occurrence of central nervous system tolerance: the decreased drug sensitivity was found to precede the central nervous system tolerance[58]. Thus, in addition to central nervous system adaptation, metabolic adaptation must be considered. Indeed, it has been shown that the rate of drug clearance from the blood is enhanced in alcoholics[59]. Of course, this could be due to a variety of factors other than ethanol, such as the congeners and the use of other drugs so commonly associated with alcoholism. Controlled studies showed, however,

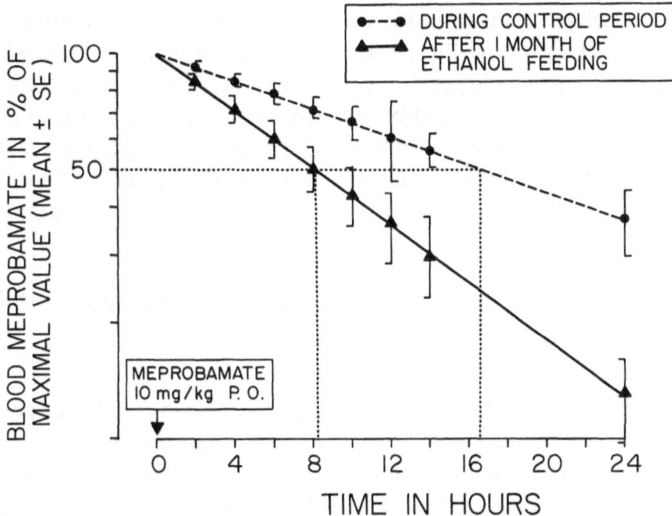

Figure 2.5 Effect of ethanol consumption on clearance of meprobamate from blood. Four volunteer alcoholics were tested before and after 1 month of ethanol ingestion; half-lives are shown by the dotted lines on x and y axes[51]

that administration of pure ethanol with non-deficient diets either to rats or man (under metabolic ward conditions) resulted in a striking increase in the rate of blood clearance of meprobamate and pentobarbital[51] (Figure 2.5). Similarly, increases in the metabolism of aminopyrine[60], tolbutamide[44] and rifamycin[61] were found. Furthermore, the capacity of liver slices from animals fed ethanol to metabolize meprobamate was also increased[51], which clearly showed that ethanol consumption affects drug metabolism in the liver itself, independent of drug excretion or distribution. Failure to verify such an effect[62] was probably due to the very low dosage of ethanol administered.

2.3.2.2 Increased CCl_4 toxicity in alcoholics

The stimulation of microsomal enzyme activities also applies to those which convert exogenous substrates to toxic compounds. For instance, CCl_4 exerts its toxicity only after conversion in the microsomes. Alcohol pretreatment remarkably stimulates the toxicity of CCl_4[63,64]. The experiments of Hasumura *et al.*[63] were carried out at a time when the ethanol had disappeared from the blood to rule out the increase of the toxicity of CCl_4 due to the presence of ethanol[65]. The potentiation of the CCl_4 toxicity by ethanol pretreatment may be accounted for by the increased production of toxic compounds of CCl_4 since the conversion of $^{14}CCl_4$ to $^{14}CO_2$ and covalent binding of CCl_4 metabolites to protein were significantly accelerated in microsomes of ethanol pretreated rats[63]. Similarly, pretreatment of rats with phenobarbital, a well-known inducer of the hepatic microsomal drug metabolizing system, increased CCl_4 hepatotoxicity[66] concomitant with an enhanced production of toxic metabolites of CCl_4[67]. Thus, the clinical observation of the enhanced susceptibility of alcoholics to the hepatotoxic effect of CCl_4[68] may be, at least in part, due to an increased activation and biotransformation of CCl_4. It is likely that a larger number of other toxic agents will be found to display a selective injurious action in the alcoholic. This side-effect is possibly an undesirable consequence of the 'adaptive' response to chronic ethanol consumption.

2.3.3 Increase in microsomal functions related to lipid metabolism

2.3.3.1 Lipid peroxidation

A microsomal pathway requiring O_2 and NADPH is also capable of generating lipid peroxides. Enhanced lipid peroxidation has been proposed as a mechanism for ethanol-induced fatty liver[69], but its role is still controversial[70–73]. The accumulation of lipid peroxide may be secondary to the lipid accumulation[74], rather than represent its cause. However, theoretically, increased activity of microsomal NADPH oxidase following ethanol consumption[75] could result in enhanced H_2O_2 production, thereby also favouring lipid peroxidation. In any event, ethanol was found to exert a sparing action on vitamin E deficiency[76] which does not favour a lipoperoxidative mechanism for chronic ethanol hepatotoxicity.

2.3.3.2 Cholesterol metabolism

The various functions of the endoplasmic reticulum include cholesterol synthesis. Increased cholesterol synthesis after ethanol[77] may have a microsomal basis akin to that after barbiturate[78] and may explain, in part, the accumulation of cholesterol ester observed in the liver after feeding of alcohol[77,79] especially with a cholesterol-free diet. When ethanol is given with cholesterol-containing diets, decreased cholesterol catabolism, evidenced by a reduction in bile-acid production and turnover after alcohol feeding, plays a major part[77]. Decreased hydrolysis of cholesterol ester may also be contributory[80]. Upon cessation of alcohol feeding, increased bile secretion occurs[81].

2.3.3.3 Alcoholic hyperlipaemia

In both man[82] and the rat[83] ethanol administration produces mild hyperlipaemia, involving especially the very low density lipoproteins. Incorporation into lipoprotein of intragastrically administered [^{3}H]palmitate and intravenously injected [^{14}C]lysine is increased[83] suggesting enhanced lipoprotein production. Fatty acids are esterified, and lipoproteins are formed in the endoplasmic reticulum. Furthermore, chronic feeding of ethanol increases hepatic lipoprotein production, even when ethanol is not present at the time of testing, which suggests an increased capacity for lipoprotein synthesis[84] (Figure 2.6). Moreover, ethanol consumption enhances the activity of hepatic

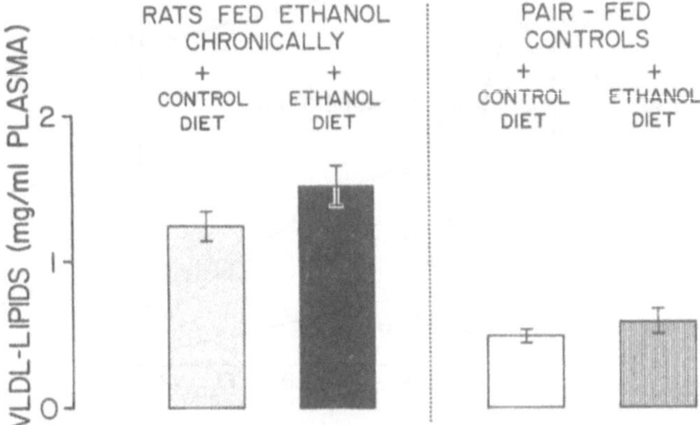

Figure 2.6 Comparison between acute and chronic ethanol administration on postprandial lipaemia in the rat. Animals were pair-fed liquid diets containing either ethanol (36 % of total calories) or isocaloric carbohydrates (controls) for 3–4 weeks. Alcohol-fed rats developed hyperlipaemia in response to a load of diet with or without ethanol; by contrast, control-fed rats did not develop hyperlipaemia in response to an acute administration of ethanol-containing diet (3 g ethanol per kg body weight). Data from Baraona *et al.*[84]

microsomal L-α-glycerophosphate acyltransferase[85]. The mechanism of the alterations of these microsomal functions produced by ethanol has not been clarified. It could be linked directly to the fact that ethanol can be oxidized at this key metabolic site. Ethanol could also induce hepatic production of lipoproteins indirectly by enhancing the availability of fatty acids either by decreasing their oxidation or by enhancing synthesis, as alluded to before. Increased glycerolipid production has indeed been found after ethanol consumption[86]. Ethanol feeding was observed to enhance the activity of glycosyltransferase in the Golgi apparatus[87] and to increase the synthesis of the protein moiety of lipoproteins[83]. In some individuals, the response is markedly exaggerated (Figure 2.7) because of a fat rich diet[88–92] or because of some underlying abnormality of lipid or carbohydrate metabolism such as a forme fruste of essential hyperlipaemia[82,93,94], pancreatitis[95], diabetes or prediabetes[82,96], or

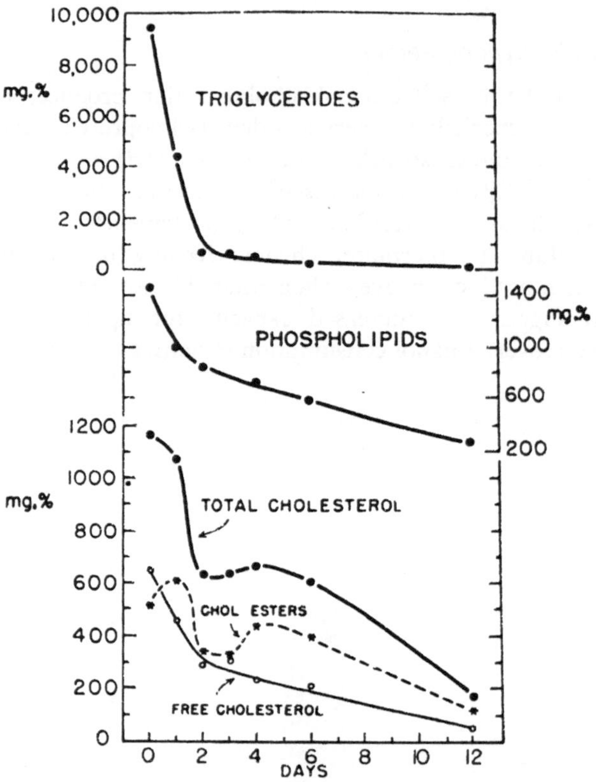

Figure 2.7 Changes in plasma lipid fractions during recovery from alcoholic hyperlipaemia[82]

an increased susceptibility to ethanol itself: indeed, whereas some subjects develop a comparable hyperlipaemia after ethanol and carbohydrate[97], others have a selective response[90]. The mechanism for the increased capacity of these patients to develop alcoholic hyperlipaemia remains unknown. Since ethanol consumption results in an increased capacity to secrete lipoproteins in response to a lipid load[84], one may wonder whether the difference in response to ethanol between some alcoholics and some individuals with type IV hyperlipaemia may be secondary, at least in part, to a difference in prior alcohol consumption.

Concerning the site of the ethanol effects, it is noteworthy that both in men and in rats, ethanol-induced hyperlipaemia results in increased concentrations of the various serum lipoprotein fractions, but the main change occurs in the lipoproteins of $d < 1.006$. In the postprandial state, this fraction includes very low density lipoproteins and chylomicrons. In patients with alcoholic hyperlipaemia, chylomicron-like particles have been observed in the fasting state[96]. In the rat rendered hyperlipaemic by ethanol feeding, the lipid/protein ratio of the $d < 1.006$ lipoproteins approaches that of chylomicrons[84]. However, the site of origin of these particles cannot be deduced with certainty from physical or chemical characteristics. Indeed, in other states of accelerated lipoprotein production, such as carbohydrate-induced hyperlipaemia, the lipid/protein ratio and particle size of the $d < 1.006$ lipoproteins increases even in the absence of dietary fat. The increase in serum lipoproteins of higher density both in man[92] and in rats[83] indicates that the hyperlipaemia is not merely of intestinal origin and that the liver participates in this process.

The possibility still remains that, after alcohol feeding, the intestine releases more lipid into the lymph, either by decreasing oxidation of fatty acids or by increasing the synthesis of lipids from sources other than dietary fat[98,99]. A decreased production of $^{14}CO_2$ from labelled fatty acids by intestinal slices after an acute load of alcohol[100] and an increased incorporation of these fatty acids into intestinal triglycerides by slices obtained from rats fed ethanol[101] have been reported. To what extent these alterations contribute to alcoholic hyperlipaemia is unknown. Mistilis and Ockner[102] have shown that intraduodenal infusion of 10 % ethanol to the fasted rat in a dose of 5 g/kg produces a mild increase in the very low density lipoprotein output in the lymph. They postulated that this increase in non-dietary lymph lipid could contribute to the hyperlipaemia, although the peak serum rise actually preceded the maximum increase in intestinal lymph lipids. Furthermore, lymph lipoproteins can derive in part from plasma lipoproteins[103]. Moreover, although a single intragastric administration of a diet containing ethanol (3 g/kg) increased both intestinal lymph flow and lipid output in rats not previously fed alcohol, postprandial hyperlipaemia was not produced under these conditions[84]. Actually, the acute load of an ethanol-containing diet did not increase lymph lipid output in rats fed alcohol for several weeks, compared to their pair-fed controls; however, marked hyperlipaemia developed in these alcohol-fed rats. Moreover, when a similar lymph lipid load was infused intravenously to alcohol-pretreated and control rats with diversion of intestinal lymph, the alcohol-fed rats developed hyperlipaemia. If lymph depletion was not prevented by intravenous replacement, hepatic and plasma lipids decreased, and alcoholic hyperlipaemia did not occur. This indicates that, although an adequate supply of dietary lipids represents a permissive factor needed to induce alcoholic hyperlipaemia in the rat, changes in lymph lipid output do not seem to play a major role in the lipaemic effect of ethanol and that the site of origin of the increased production of serum lipoprotein is a non-intestinal one, most likely hepatic. Similarly, the contribution of lymph lipids to the steatosis appears to be a minor one[104].

The mechanism for the increase in lipids other than triglycerides in the course of alcoholic hyperlipaemia remains unknown. This is due partly to the fact that the role of cholesterol and phospholipids in serum lipoproteins has not been clarified. The changes in the plasma concentration of these lipids could be a reflection of variations in the mass of serum lipoprotein secondary to changes in triglyceride transport. As discussed before, ethanol also increases cholesterogenesis in the liver[77] and in the small intestine[105].

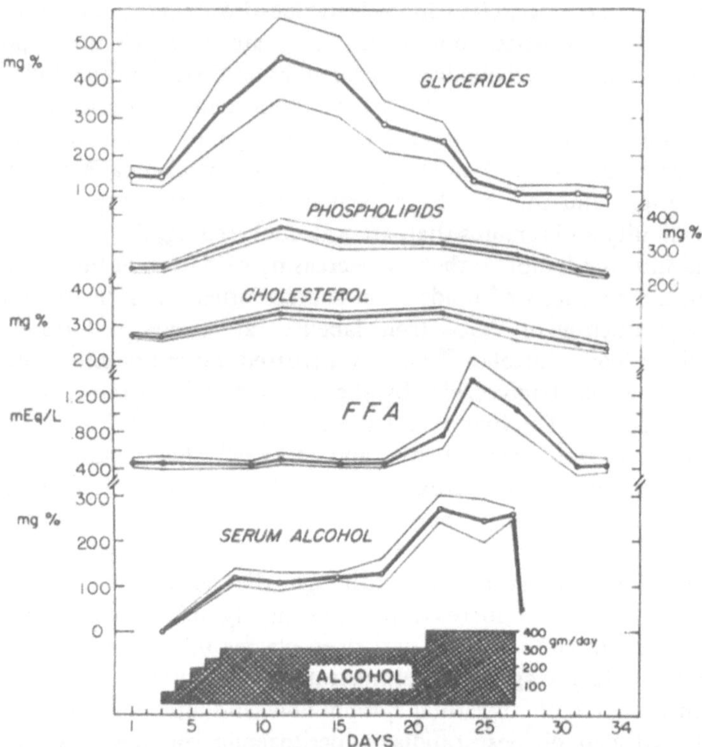

Figure 2.8 Effect of prolonged alcohol intake on serum lipids in seven chronic alcoholic individuals (average results ± SE of the mean)[79]

After the initial development of fatty liver associated with hyperlipaemia, the blood lipids return towards normal[79] (Figure 2.8). Progressive deterioration of liver function, including lipoprotein production and secretion, could be responsible, and may secondarily aggravate fat accumulation in the liver. Indeed, high concentrations of ethanol exert depressive effects on lipoprotein secretion (contrasting to the adaptive response to the lower ones) which may be a reflection of a hepatotoxic effect and will be discussed in the following section.

2.3.4 Miscellaneous changes in microsomal functions

Hepatic microsomes are responsible for a large number of metabolic functions some of which have been found to be affected by either acute or chronic ethanol consumption. For instance, some researchers[106] report that ethanol prevents hyperbilirubinaemia of the newborn, an effect attributed to induction of microsomal uridine-diphosphate-glucuronyl transferase[107]. Others found no bilirubin change[108,109]; in any event, practical applications are limited by possible toxic effects of ethanol on the fetus (fetal alcohol syndrome).

As discussed before, alcohol ingestion may also severely affect glucose metabolism. Contrasting with the lack of effect of other microsomal inducers on microsomal glucose-6-phosphatase, both short[110] and long term[111] ethanol feeding significantly increased this activity. Another study[112] failed to reveal such an effect, but this may have been due to the diet used. Indeed, as discussed elsewhere[111], diets high in fructose or sucrose increase glucose-6-phosphatase activity. Fitch and Chaikoff[113] pointed out the importance of the type of carbohydrate: a 60 % fructose diet increased glucose-6-phosphatase activity, but a 60 % glucose diet did not. In the study of Ishii *et al.*[111] the carbohydrate preparation used (Dextri-Maltose), is broken down to glucose, and was expected not to interfere with the assessment of the effect of ethanol on glucose-6-phosphatase activity, whereas in the study of Carter and Isselbacher[112] sucrose was used, and it provided 41 % of total calories in the control diet, but only 5 % in the ethanol diet. This difference may account for a high glucose-6-phosphatase activity in control animals and an apparent lack of ethanol effect. Thus, when the carbohydrate content is taken into account, it is clear that ethanol feeding increases glucose-6-phosphatase activity, but the significance of this effect with regard to carbohydrate metabolism has not been established.

2.4 INJURIOUS MANIFESTATIONS OF THE ALTERATIONS OF LIVER METABOLISM ASSOCIATED WITH ALCOHOLISM

In its milder form, alcoholic liver disease is characterized by accumulation of excess fat in the liver, so-called fatty liver. When a number of liver cells die and this necrosis causes inflammation, one is dealing with alcoholic hepatitis, a more severe form of alcoholic liver injury associated with a mortality ranging from 10–30 % depending on the series. Eventually, scarring by fibrous tissue occurs and its excess distorts the normal architecture of the liver, fibrous bands dissect the organ and alter its function. The term cirrhosis characterizes this more severe, irreversible form of alcoholic liver injury.

Because the fatty liver is a very common complication of alcoholism and usually fully reversible, it has been considered as benign. However, already at the fatty liver stage, signs of hepatic injury are evident particularly in the mitochondria and in the capacity of the liver to export proteins. One must therefore wonder whether the fatty liver must be considered as a serious condition which in predisposed individuals may be a precursor to the hepatitis and cirrhosis. Furthermore it has now become clear that the entire spectrum of alcohol-induced liver injury can be attributed to ethanol itself, in part, through the metabolic derangements produced by this compound, rather than to the malnutrition associated with alcoholism which was originally thought to be exclusively the cause of liver injury observed in the alcoholic.

2.4.1 Alcoholic fatty liver

2.4.1.1 Origin and mechanisms of fat deposition in the liver

Figure 2.9 illustrates the main mechanisms whereby fatty liver can develop, namely excessive supply of lipids to the liver or interference with lipid disposition. As shown in Figure 2.9, lipids which accumulate in the liver can originate from three main sources: dietary lipids, which reach the bloodstream

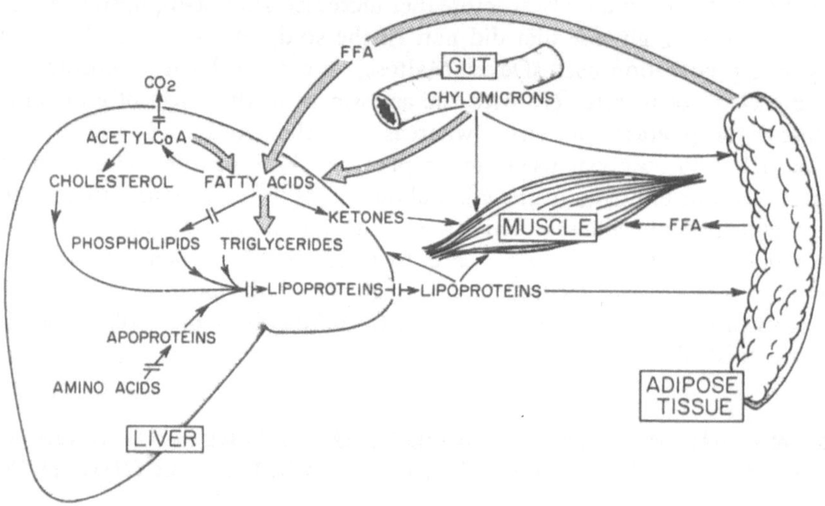

Figure 2.9 Possible mechanisms of fatty liver production through either increase (→) or decrease (⊣⊢→) of lipid transport and metabolism

as chylomicrons, adipose tissue lipids, which are transported to the liver as free fatty acids (FFA), and lipids synthesized in the liver itself. These fatty acids of various sources can accumulate in the liver because of a large number of metabolic disturbances, represented schematically in Figure 2.9. The four major disturbances which have been proposed are (a) increased peripheral fat mobilization, (b) decreased hepatic lipoprotein release, (c) decreased lipid oxidation in the liver, and (d) enhanced hepatic lipogenesis. Depending on the experimental conditions, any of the three sources and the four mechanisms can be implicated.

During consumption of ethanol with lipid-containing diets, the fatty acids which accumulate in the liver are derived primarily from dietary fatty acids, whereas when ethanol is given with a low fat diet endogenously synthesized fatty acids are deposited in the liver[21–23]. Some of these effects can be considered as consequences of the metabolism of ethanol in the liver. Depending on the metabolic state of the animal both decreased lipid oxidation and enhanced lipogenesis can be linked to ethanol oxidation and the associated increased generation of NADH as discussed before in this chapter (section 2.2.1.2).

In *fasted* rats, ethanol did not stimulate fatty acid synthesis[114]. Moreover, in rats given one large, *sublethal dose* of ethanol, it was observed that fatty acids resembling those of adipose tissue accumulate in the liver[22,115]. Experimental procedures or agents which reduce the normal rate of peripheral fat mobilization, i.e. adrenalectomy, spinal cord trans-section, or ganglioplegic drugs, prevent or decrease this type of hepatic fat accumulation[115–117]. More direct approaches, however, such as studies in rats with prelabelled epididymal fat pads yielded conflicting information, with evidence for increased[118] or unchanged[119] fatty acid mobilization. Similarly, in rats, one large dose of ethanol has been reported to result in increased[115,120] or unchanged[121] circulating levels of free fatty acids. In man, even with amounts of ethanol as large as 300 g/day, the concentration of circulating free fatty acids did not increase; it rose only after ingestion of very large doses of ethanol (400 g/day)[79] (see Figure 2.8). In short-term studies, ethanol administration produced a fall in the level of circulating free fatty acids in man[2,122] with reduced peripheral venous–arterial differences in free fatty acids[2], decreased free fatty acid turnover[123] and concomitant reduction in circulating glycerol[124]. This effect of ethanol upon free fatty acid mobilization from adipose tissue was found to be mediated by acetate[125] (Figure 2.10). Acetate is the end product of ethanol metabolism in the liver (see Figure 2.1) and is released into the bloodstream. Since stressful doses of ethanol probably both stimulate fatty acid mobilization (via catecholamine release) and depress it (via the acetate produced), the net effect may depend upon the particular experimental conditions. This may account for some of the apparent contradictions of the literature.

Actually, whether enhanced peripheral fat mobilization is responsible for hepatic fat accumulation after one large sublethal dose of ethanol in the rat is of little clinical relevance after *chronic* ethanol consumption. Under the latter conditions, the fatty acids deposited in the liver do not derive primarily from adipose tissue[21,22].

Thus, the main event leading to the development of the alcoholic fatty liver can be summarized as follows: ethanol, which has an almost 'obligatory' hepatic metabolism, replaces the fatty acids as a normal fuel for the hepatic mitochondria. This results in fatty acid accumulation, directly because of decreased lipid oxidation and indirectly because one way for the liver to dispose of excess hydrogen generated by ethanol oxidation is to synthesize more lipids. Fatty acids derived from adipose tissue accumulate in the liver only when very large amounts of ethanol are given. The lipids increase in the liver despite the fact that the transport mechanism via release of lipoproteins from the liver into the blood stream is stimulated by ethanol, at least during the initial state of intoxication.

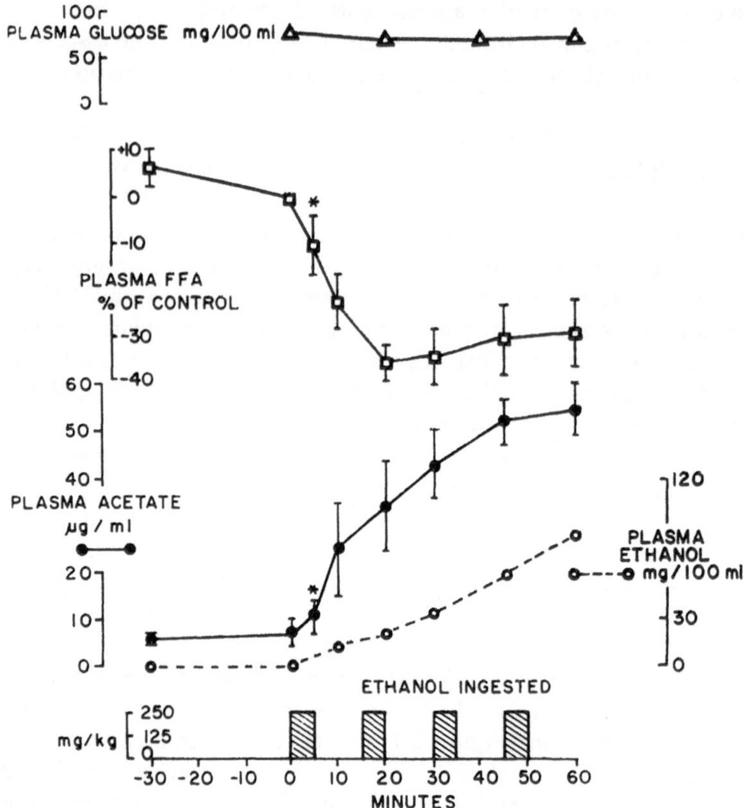

Figure 2.10 Effect of oral administration of sodium acetate on plasma glucose (△), free fatty acids (□), and acetate (●). Points represent average values for five volunteers. Variation is expressed as SEM. Plasma FFA at zero time averaged 572 ± 91 μeq/l[125]

2.4.1.2 Alcohol as a direct cause of the fatty liver

Each gram of ethanol provides 7.1 calories which means that 586 ml (20 oz) of 86 proof (43 %v/v) beverage represents about 1500 calories or a half of two-thirds of the normal daily caloric requirement. Therefore, the alcoholic has a much reduced demand for food to fulfill his caloric needs. Since alcoholic beverages do not contain significant amounts of protein, vitamins and minerals, the intake of these nutrients may become readily borderline or insufficient. Economic factors may also reduce the consumption of nutrient-rich food by the alcoholic. In addition to acting as 'empty' or 'naked' calories, alcohol can result in malnutrition by interfering with the normal processes of food digestion and absorption[126]. For all these reasons, deficiency diseases readily develop in the alcoholic. In rodents, severely deficient diets result in liver damage even in the absence of alcohol. Extrapolation from these animal results to man led to the belief that in alcoholics, the liver disease is due not to ethanol but solely to the nutritional deficiencies and that given an adequate diet alcohol is merely acting by its caloric contribution and that it is not more toxic than a similar caloric load derived from fats or starches[127]. This opinion prevailed, despite some statistical evidence gathered both in France[128] and in Germany[129] which indicated that the incidence of liver disease correlated with the amount of alcohol consumed rather than with deficiencies in the diet. A major challenge to the concept of the exclusively nutritional origin of alcoholic liver disease arose from an improvement of the method of alcohol feeding to experimental animals. Indeed, when the conventional alcohol feeding procedure is used, namely when ethanol is given as part of the drinking water, rats usually refuse to take a sufficient amount of ethanol to develop liver injury, if the diet is adequate. This aversion of rats to ethanol was counteracted by the introduction of the new technique of feeding of ethanol as part of a nutritionally adequate totally liquid diet[79,130,131]. With this procedure, ethanol intake was sufficient to produce a fatty liver despite an adequate diet. This technique is now widely adopted for the study of the pathogenesis of the fatty liver in the rat. In addition to the fatty liver, ethanol dependence developed in these rats, as witnessed by typical withdrawal seizures after cessation of alcohol intake[132].

Having established an etiological role for ethanol in the pathogenesis of the experimental fatty liver, the question of its importance for the development of human pathology remained. To determine whether ingestion of alcohol, in amounts comparable to those consumed by chronic alcoholics, is capable of injuring the liver even in the absence of dietary deficiencies, volunteers (with or

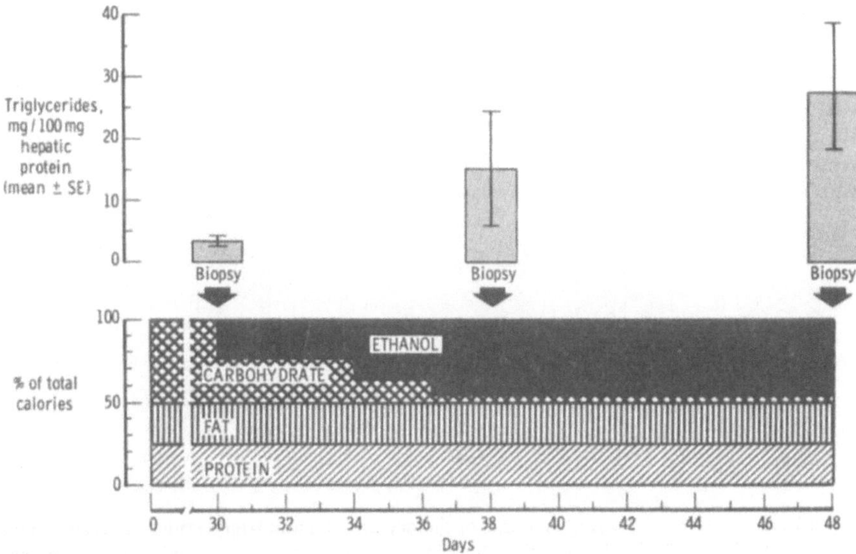

Figure 2.11 Effect of ethanol on hepatic triglycerides in five volunteers given a high-protein, low-fat diet[320]

without a history of alcoholism) were given a variety of non-deficient diets under metabolic ward conditions, with ethanol either as a supplement to the diet or as an isocaloric substitution for carbohydrates[45,79,130]. In all these individuals, ethanol administration resulted in fatty liver development which was evident on both morphological examination and by direct measurement of the lipid content of the liver biopsies which revealed a rise in triglyceride concentration up to 15-fold (Figure 2.11).

2.4.1.3 The influence of dietary factors

(*a*) *Role of dietary fat* — As discussed before, alcohol ingestion leads to deposition in the liver of dietary fat. This observation prompted an investigation into the role of the amount and kind of dietary fat in the pathogenesis of alcohol-induced liver injury. Rats were given liquid diets containing a normal amount of protein for rodents (18 % of total calories), with varying amounts of fat. Reduction in dietary fat to a level of 25 % (or less) of total calories was accompanied by a significant decrease in the steatosis induced by ethanol[133] (Figure 2.12). The importance of dietary fat was confirmed in volunteers: for a given alcohol intake, much more steatosis developed with diets of normal fat content than with a low fat diet[21]. In addition to the amount, the chain length of the dietary fatty acid is also important for the degree of fat deposition in the liver after alcohol feeding. Replacement of dietary triglycerides containing long-chain fatty acids (LCT) by fat containing medium-chain fatty acids (MCT)

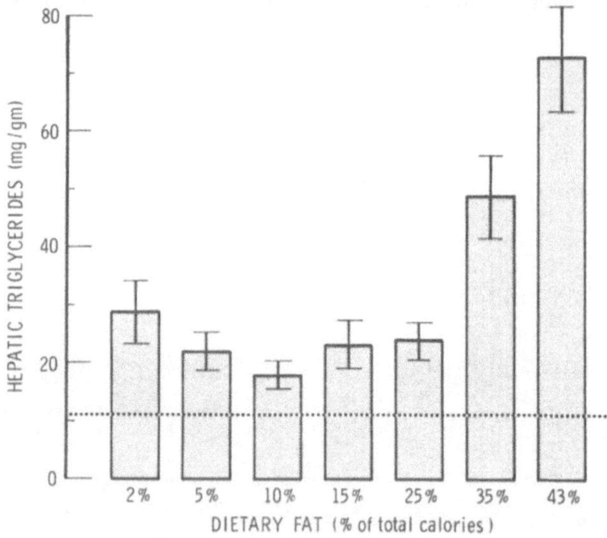

Figure 2.12 Effect of varying amounts of dietary fat. Hepatic triglycerides in seven groups of rats given ethanol (36 % of calories) with a diet of normal protein (18 % of calories). Average hepatic triglyceride concentration in the control animals is indicated by a dotted line[133]

markedly reduced the capacity of alcohol to produce a fatty liver in rats[14]. The propensity of medium-chain fatty acids to oxidation rather than to esterification most likely explains the reduction in alcoholic steatosis upon replacement of dietary long-chain fatty acids by medium-chain fatty acids.

(*b*) *Role of protein and lipotropic factors* (*choline and methionine*) — In perfused livers, ethanol was shown to increase choline uptake[134] but this was found to be unrelated to lipid accumulation[135]. In growing rats, deficiencies in dietary protein and lipotropic factors (choline and methionine) can produce fatty liver[127] but primates are far less susceptible to protein and lipotrope deficiency than rodents[136]. Clinically, treatment with choline of patients suffering from alcoholic liver injury has been found to be ineffective in the face of continued alcohol abuse[137] and, experimentally, massive supplementation with choline failed to prevent fatty liver produced by alcohol in volunteer subjects[138]. This is not surprising, since there is no evidence that a diet which is deficient in choline is deleterious to adult man. Unlike rat liver, human liver contains very little choline oxidase activity which may explain the species difference with regard to choline deficiency. The phospholipid content of the liver represents another key difference between the ethanol and choline deficiency fatty liver. After the administration of ethanol, hepatic phospholipids increase[130] whereas in the fatty liver produced by choline deficiency, they decrease[139]. Moreover, orotic acid which prevents the phospholipid decrease and the development of fatty liver due to choline deficiency, had no such effects after ethanol[140]. Furthermore, hepatic ATP decreased after chronic ethanol feeding[141–143] but was unaffected in choline deficiency[144]. Conversely, hepatic carnitine is decreased by choline deficiency[145] but increased after ethanol feeding[146]. Moreover, ethanol-induced fatty liver is associated with increased circulatory lipoproteins and enhanced incorporation of [^{14}C]lysine in lipoproteins[83], whereas the opposite occurs with choline deficiency[147]. Ultrastructurally, the lesions also differ[43,148]. Thus, hepatic injury induced by choline deficiency appears to be primarily an experimental disease of rats with little, if any, relevance to alcoholic liver injury particularly in humans. Even in the rats, massive choline supplementation failed to prevent fully the ethanol-induced lesion, whether alcohol was administered acutely[149] or chronically[150]. Alcohol has been reported to either aggravate[151] or attenuate[152] choline-induced liver injury.

Protein deficiency may affect the liver but this has not yet been clearly delineated in human adults. In children, protein deficiency leads to steatosis, one of the manifestations of kwashiorkor. In adolescent baboons, however, protein restriction to 7 % of total calories (as part of a low fat diet, 14 % of calories) did not result in liver injury on either biochemical analysis or light and electronmicroscopic examination even after 19 months[153]. Conversely, an excess of protein was not capable of preventing ethanol from producing fat accumulation in human volunteers, as illustrated in Figure 2.11. In that study, dietary protein represented 25 % of total calories, or two and a half times the recommended amount. Thus, even in the absence of protein deficiency, ethanol is capable, in man, of producing striking changes in the liver. Severe protein deficiency (4 % of total calories) also produced steatosis in the baboon[153]. Similar lesions were reported in the rhesus monkey[154]. When protein deficiency is present, it could potentiate the effect of ethanol. Indeed administration of ethanol with a diet deficient in protein and lipotropic factors had more pronounced effects than that of either factor alone[23,155], at least in rodents.

The ultrastructural abnormalities produced by protein deficiency, however,[156,157] differ from those resulting from alcohol[43,158]. Furthermore, clinical protein malnutrition is associated with characteristic plasma amino acid abnormalities, including a depression of branched-chain amino acids[159]. The alcohol-induced liver injury in the well-fed baboon was associated with opposite amino acid changes[160]. Of course, plasma amino acid abnormalities in chronic alcoholism may reflect a complex interaction of many factors: nutrition, alcoholic liver disease, alcohol-induced injury in other organs and associated disease states. The frequent concurrence of chronic alcoholism and nutritional deficiency makes the separation of these variables especially difficult. However, branched-chain amino acids (BCAA) and α-amino-n-butyric acid (AANB) were found to be increased 2–3-fold and 7-fold respectively in the plasma of baboons fed alcohol as 50 % of total calories[160]. These amino acids are all depressed when measured in protein deficiency. Following intestinal bypass for obesity, decreased absorption of dietary protein is observed[161]. In such patients, plasma BCAA, phenylalanine, threonine and lysine are decreased while plasma serine and glycine, both non-essential amino acids, are increased.

In a limited number of patients studied at the Bronx Veterans Administration Hospital with a diagnosis of chronic alcoholism and alcoholic liver disease, plasma amino acid patterns similar to those described in patients by Zinneman *et al.*[162], Ning *et al.*[163], and Siegel *et al.*[164] were found with depressions of BCAA, normal levels of AANB and slight depressions of plasma proline[165]. The increased AANB relative to BCAA was considered characteristic of changes of plasma amino acids in alcoholic liver disease[165]. The AANB/BCAA ratio was altered independently of malnutrition and degree of liver injury and it correlated well with various criteria of alcoholism.

Possible interactions of ethanol and protein nutrition were suggested by the observation that ethanol feeding increases the activities of hepatic cystathionine synthetase and S-methyl-tetrahydrofolate homocysteine methyltransferase, which may impair mechanisms for methionine conservation in protein deficiency[166]. To what extent such abnormalities contribute to the ethanol-induced liver lesions remains to be assessed.

2.4.2 Transitional lesions from alcohol fatty liver to hepatitis

2.4.2.1 Accumulation of proteins in the alcoholic fatty liver and impairment of lipoprotein and protein export

Recent studies have indicated that in addition to fat accumulation, the alcoholic fatty liver is characterized by striking deposition of protein[167]. In the early stages of fatty liver development, this protein accumulation was found to be as important quantitatively as that of fat and contributed to a similar extent to the hepatomegaly which developed after chronic alcoholism (Figure 2.13).

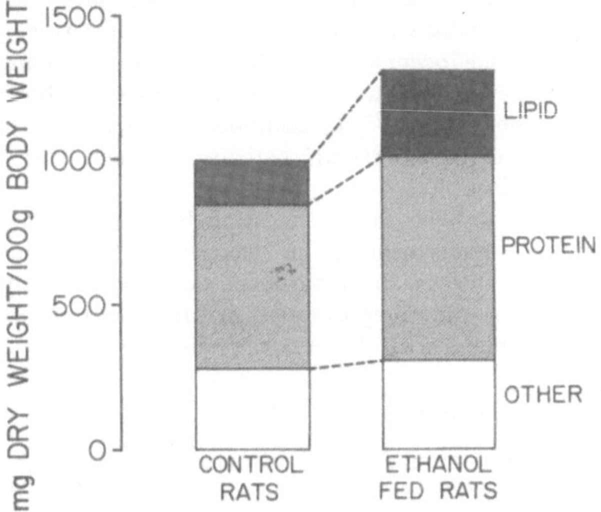

Figure 2.13 Effect of ethanol feeding on hepatic dry weight, lipid and protein contents[167]

Although increasing organelle proteins (mitochondria and microsomes) do contribute to the total increase, the major fraction of the proteins is deposited in the cytosol. The nature of all the proteins which accumulate in the cytosol have not been elucidated and up to now, increases were found in export proteins such as albumin and transferrin[168] but not in constituent proteins of the cytosol. This observation led to the hypothesis that one of the early lesions induced by chronic alcoholism may be the interference with the capacity of the liver to export proteins. Consistent with this concept was the finding of a decrease in hepatic microtubulin believed to be implicated in the export of proteins from the liver[168] and delayed serum albumin labelling after administration of labelled amino acids[168]. The retention of protein may be responsible for the 'ballooning' of the hepatocytes, a common morphological alteration found in alcoholic liver injury, and the decrease in plasma transferrin in alcoholics with or without cirrhosis[169].

In addition to protein release, lipoprotein secretion is also affected. Contrasting with the hyperlipaemia, which is commonly associated with the administration of moderate to large amounts of ethanol, an extremely high dose has been reported to decrease serum triglycerides[170], very low density lipoproteins[171], high density lipoproteins[172], and the incorporation of glucosamine into the carbohydrate moiety of serum lipoproteins[173] in the rat.

In volunteers, chronic ethanol administration resulted in initial hyperlipaemia[79]. However, blood lipid content declined after 2–3 weeks (see Figure 2.8), implying that lipoprotein output falls with progressing alcoholic liver disease. This concept is supported by the study of Marzo *et al.*[174] who correlated serum lipids with the histological stage in 90 alcoholics. Peak serum lipid values were found during the stage of fatty metamorphosis. During the succeeding stages of steatosis and interstitial chronic hepatitis, a progressive decrease in serum lipids occurred. The decrease was predominantly in the triglyceride and cholesterol fractions. In well-established cirrhosis, circulating lipoproteins are generally low[175]. In addition, α-lipoproteins are absent by electrophoresis in sera from cirrhotic patients[176], which illustrates another lipoprotein abnormality.

The progression of liver injury to alcoholic hepatitis in primates is associated with an enhancement of the steatosis[177]. Our preliminary observations also indicate that serum lipoproteins decrease with advancing liver damage[178], suggesting the disappearance of the compensatory role that alcoholic hyperlipaemia exerts on the development of fatty liver.

2.4.2.2 Alterations in protein synthesis

After chronic alcohol consumption, the membranes of the rough endoplasmic reticulum (RER) appear decreased on electronmicroscopy[43,45,158,179], and this reduction has now been substantiated by chemical fractionation[47]. One of the main functions of the rough endoplasmic reticulum is protein synthesis. The subject of the interaction of ethanol with protein synthesis is complex and not fully elucidated, especially after chronic ethanol consumption. The effects may actually differ after acute and chronic ethanol administration. The administration of a single dose of ethanol to rats and the incubation of liver tissue in ethanol-containing media generally result in inhibitory effects on the production of liver and plasma proteins. Sometimes, these acute effects can be attributed to a direct action of high ethanol concentration[180,181] or they depend on the route of administration[182]. In other experimental situations, in which the ethanol concentrations achieved are compatible with moderate intoxication, the inhibitory effects appear to be associated with a relative lack of amino acids[185–187]: this inhibition of hepatic production of plasma proteins mimics that of fasting, is aggravated by fasting and is abolished by amino acid supplementation[183–186]. A third experimental situation in which ethanol was shown to exert inhibitory effects on protein synthesis was obtained when liver slices (from fed or fasted rats) were incubated in a medium containing ethanol and only trace amounts of amino acids[187]. The decreased incorporation of amino acid into the liver protein could result from reduced uptake[188–190] and/or decreased synthesis. Chronic ethanol consumption has been reported to be accompanied by enhanced liver protein synthesis[180,191]. Only when ethanol feeding was associated with obvious signs of undernutrition was decreased protein production observed[192,193]. Under those conditions, ethanol feeding failed to sustain body growth and did not produce fatty liver and hepatic enlargement. Those results, therefore, are not directly relevant to the prevailing clinical situation of the alcoholic characterized by fatty liver and hepatomegaly. However, this clinical combination of fatty liver and hepatomegaly was reproduced when we administered ethanol in liquid diets[130,131]. As discussed before, the hepatomegaly is due to the retention of both fat and protein. Alteration of protein synthesis under these conditions is still being investigated.

2.4.2.3 Development of mitochondrial injury

In addition to the alterations of the rough endoplasmic reticulum, alcoholics are known to have profound hepatic mitochondrial changes[194] which are associated with increased serum activity of the intramitochondrial enzyme glutamate dehydrogenase[195]. From these observations, however, it was impossible to assess whether the mitochondrial changes were a direct result of chronic ethanol intake or were secondary to other factors such as dietary deficiencies. Recent studies have incriminated alcohol itself as the responsible agent and have clarified some functional counterparts of the ultrastructural lesions.

(*a*) *Ultrastructural changes of mitochondria* — Chronic alcohol consumption results in striking mitochondrial alterations which include swelling and disfiguration of mitochondria, disorientation of the cristae, and intramitochondrial crystalline inclusions[194,196]. Similarly, in the rat, isocaloric substitution of ethanol for carbohydrate in otherwise adequate diets leads to enlargement and alterations of the configurations of the mitochondria[43] indicating that ethanol itself or one of its metabolites causes the alterations rather than dietary deficiencies. Mitochondrial changes similar to those seen in chronic alcoholics were also produced by isocaloric substitution of ethanol for carbohydrate in baboons[153] and in man, both in alcoholics[45,158] and in non-alcoholics[138]. Degenerated mitochondria were conspicuous and the debris of these degraded organelles was also found within autophagic vacuoles and residual vacuolated bodies[179]. The striking structural changes of the mitochondria are associated with corresponding functional abnormalities.

(*b*) *Alterations of mitochondrial functions; alcoholic ketoacidosis* — These injured mitochondria have a reduction in cytochrome a and b content[197] and in succinic dehydrogenase activity[197,198] although in one study[199] succinic dehydrogenase activity measured in total liver homogenates was reported to be increased in ethanol-fed rats. The respiratory capacity of the mitochondria was found to be depressed[200–203] using pyruvate succinate and acetaldehyde as substrates. Oxidation of other substrates was also found to be reduced in mitochondria of ethanol-fed rats, except for α-glycerophosphate, the oxidation of which was reported by some to be increased[204] or unchanged[205], whereas others found it to be decreased[202].

Oxidative phosphorylation was found to be selectively altered at site I[206]. Since the structural changes of the mitochondria persist, the question arose as to whether these in turn could be responsible for some alterations in lipid metabolism beyond those which were attributed to the altered redox change. The first indication that ethanol consumption may result in more persistent metabolic changes came from the observation that alcohol ingestion is associated with a progressive increase in ketonaemia and ketonuria, which was most pronounced in the fasting[207]. The ketonaemia may aggravate the acidosis of the hyperlactacidaemia[79], and on occasion may lead to severe alcoholic ketoacidosis[208,209]. The capacity for ethanol to produce ketonaemia was found to be greater than that of fat itself, provided however that fat was present in the diet. Thus, fat seems to play a permissive role[207]. Mitochondria obtained from ethanol-fed rats, when incubated *in vitro*, even in the absence of ethanol, display decreased capacity to oxidize fatty acids, but enhanced β-oxidation which is possibly responsible for the increased ketogenesis[210]. Decreased fatty acid oxidation, whether as a function of the reduced citric acid cycle activity (secondary to the altered redox potential) as discussed before, or whether as a consequence of permanent changes in mitochondrial structure (as emphasized in this paragraph) offers the most likely explanation for the deposition of fat in the liver after chronic alcohol ingestion, especially fat derived from the diet[21–24]. It is noteworthy that high concentrations of acetaldehyde, the product of ethanol metabolism, mimic the defects produced by chronic ethanol consumption on oxidative phosphorylation at site I[211]. One may wonder to what extent chronic exposure to acetaldehyde is the cause for the defect observed after chronic ethanol consumption. Alterations of acetaldehyde metabolism associated with alcoholism have been discussed in Chapter 1. As has been pointed out, alcoholics may exhibit higher acetaldehyde levels than non-alcoholics for a given ethanol load and blood level. It is therefore not unreasonable to speculate that exposure to high acetaldehyde levels may in turn affect mitochondrial function and result in the vicious cycle depicted in Figure 1.8 in Chapter 1.

There are of course other possible mechanisms for increased acetaldehyde levels and aggravation of mitochondrial injury. Several studies of blood acetaldehyde levels following oral ingestion of various alcoholic beverages have been performed. Majchrowicz and Mendelson[212] showed that acetaldehyde levels in the blood of chronic alcoholic patients were higher after bourbon whisky ingestion than after grain ethyl alcohol and attributed this difference to the acetaldehyde content of the bourbon. Truitt[213] followed levels of acetaldehyde after oral administration of vodka that resulted in modest elevations of blood ethanol; slightly higher levels of acetaldehyde were found in alcoholic subjects when compared with non-alcoholics. However, Freund[214] could find no measurable amounts of serum acetaldehyde after oral ingestion of an aqueous acetaldehyde solution 10 times in excess of the concentration found in most bourbons.

Since the amount of acetaldehyde in even the 'dirtiest' of alcoholic beverages is about one-thousandth the amount produced by ethanol oxidation in the liver, it is probably not the acetaldehyde in the beverage that leads to higher blood acetaldehyde levels after ingestion, but more likely an effect of other congeners of the beverages. These congeners may somehow interfere with acetaldehyde metabolism initiating a vicious cycle of mitochondrial impairment which further decreases acetaldehyde catabolism. For example, Rubenstein *et al.*[215] found that pyrogallol (1 and 10 mM concentrations), a metabolic product of gallic acid found in tannins, inhibits rat liver aldehyde dehydrogenase activity *in vitro*. *In vivo*, Collins *et al.*[216] have shown that pyrogallol (250 mg/kg, i.p.) increases acetaldehyde blood levels in rats when it is given 1 h before ethanol (3 g/kg i.p.). Higher aliphatic aldehydes were found to inhibit mitochondrial acetaldehyde metabolism[217]. Thus elevated acetaldehyde levels following ingestion of alcoholic beverages (discussed above) when compared with acetaldehyde levels following an ethanol–acetaldehyde mixture suggest an effect of congeners on acetaldehyde metabolism. When taken in relatively moderate amounts for a short period of time, the congener content of alcoholic beverages did not appear to affect the degree of steatosis[218], but the effects of higher amounts of congeners in conjunction with a greater alcohol intake over a longer period of time have not been extensively studied. Some evidence was recently presented that prolonged consumption of whisky might exert more strikingly undesirable effects on the liver than pure ethanol[219], and that certain alcoholic beverages, particularly brandy, were more toxic to liver cell cultures than pure ethanol[220].

2.4.2.4 Various effects of alcohol upon liver and serum enzymes

Alcohol abuse is often associated with reciprocal liver and serum enzyme changes which again illustrates the hepatotoxicity of ethanol and suggests that parenchymal injury often complicates so-called 'simple fatty liver'. Indeed, serum isocitric dehydrogenase and ornithine carbamyltransferase activities increased after ethanol ingestion[221], whereas hepatic isocitric dehydrogenase was reduced[222]. Serum glutamyl transpeptidase activity was commonly found increased in alcoholics[223–226], probably as a non-specific witness of liver injury, since this enzyme is increased in many types of liver diseases[227]. In man, serum transaminases are also increased after ethanol administration[138,228], reflecting either liver or muscle damage, or both. In rats given ethanol, hepatic glutamic–pyruvic transferase activity was also found to be decreased[229]. Hepatic tryptophan oxygenase increased after acute ethanol administration *in vivo*[230,231], but decreased after chronic ethanol consumption[231], or when isolated livers were perfused with ethanol *in vitro*[232]. The latter effect may be secondary to the acidosis produced by ethanol[232]. Hepatic glucagon-responsive adenyl cyclase (but not the epinephrine-responsive component) is activated by ethanol[233]. Hepatic coenzyme A was found to be reduced after ethanol by some[234] but not by others[235,236].

2.4.2.5 Alterations of the immune system in alcoholic liver injury

Serum immunoglobulins are usually increased in patients with alcoholic liver disease[237] and they include some autoantibodies[238]. In the last few years an increased body of evidence suggests that lymphocytes play an important role in tissue-damaging immune reactions and autoimmunity. A cell-mediated mechanism has also been implicated in some chronic liver diseases. Changes in cellular immunity that have been documented in chronic alcoholic liver disease include loss of delayed hypersensitivity[239], decreased 'active' T rosette formation[240], decreased lymphocyte response to phytohaemagglutinin[241], and a pronounced decrease in peripheral blood T lymphocytes in patients with alcoholic hepatitis[242], suggesting that there is a basic impairment in cell-mediated immunity in alcoholic liver diseases. The pathogenic role of the stimulation of lymphocytic transformation by ethanol in patients with alcoholic hepatitis[243] has not been clarified; it is relatively non-specific since ethanol produces a similar change in patients with chronic active hepatitis[243]. The observation of increased *in vitro* lymphocytic transformation in response to Australian antigen in patients with chronic alcoholic liver disease[244] is intriguing. In rats fed ethanol for three months, a delayed hypersensitivity to dinitrochlorobenzene was found[245]. However, it is not known whether immunological reactions actually play any role in the induction and perpetuation of alcoholic liver diseases. An altered cell-mediated immunity to liver antigens has been described in patients with alcoholic hepatitis using either autologous liver[243], normal human liver[246], or alcoholic hyaline[247]. Finally it has recently been shown that lymphocytes from baboons with alcoholic hepatitis are cytotoxic against autologous liver cells in tissue culture[248]. These observations suggest that immunological mechanisms may be involved in the perpetuation of hepatic damage produced by alcohol, and while they do not provide direct support for this possibility they justify further investigation directed at determining the role of immunological factors in the development and progression of alcoholic liver disease, keeping in mind however that ethanol has more than one effect on the human immune system, as demonstrated by the inhibition, by alcohol, of bone marrow granulocyte colonies[249]. Other bone marrow effects of alcohol are discussed in Chapter 8.

2.4.3 Alcoholic hepatitis and cirrhosis

It has been known for a long time that alcoholics may display liver complications of a varying degree of severity ranging from the still reversible fatty liver to the alcoholic hepatitis and finally irreversible cirrhosis. It is generally believed that alcoholic cirrhosis (characterized by extensive scarring or fibrosis) may be, at least in part, a consequence of the necrosis and inflammation associated with the alcoholic hepatitis. Whether the fatty liver is a precursor for the hepatitis has been less well accepted (Figure 2.14). As has

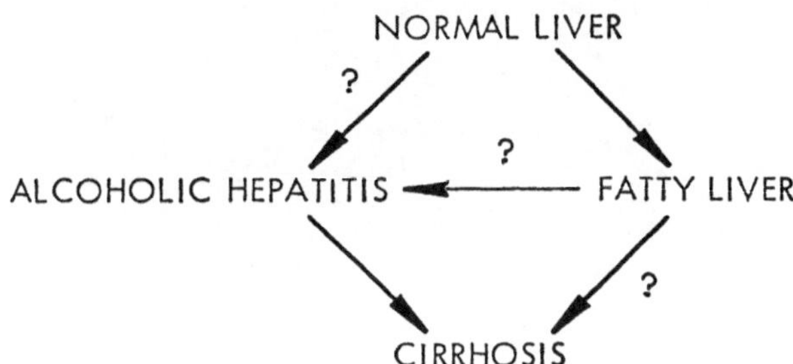

Figure 2.14 Possible links between the three types of liver injury in the alcoholic

been pointed out, although hepatic fat accumulation by itself may be harmless, it reflects a severe metabolic disturbance in the liver. It is possible that this disturbance, when exaggerated, may eventually engender irreversible damage of the hepatocyte possibly through one of the mechanisms described under 'transitional lesions from fatty liver to alcoholic hepatitis'. Necrosis in turn could lead to inflammation, resulting in alcoholic hepatitis. Indeed, comparable electronmicroscopic changes of the mitochondria accompany alcoholic hepatitis[194] and the fatty liver, as described before (section 2.4.2.3). Alteration of the rough endoplasmic reticulum was also found in patients with alcoholic hepatitis[194]. Although the alcoholic fatty liver is not an inflammatory condition, and is distinguishable from alcoholic hepatitis by light microscopy, the remarkable similarity of the ultrastructural features in the hepatocytes suggests that the former may represent the precursor of the latter. Other fatty livers, however, such as that of kwashiorkor, do not undergo transformation to cirrhosis[250]. Moreover, rats fed alcohol in liquid diets, though they get a fatty liver, do not develop the more severe forms of liver injury seen in alcoholics, namely hepatitis and cirrhosis. We wondered therefore whether this failure might be due to the fact that in the rat, even when alcohol is given as part of a liquid diet, its intake does not exceed 36 % of total calories which corresponds to moderate consumption in man. Of potential importance was also the fact that whereas in the human, development of cirrhosis requires 5 to 20 years of steady drinking, the rat only lives about 2 years. To overcome this difficulty, we turned to the baboon, a species which is long-lived and phylogenetically closer to man than the rat. First, baboons were given a dose of ethanol similar to that of the rat (that is, 36 % of total calories) and again a fatty liver developed but no hepatitis or cirrhosis[153]. The dose of alcohol was then increased to 50 % of the total calories, taking advantage of the liquid diet technique first developed in the

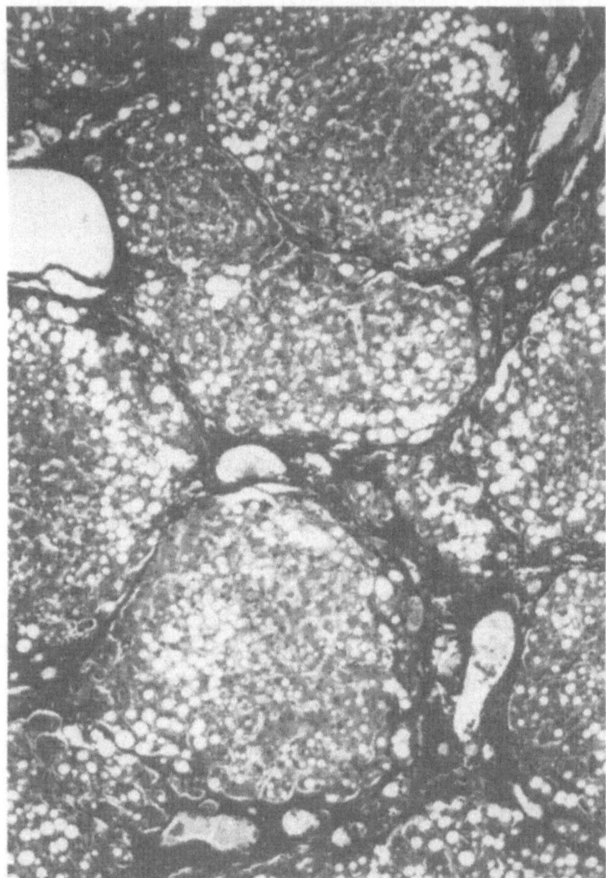

Figure 2.15 Cirrhosis in a baboon fed alcohol for 4 years. Fat is regularly distributed through hepatic nodules surrounded by connective tissue septa (chromotrope-aniline blue; ×60[177])

rat and now applied to the baboon[177]. With this diet alcohol intake was sufficient to result in periods of obvious inebriation. Upon interruption of alcohol administration, some withdrawal symptoms (such as seizures) were observed. These experiments are still in progress but at the writing of this chapter the following results have been observed[251]: 16 baboons fed the isocaloric control diet retained normal livers, whereas the animals given ethanol all developed excessive fat accumulation. In addition, five showed mild alcoholic hepatitis, and in six baboons studied for 2–4 years cirrhosis evolved (Figure 2.15). The diagnosis of alcoholic hepatitis was based on necrosis and inflammation; although sometime present, alcoholic hyaline of Mallory was not a required feature.

Alcoholic hyaline is considered characteristic (especially when centrolobular) of alcoholic hepatitis. By electronmicroscopy, however, it is also observed in primary biliary cirrhosis[252–254], hepatocellular carcinoma[255], Indian childhood cirrhosis[256], after griseofulvin treatment[257], and in extrahepatic tissues[258]. Moreover, hyaline is not necessary for diagnosis of alcoholic hepatitis[259,260]. Ultrastructurally, Mallory material is fibrillar[261–265], not bound by a limiting membrane and bears no resemblance to giant mitochondria[266] or any other subcellular organelle. Three fibrillar arrangements have been delineated. Fibrils may be arranged parallel to one another (type I) or have a random orientation (type II). In type III hyaline, fibrillar material may be part of a subcellular contractile system[266] but this is may represent degenerative forms of type I[266]. There is no concensus regarding the origin of the fibrillar material in alcohol hepatitis. Investigators have both found[261,267–269] and not found[253,263,266] a relationship between hyaline material and contiguous cell organelles. Recent data suggest that the fibrillar material may be part of a subcellular contractile system[266] but this is also controversial[269].

It has been widely postulated that the hepatitis, through the necrosis and inflammation, may in turn initiate scarring (or fibrosis), and, eventually cirrhosis. The earliest deposition of fibrous tissue appears to occur in the central zones of the hepatic lobule leading to what has been called 'central hyaline sclerosis', a lesion commonly associated with alcoholic hepatitis[270]. The appearance of this lesion appears to bridge the gap between alcoholic hepatitis and cirrhosis, and supports the theory that one is a precursor of the other. Similar lesions were present already at the fatty liver stage in the baboons fed alcohol. The magnitude of central hyaline sclerosis correlated with the degree of portal hypertension[271]. Thus, for the first time an experimental model has now been developed[177] which reproduces all the liver lesions observed in the alcoholic namely the fatty liver, the hepatitis and the cirrhosis[251].

These findings are significant, both with regard to the understanding of the pathogenesis of alcoholic liver injury and to its treatment. The experimental reproduction of the lesions of alcoholic hepatitis, and the demonstration for the first time in an experimental model, of its transition to cirrhosis supports the hypothesis that alcoholic hepatitis is a precursor of the cirrhotic lesion. Moreover, this study shows that animals which display fatty liver with a moderate alcohol intake developed hepatitis and cirrhosis when the alcohol content of the diet was increased; this supports the possibility that the fatty liver may be a precursor state for the hepatitis and cirrhosis. In addition, it was found that already in the fatty liver phase there was an increase in chemically detectable collagen, the protein which is the hallmark for the fibrosis characteristic of cirrhosis[6] and central sclerosis[271]. This was associated with enhanced activity of peptidylproline hydroxylase, an enzyme active in the initial step of fibrogenesis[6]. Increased activity of this enzyme was confirmed in livers of alcoholics[272,273]. This was associated with increased urinary hydroxyproline excretion in the case of alcoholic hepatitis[274].

Not all baboons fed ethanol progressed to cirrhosis; similarly, not all alcoholics develop this complication: the incidence varies depending on duration and dose of alcohol intake[275]. Regardless of possible predisposing factors, the baboon study clarifies the respective role of malnutrition and alcohol itself in the pathogenesis of the alcoholic hepatitis and cirrhosis. As discussed before, the fatty liver can be produced by ethanol *per se* in the absence of dietary deficiencies[45,79,130,138]. We now find that this also applies to the hepatitis and the cirrhosis. It is noteworthy that although fibrosis and cirrhosis have been produced before in subhuman primates after the feeding of deficient diet lacking in protein and/or choline[136,148,276] these animals did not develop hepatitis, a rather characteristic stage in alcoholic liver injury. Under different experimental conditions protein deficiency actually protected against carbon tetrachloride-induced cirrhosis[277], and diminished experimental fibroplasia in the rat[278]. In any event, one may conclude from our studies that despite the evidence produced before indicating that malnutrition can cause liver damage, alcohol itself is an indispensable etiological agent for the development of the typical complications observed in the alcoholic. An important corollary of this finding is the fact that adequate diet did not prevent the development of the alcoholic lesions. The therapeutic implication of this observation is that alcoholics cannot fully prevent the development or the aggravation of liver injury by maintaining an adequate diet unless they also control the degree of alcohol intake. It has been shown in the past by others and our own group that alcohol ingestion results in impaired digestion and malabsorption and that it produces intestinal injury. These aspects are discussed in detail by Baraona and Lindenbaum in Chapter 3 of this book. It is unlikely however that the effects described are of sufficient magnitude to offset the large excess of nutrients present in our baboon diet. Moreover, preliminary studies have indicated the absence of protein and fat malabsorption under our experimental conditions (Lindenbaum and Lieber, unpublished observation). Moreover, the increase in plasma BCAA found in these baboons[160] contrasts with the reduction after protein malnutrition[159] as mentioned before. The possibility that nutritional deficiencies may potentiate the effect of alcohol is presently being investigated in the baboon, since such a phenomenon was observed for the fatty liver in the rat[23]. Whether this applies to clinical conditions and particularly the development of cirrhosis is less clear.

Epidemiological studies of Lelbach[129,275] did not detect dietary insufficiency as a precondition for alcoholic cirrhosis: the incidence of cirrhosis correlated with the amount of alcohol consumed, not with history of dietary deficiencies; similar results were observed in France by Pequignot[128]. Recently, some have even suggested a lowered incidence of cirrhosis with dietary insufficiency[279], whereas others reached the opposite conclusion[280].

In our present state of knowledge, one is justified in stressing the importance of correcting nutrient deficiencies in the alcoholic who, as illustrated in Figure 2.16, is prone to malnutrition because of his poor diet (primary malnutrition) and also because ethanol alters the gastrointestinal tract and affects absorption and digestion, as discussed in Chapter 3 (secondary malnutrition). Moreover, malnutrition by itself alters intestinal functions (ter-

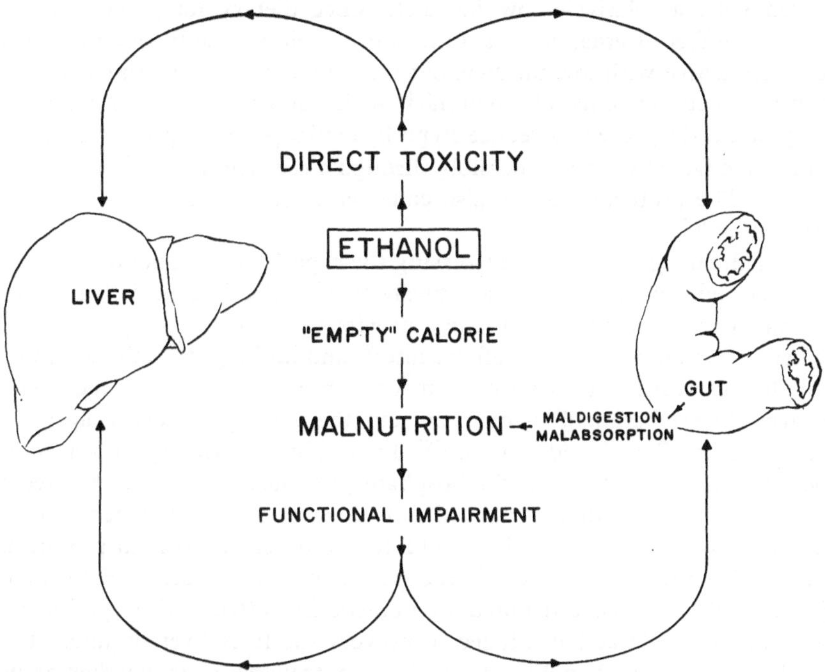

Figure 2.16 Interaction of direct toxicity of ethanol on liver and gut with malnutrition secondary to dietary deficiencies, maldigestion, and malabsorption[321]

tiary malnutrition). Ethanol may also deplete the liver of vitamins[281] and acetaldehyde, as discussed in the first chapter, may promote the breakdown of activated pyridoxine (quaternary malnutrition).

Thus, although ethanol has to be considered as a primary etiological agent in the development of alcoholic liver injury, malnutrition, which may play a potentiating role, and is often present in the alcoholic, should be corrected when associated with deficiency states. Other therapeutic interventions are essentially of an experimental nature; they often lack clinical validation and emphasize fatty liver prevention, as discussed in the next section.

2.5 PREVENTION AND TREATMENT OF ALCOHOLIC LIVER INJURY, PRIMARILY THE FATTY LIVER

As already mentioned, decreasing dietary fat[21,22,133] or replacing it with medium-chain triglycerides[150] reduces the capacity of ethanol to produce a fatty liver. Differences in dietary fat may explain some of the discrepancies in reports concerning the effect of antioxidants which reduced or prevented hepatic steatosis in some studies[282,283] but not in others[150]. The negative results were obtained with diets containing 43 % total calories as fat (an amount comparable to that of the average U.S. diet), whereas partial protection was observed with a relatively low fat diet. Since dietary fat potentiated the steatogenic effect of ethanol, it is quite conceivable that antioxidants may be moderately active with low fat diets but incapable of counteracting the much stronger effects of ethanol combined with dietary fat. Chlorophenoxyisobutyrate, a drug used to reduce hyperlipaemia, partially protected against the alcoholic fatty liver[284,285], possibly through a reduction in glycerolipid formation[286]. The protective action also could be related to the abolition of the redox change[287].

Among the drugs capable of decreasing the capacity of ethanol to produce a fatty liver, one must list the barbiturates[288,289], nicotinic acid[290] and antihistamine derivatives[291]. Asparagine, previously reported as protective[292], now has been found ineffective after acute[293] and prolonged[150] ethanol intake. To the list of measures previously reported to prevent fatty liver produced by one large dose of ethanol[294], one can add the β-sympathicolytic agents[295], pyridyncarbinol[296], and cold exposure[297]. In rats, hyperbaric oxygen was found to be protective[298]. Adenosine triphosphate previously has been reported to protect against acute ethanol-induced fatty liver[299]. However, when given in moderate amounts, it restored liver ATP levels to normal without preventing the ethanol-induced fatty liver[300]; the partial protection afforded by much larger doses[299] may be attributed to non-specific effects. Chlorpromazine, which inhibits ADH activity, failed to prevent the fatty liver produced by a single large dose of ethanol[301]. There is a controversy over whether or not pyrazole, another ADH inhibitor prevents the fatty liver produced by a single large dose of ethanol: some found no reduction[302] whereas others found prevention[303,304]; the difference is perhaps due to the dose of the drug[305] or the sex of the animal[306] used. Though some acute effects of ethanol on lipid metabolism were prevented by pyrazole[307], the effects of this drug on the consequences of chronic ethanol ingestion were inconclusive[308], a not unexpected result in view of the hepatotoxicity of pyrazole[309]. A derivative of pyrazole, 3,5-dimethyl pyrazole, was shown to reduce the fatty liver resulting from a single large dose of ethanol by blocking free fatty acid mobilization from adipose tissue[310].

Anabolic steroids were reported to be ineffective by some[311] but not by others[312,313] in accelerating the disappearance of fat from the alcoholic fatty liver.

Controlled, therapeutic trials of alcoholic hepatitis using glucocorticoids have generally been disappointing[313–316]. However, Helman and co-workers[317] found that steroids increased the survival rate but did not prevent progression to cirrhosis in a selected group of very ill patients with hepatic encephalopathy. The efficacy of prednisolone (40 mg/day) was attributed to increased appetite and caloric intake. In a follow-up study[318] prednisolone was compared with caloric supplementation in the treatment of alcoholic hepatitis complicated by encephalopathy. Caloric supplementation (1600 calories/day via various routes) by itself was associated with 0 % (0/6) survival whereas 71 % (5/7) patients treated with prednisolone recovered from the acute episode. Thus, the efficacy of steroids cannot be attributed to its effect on nutrition alone.

Preliminary observations with d-penicillamine therapy in acute alcoholic liver disease suggests possible beneficial effects; confirmation on a larger population sample will be needed, however[319].

In conclusion, at the present time outcome of therapy of the severe stages of alcoholic liver injury is disappointing, but best results are obtained by prophylaxis and early detection with treatment at fully reversible initial stages.

References

1. Lieber, C. S. and Davidson, C. S. (1962). Some metabolic effects of ethyl alcohol. *Am. J. Med.*, **33**, 319
2. Lieber, C. S., Leevy, C. M., Stein, S. W., George, W. S., Cherrick, G. R., Abelmann, W. H. and Davidson, C. S. (1962). Effect of ethanol on plasma free fatty acids in man. *J. Lab. Clin. Med.*, **59**, 826
3. Lieber, C. S., Jones, D. P., Losowsky, M. S. and Davidson, C. S. (1962). Interrelation of uric acid and ethanol metabolism in man. *J. Clin. Invest.*, **41**, 1863
4. Olin, J. S., Devenyi, P. and Weldon, K. L. (1973). Uric acid in alcoholics. *Q. J. Stud. Alc.*, **34**, 1202
5. Newcombe, D. S. (1972). Ethanol metabolism and uric acid. *Metabolism*, **21**, 1193
6. Feinman, L. and Lieber, C. S. (1972). Hepatic collagen metabolism: effect of alcohol consumption in rats and baboons. *Science*, **176**, 795
7. Nikkila, E. A. and Ojala, K. (1963). Role of hepatic L-α-glycerophosphate and triglyceride synthesis in production of fatty liver by ethanol. *Proc. Soc. Exp. Biol. Med.*, **113**, 814
8. Johnson, O. (1974). Influence of the blood ethanol concentration on the acute ethanol-induced liver triglyceride accumulation in rats. *Scand. J. Gastroenterol.*, **2**, 207
9. Lieber, C. S. and Schmid, R. (1961). The effect of ethanol on fatty acid metabolism: stimulation of hepatic fatty acid synthesis *in vitro*. *J. Clin. Invest.*, **40**, 394
10. Gordon, E. R. (1972). Effect of an intoxicating dose of ethanol on lipid metabolism in an isolated, perfused rat liver. *Biochem. Pharmacol.*, **21**, 2991
11. Guynn, R. W., Veloso, D., Harris, R. I., Lawson, J. W. R. and Veech, R. L. (1973). Ethanol administration and the relationship of malonyl-coenzyme A concentrations to the rate of fatty acid synthesis in rat liver. *Biochem. J.*, **136**, 639
12. Arakawa, M., Taketomi, S., Furuno, K., Matsuo, T., Iwatsuka, H. and Suzuoki, Z. (1975). Metabolic studies on the development of ethanol-induced fatty liver in KK-Ay mice. *J. Nutr.*, **105**, 1500

13. Forsander, O. A., Maenpaa, P. H. and Salaspuro, M. P. (1965). Influence of ethanol on the lactate/pyruvate and β-hydroxybutyrate/acetoacetate ratios in rat liver experiments. *Acta Chem. Scand.*, **19**, 1770
14. Lieber, C. S., Lefevre, A., Spritz, N., Feinman, L. and DeCarli, L. M. (1967). Difference in hepatic metabolism of long- and medium-chain fatty acids: the role of fatty acid chain length in the production of the alcoholic fatty liver. *J. Clin. Invest.*, **46**, 1451
15. Ontko, J. A. (1973). Effects of ethanol on the metabolism of free fatty acids in isolated liver cells. *J. Lipid Res.*, **14**, 78
16. Williamson, J. R., Scholz, R., Browning, E. T., Thurman, R. G. and Fukami, M. H. (1969). Metabolic effects of ethanol in perfused rat liver. *J. Biol. Chem.* **244**, 5044.
17. Fritz, I. B. (1961). Factors influencing the rates of long-chain fatty acid oxidation and synthesis in mammalian systems. *Physiol. Rev.*, **41**, 52
18. Blomstrand, R., Kager, L. and Lantto, O. (1973). Studies on the ethanol-induced decrease of fatty acid oxidation in rat and human liver slices. *Life Sci.*, **13**, 1131
19. Fischel, P. and Oette, K. (1974). Experimentell Untersuchungen an menschlichen Leberpunktaten und Rattenleberschnitten zur Oxidation von Fettsäuren mit unterschiedlicher Kettenlänge und unterschiedlicher Zahl von Doppelbindungen. *Res. Exp. Med.*, **163**, 1
20. Blomstrand, R. and Kager, L. (1973). The combustion of triolein-1-^{14}C and its inhibition by alcohol in man. *Life Sci.*, **13**, 113
21. Lieber, C. S. and Spritz, N. (1966). Effects of prolonged ethanol intake in man: role of dietary, adipose, and endogenously synthesized fatty acids in the pathogenesis of the alcoholic fatty liver. *J. Clin. Invest.*, **45**, 1400
22. Lieber, C. S., Spritz, N. and DeCarli, L. M. (1966). Role of dietary, adipose and endogenously synthesized fatty acids in the pathogenesis of the alcoholic fatty liver. *J. Clin. Invest.*, **45**, 51
23. Lieber, C. S., Spritz, N. and DeCarli, L. M. (1969). Fatty liver produced by dietary deficiencies: its pathogenesis and potentiation by ethanol. *J. Lipid Res.*, **10**, 283
24. Mendenhall, C. L. (1972). Origin of hepatic triglyceride fatty acids: quantitative estimation of the relative contribution of linoleic acid by diet and adipose tissue in normal and ethanol-fed rats. *J. Lipid Res.*, **13**, 177
25. Forney, R. B. and Hughes, F. W. (1968). *Combined Effects of Alcohol and Other Drugs*, p. 124. Springfield, Illinois: Charles C. Thomas
26. Soehring, K. and Schuppel, R. (1966). Wechselwirkungen zwischen Alkohol und Arzneimittein. *Deutsch Med. Wochenschr.*, **91**, 1892
27. Rubin, E. and Lieber, C. S (1968). Hepatic microsomal enzymes in man and rat: induction and inhibition by ethanol. *Science*, **162**, 690
28. Ariyoshi, T., Takabatake, E. and Remmer, H. (1970). Drug metabolism in ethanol-induced fatty liver. *Life Sci.* (*Part II*), **9**, 361
29. Schüppel, R. (1971). Wirkungen von Alkohol auf den Arzneistoffwechsel. In W. Gerök, K. Sickinger and H. H. Hennekeuser, eds. *Alcohol and the Liver*, p. 227. New York: Schattauer Verlag
30. Rubin, E., Gang, H., Misra, P. S. and Lieber, C. S. (1970). Inhibition of drug metabolism by acute ethanol intoxication. A hepatic microsomal mechanism. *Am. J. Med.*, **49**, 801
31. Cohen, G. M. and Mannering, G. J. (1973). Involvement of a hydrophobic site in the inhibition of the microsomal *p*-hydroxylation of aniline by alcohols. *Molec. Pharmacol.*, **9**, 383
32. Cinti, D. L., Grundin, R. and Orrenius, S. (1973). The effect of ethanol on drug oxidations *in vitro* and the significance of ethanol-cytochrome P-450 interaction. *Biochem. J.*, **134**, 367
33. Cohen, B. S. and Estabrook, R. W. (1971). Microsomal electron transport reactions. III. Cooperative interactions between reduced diphosphopyridine nucleotide and reduced triphosphopyridine nucleotide-linked reactions. *Arch. Biochem. Biophys.*, **143**, 54
34. Whitehouse, L. W., Paul, C. J., Coldwell, B. B. and Thomas, B. H. (1975). Effect of ethanol on diazepam distribution in rat. *Res. Commun. Chem. Path. Pharmacol.*, **12**, 221

35. Hildebrandt, A. G., Speck, M. and Roots, I. (1974). The effects of substrates of mixed function oxidase on ethanol oxidation in rat liver microsomes. *Naunyn-Schmiedeberg's Arch. Pharmacol.*, **281**, 371
36. Grundin, R. (1975). Metabolic interaction of ethanol and alprenolol in isolated liver cells. *Acta Pharmacol. Toxicol.*, **37**, 185
37. Sutherland, V. C., Burbridge, T. N., Adams, J. E. and Simon, A. (1960). Cerebral metabolism in problem drinkers under the influence of alcohol and chlorpromazine hydrochloride. *J. Appl. Physiol.*, **15**, 189
38. Voas, R. B. (1973). Alcohol as an underlying factor in behavior leading to fatal highway crashes. In M. E. Chafetz, ed. *Proceedings of the First Annual Alcoholism Conference of the National Institute on Alcohol Abuse and Alcoholism*, p. 324. Washington, D.C.: DHEW Publ. (NIH) 74-675, U.S. Government Printing Office
39. Truitt, E. B. and Duritz, G. (1966). The role of acetaldehyde in the actions of ethanol. In R. P. Maickel, ed. *Biochemical Factors in Alcohol*, p. 61. New York: Pergamon Press
40. Marjanen, L. (1972). Intracellular localization of aldehyde dehydrogenase in rat liver. *Biochem. J.*, **127**, 633
41. Grunnet, N. (1973). Oxidation of acetaldehyde by rat liver mitochondria in relation to ethanol oxidation and the transport of reducing equivalents across the mitochondrial membrane. *Eur. J. Biochem.*, **35**, 236
42. Iseri, O. A., Gottlieb, L. S. and Lieber, C. S. (1964). The ultrastructure of ethanol-induced fatty liver. *Fed. Proc.*, **23**, 579
43. Iseri, O. A., Lieber, C. S. and Gottlieb, L. S. (1966). The ultrastructure of fatty liver induced by prolonged ethanol ingestion. *Am. J. Pathol.*, **48**, 535
44. Carulli, N., Manenti, F., Gallo, M. and Salvioli, G. F. (1971). Alcohol–drugs interaction in man: alcohol and tolbutamide. *Eur. J. Clin. Invest.*, **1**, 421
45. Lieber, C. S. and Rubin, E. (1968). Alcoholic fatty liver in man on a high protein and low fat diet. *Am. J. Med.*, **44**, 200
46. Rubin, E., Hutterer, F. and Lieber, C. S. (1968). Ethanol increases hepatic smooth endoplasmic reticulum and drug-metabolizing enzymes. *Science*, **159**, 1469
47. Ishii, H., Joly, J.-G. and Lieber, C. S. (1973). Effect of ethanol on the amount and enzyme activities of hepatic rough and smooth microsomal membranes. *Biochim. Biophys. Acta*, **291**, 411
48. Kater, R. M. H., Carulli, N. and Iber, F. L. (1969). Differences in the rate of ethanol metabolism in recently drinking alcoholic and nondrinking subjects. *Am. J. Clin. Nutr.*, **22**, 1608
49. Ugarte, G., Pereda, T., Pino, M. E. and Iturriaga, H. (1972). Influence of alcohol intake, length of abstinence and meprobamate on the rate of ethanol metabolism in man. *Q. J. Stud. Alc.*, **33**, 698
50. Lieber, C. S. and DeCarli, L. M. (1970). Hepatic microsomal ethanol oxidizing system: *in vitro* characteristics and adaptive properties *in vivo*. *J. Biol. Chem.*, **245**, 2505
51. Misra, P. S., Lefevre, A., Ishii, H., Rubin, E. and Lieber, C. S. (1971). Increase of ethanol, meprobamate and pentobarbital metabolism after chronic ethanol administration in man and in rats. *Am. J. Med.*, **51**, 346
52. Tobon, F. and Mezey, E. (1971). Effect of ethanol administration on hepatic ethanol and drug-metabolizing enzymes and on rates of ethanol degradation. *J. Lab. Clin. Med.*, **77**, 110
53. Joly, J.-G., Ishii, H., Teschke, R., Hasumura, Y. and Lieber, C. S. (1973). Effect of chronic ethanol feeding on the activities and submicrosomal distribution of reduced nicotinamide adenine dinucleotide phosphate (NADPH)-cytochrome P-450 reductase and the demethylases for aminopyrine and ethyl-morphine. *Biochem. Pharmacol.*, **22**, 1532
54. Powis, G. (1975). Effect of a single oral dose of methanol, ethanol and propan-2-ol on the hepatic microsomal metabolism of foreign compounds in the rat. *Biochem. J.*, **148**, 269

55. Luoma, P. and Vorne, M. (1973). The combined effect of ethanol and phenobarbital on the activities of hepatic drug metabolizing enzymes in rats. *Acta Pharmacol. Toxicol.*, **33,** 442
56. Lu, A. Y. H., Junk, K. W. and Coon, M. J. (1969). Resolution of the cytochrome P-450 containing w-hydroxylation system of liver microsomes into three components. *J. Biol. Chem.*, **244,** 3714
57. Kalant, H., Khanna, J. M. and Marshman, J. (1970). Effect of chronic intake of ethanol on pentobarbital metabolism. *J. Pharmacol. Exper. Ther.*, **175,** 318
58. Ratcliffe, F. (1969). The effect of chronic ethanol administration on the responses to amylobarbitone sodium in the rat. *Life Sci.*, **8,** 1051
59. Kater, R. M. H., Roggin, G., Tobon, F., Zieve, P. and Iber, F. L. (1969). Increased rate of clearance of drugs from the circulation of alcoholics. *Am. J. Med. Sci.*, **258,** 35
60. Vesell, E. S., Page, J. G. and Passananti, G. T. (1971). Genetic and environmental factors affecting ethanol metabolism in man. *Clin. Pharmacol. Ther.*, **12,** 192
61. Grassi, G. G. and Grassi, C. (1975). Ethanol–antibiotic interactions at hepatic level. *J. Clin. Pharmacol. Biopharmacol.*, **11,** 216
62. Ioannides, C., Lake, B. G. and Parke, D. V. (1975). Enhancement of hepatic microsomal drug metabolism *in vitro* following ethanol administration. *Xenobiotica*, **5,** 665
63. Hasumura, Y., Teschke, R. and Lieber, C. S. (1974). Increased carbon tetrachloride hepatotoxicity, and its mechanism, after chronic ethanol consumption. *Gastroenterology*, **66,** 415
64. Maling, H. M., Stripp, B., Sipes, I. G., Highman, B., Saul, W. and Williams, M. A. (1975). Enhanced hepatotoxicity of carbon tetrachloride, thioacetamide, and dimethyl-nitrosamine by pretreatment of rats with ethanol and some comparisons with potentiation by isopropanol. *Toxicol. Appl. Pharmacol.*, **33,** 291
65. Traiger, G. J. and Plaa, G. L. (1972). Relationship of alcohol metabolism to the potentiation of CCl_4 hepatotoxicity induced by aliphatic alcohols. *J. Pharmacol. Exper. Ther.*, **183,** 481
66. Garner, R. C. and McLean, A. E. M. (1969). Increased susceptibility to carbon tetrachloride poisoning in the rat after pretreatment with oral phenobarbitone. *Biochem. Pharmacol.*, **18,** 645
67. Diaz Gomez, M. I., Castro, J. A., de Ferreyra, E. C., D'Acosta, N. and de Castro, C. R. (1973). Irreversible binding of ^{14}C from $^{14}CCl_4$ to liver microsomal lipids and proteins from rats pretreated with compounds altering microsomal mixed function oxygenase activity. *Toxicol. Appl. Pharmacol.*, **25,** 534
68. Moon, H. D. (1950). The pathology of fatal carbon tetrachloride poisoning with special reference to the histogenesis of the hepatic and renal lesions. *Am. J. Pathol.*, **26,** 1041
69. DiLuzio, N. R. and Hartman, A. D. (1967). Role of lipid peroxidation in the pathogenesis of the ethanol-induced fatty liver. *Fed. Proc.*, **26,** 1436
70. Hashimoto, S. and Recknagel, R. O. (1968). No chemical evidence of hepatic lipid peroxidation in acute ethanol toxicity. *Exper. Molec. Pathol.*, **8,** 225
71. Scheig, R. and Klatskin, G. (1969). Some effects of ethanol and carbon tetrachloride on lipoperoxidation in rat liver. *Life Sci.*, **8,** 855
72. Bunyan, J. Cawthorne, M. A., Diplock, A. T. and Green, J. (1969). Vitamin E and hepatotoxic agents. 2. Lipid peroxidation and poisoning with orotic acid, ethanol and thioacetamide in rats. *Br. J. Nutr.*, **23,** 309
73. Comporti, M., Burdino, E. and Raja, F. (1971). Fatty acid composition of mitochondrial and microsomal lipids of rat liver after acute ethanol intoxication. *Life Sci.*, **10,** 855
74. Bloom, R. J. and Westerfield, W. W. (1971). The thiobarbituric acid reaction in relation to fatty livers. *Arch. Biochem. Biophys.*, **145,** 669
75. Lieber, C. S. and DeCarli, L. M. (1970). Reduced nicotinamide-adenine dinucleotide phosphate oxidase: activity enhanced by ethanol consumption. *Science*, **170,** 78

76. Levander, O. A., Morris, V. C., Higgs, D. J. and Varma, R. N. (1973). Nutritional interrelationships among vitamin E selenium, antioxidants and ethyl alcohol in the rat. *J. Nutr.*, **103**, 536
77. Lefevre, A. F., DeCarli, L. M. and Lieber, C. S. (1972). Effect of ethanol on cholesterol and bile acid metabolism. *J. Lipid Res.*, **13**, 48
78. Schoenfield, L. J., Bonorris, G. G. and Ganz, P. (1973). Induced alterations in the rate-limiting enzymes of hepatic cholesterol and bile acid synthesis in the hamster. *J. Lab. Clin. Med.*, **82**, 858
79. Lieber, C. S., Jones, D. P., Mendelson, J. and DeCarli, L. M. (1963). Fatty liver, hyperlipemia and hyperuricemia produced by prolonged alcohol consumption, despite adequate dietary intake. *Trans. Ass. Am. Physicians*, **76**, 289
80. Takeuchi, N., Ito, M. and Yamamura, Y. (1974). Esterification of cholesterol and hydrolysis of cholesteryl ester in alcohol-induced fatty liver of rats. *Lipids*, **9**, 353
81. Maddrey, W. C. and Boyer, J. L. (1973). The acute and chronic effects of ethanol administration on bile secretion in the rat. *J. Lab. Clin. Med.*, **82**, 215
82. Losowsky, M. S., Jones, D. P., Davidson, C. S. and Lieber, C. S. (1963). Studies of alcoholic hyperlipemia and its mechanism. *Am. J. Med.*, **35**, 794
83. Baraona, E. and Lieber, C. S. (1970). Effects of chronic ethanol feeding on serum lipoprotein metabolism in the rat. *J. Clin. Invest.* **49**, 769
84. Baraona, E., Pirola, R. C. and Lieber, C. S. (1973). The pathogenesis of postprandial hyperlipemia in rats fed ethanol-containing diets. *J. Clin. Invest.*, **52**, 296
85. Joly, J.-G., Feinman, L., Ishii, H. and Lieber, C. S. (1973). Effect of chronic ethanol feeding on hepatic microsomal glycerophosphate acyltransferase activity. *J. Lipid Res.*, **14**, 337
86. Mendenhall, C. L., Bradford, R. H. and Furman, R. H. (1969). Effect of ethanol on glycerolipid metabolism in rat liver. *Biochim. Biophys. Acta*, **187**, 501
87. Gang, H., Lieber, C. S. and Rubin, E. (1973). Ethanol increases glycosyl transferase activity in the hepatic Golgi apparatus. *Nature (New Biology)*, **243**, 123
88. Barboriak, J. J. and Meade, R. C. (1968). Enhancement of alimentary lipemia by preprandial alcohol. *Am. J. Med. Sci.*, **255**, 245
89. Brewster, A. C., Lankford, H. G., Schwartz, M. G. and Sullivan, J. F. (1966). Ethanol and alimentary lipemia. *Am. J. Clin. Nutr.*, **19**, 255
90. Kudzma, D. J. and Schonfeld, G. (1971). Alcoholic hyperlipidemia: induction by alcohol but not by carbohydrate. *J. Lab. Clin. Med.*, **77**, 384
91. Verdy, M. and Gattereau, A. (1967). Ethanol, lipase activity and serum-lipid level. *Am. J. Clin. Nutr.*, **20**, 997
92. Wilson, D. E., Schreibman, P. H., Brewster, A. C. and Arky, R. A. (1970). The enhancement of alimentary lipemia by ethanol in man. *J. Lab. Clin. Med.*, **75**, 264
93. Mendelson, J. H. and Mello, N. K. (1973). Alcohol-induced hyperlipidemia and beta lipoproteins. *Science*, **180**, 1372
94. Ginsberg, H., Olefsky, J., Farquhar, J. W. and Reaven, G. M. (1974). Moderate ethanol ingestion and plasma triglyceride levels. *Ann. Intern. Med.* **80**, 143
95. Kessler, J. I., Miller, M., Barza, D. and Mishkin, S. (1967). Hyperlipemia in acute pancreatitis. Metabolic studies in a patient and demonstration of abnormal lipoprotein–triglyceride complexes resistant to the action of lipoprotein lipase. *Am. J. Med.*, **42**, 968
96. Chait, A., February, A. W., Mancini, M. and Lewis, B. L. (1972). Clinical and metabolic study of alcoholic hyperlipidaemia. *Lancet*, **ii**, 62
97. Fry, M. M., Spector, A. A., Connor, S. L. and Connor, W. E. (1973). Intensification of hypertriglyceridemia by either alcohol or carbohydrate. *Am. J. Clin. Nutr.*, **26**, 798
98. Windmueller, H. G. and Levy, R. I. (1968). Production of β-lipoprotein by intestine in the rat. *J. Biol. Chem.*, **243**, 4878

99. Ockner, R. K., Hughes, F. B. and Isselbacher, K. J. (1969). Very low density lipoproteins in intestinal lymph: origin, composition and role in lipid transport in the fasting state. *J. Clin. Invest.*, **48,** 2079
100. Baraona, E., Pirola, R. C. and Lieber, C. S. (1975). Acute and chronic effects of ethanol on intestinal lipid metabolism. *Biochim. Biophys. Acta,* **388,** 19
101. Carter, E. A., Drummey, G. D. and Isselbacher, K. J. (1971). Ethanol stimulates triglyceride synthesis by the intestine. *Science,* **174,** 1245
102. Mistilis, S. P. and Ockner, R. K. (1972). Effects of ethanol on endogenous lipid and lipoprotein metabolism in small intestine. *J. Lab. Clin. Med.,* **80,** 34
103. Windmueller, H. G., Herbert, P. N. and Levy, R. L. (1973). Biosynthesis of lymph and plasma lipoprotein apoproteins by isolated perfused rat liver and intestine. *J. Lipid Res.,* **14,** 215
104. Ockner, R. K., Mistilis, S. P., Peppenhausen, R. B. and Stiehl, A. F. (1973). Ethanol-induced fatty liver: effect of intestinal lymph fistula. *Gastroenterology,* **64,** 603
105. Middleton, W. R. J., Carter, E. A., Drummey, G. D. and Isselbacher, K. J. (1971). Effect of oral ethanol administration on intestinal cholesterogenesis in the rat. *Gastroenterology,* **60,** 880
106. Waltman, R., Bonura, F., Nigrin, G. and Pipat, C. (1969). Ethanol in prevention of hyperbilirubinaemia in the newborn. *Lancet,* **ii,** 1265
107. Ideo, G., DeFranchis, R., Del Ninno, E. and Dioguardi, N. (1971). Ethanol increases liver uridine-diphosphate-glucuronyltransferase. *Experientia,* **27,** 24
108. Okolicsanyi, L., Cartei, G. and Naccarato, R. (1972). Effects of ethanol on Gilbert's hyperbilirubinaemia. *Lancet,* **i,** 450
109. Jouppila, P., Koivisto, M. and Suonio, S. (1973). Ethanol in the prevention of neonatal hyperbilirubinaemia. *Acta Paediat. Scand.,* **63,** 501
110. Nelson, P., Tan, W. C., Wagle, S. R. and Ashmore, J. (1967). Hepatic metabolism and enzyme activity in acute ethanol administration. *Biochem. Pharmacol.,* **16,** 1813
111. Ishii, H., Joly, J.-G. and Lieber, C. S. (1973). Increase of microsomal glucose-6-phosphatase activity after chronic ethanol administration. *Metabolism,* **22,** 799
112. Carter, E. A. and Isselbacher, K. J. (1971). The role of microsomes in the hepatic metabolism of ethanol. *Ann. N.Y. Acad. Sci.,* **179,** 282
113. Fitch, W. W. and Chaikoff, I. L. (1960). Extent and patterns of adaptation of enzyme activities in liver of normal rats fed diets high in glucose and fructose. *J. Biol. Chem.,* **235,** 554
114. Olivecrona, T., Hernell, O., Johnson, O., Fex, G., Wallinder, L. and Sandgren, O. (1972). Effect of ethanol on some enzymes inducible by fat-free refeeding. *Q. J. Stud. Alc.,* **33,** 1
115. Brodie, B. B., Butler, W. M., Horning, M. G., Maickel, R. P. and Maling, H. M. (1961). Alcohol-induced triglyceride deposition in liver through derangement of fat transport. *Am. J. Clin. Nutr.* **9,** 432
116. Mallov, S. (1957). Effect of adrenalectomy on ethanol and fat metabolism in the rat. *Am. J. Physiol.,* **189,** 428
117. Rebouças, G. and Isselbacher, K. J. (1961). Studies on the pathogenesis of the ethanol-induced fatty liver. I. Synthesis and oxidation of fatty acids by the liver. *J. Clin. Invest.,* **40,** 1355
118. Kessler, J. I. and Yalovsky-Mishkin, S. (1966). Effect of ingestion of saline, glucose, and ethanol on mobilization and hepatic incorporation of epididymal pad palmitate-1-^{14}C in rats. *J. Lipid Res.,* **7,** 772
119. Poggi, M. and Di Luzio, N. R. (1964). The role of liver and adipose tissue in the pathogenesis of the ethanol-induced fatty liver. *J. Lipid Res.,* **5,** 437
120. Mallov, S. (1961). Effect of ethanol intoxication on plasma-free fatty acids in the rat. *Q. J. Stud. Alc.,* **22,** 250

121. Elko, E. E., Wooles, W. R. and Di Luzio, N. R. (1961). Alterations and mobilization of lipids in acute ethanol-treated rats. *Am. J. Physiol.*, **201,** 923
122. Jones, D. P., Losowsky, M. S., Davidson, C. S. and Lieber, C. S. (1963). Effects of ethanol on plasma lipids in man. *J. Lab. Clin. Med.*, **62,** 675
123. Jones, D. P., Perman, E. S. and Lieber, C. S. (1965). Free fatty acid turnover and triglyceride metabolism after ethanol ingestion in man. *J. Lab. Clin. Med.*, **66,** 804
124. Feinman, L. and Lieber, C. S. (1967). Effect of ethanol on plasma glycerol in man. *Am. J. Clin. Nutr.*, **20,** 400
125. Crouse, J. R., Gerson, C. D., DeCarli, L. M. and Lieber, C. S. (1968). Role of acetate in the reduction of plasma-free fatty acids produced by ethanol in man. *J. Lipid Res.*, **9,** 509
126. Lindenbaum, J., and Lieber, C. S. (1975). Effects of chronic ethanol administration on intestinal absorption in man in the absence of nutritional deficiency. *Ann. N.Y. Acad. Sci.*, **252,** 228
127. Best, C. H., Hartroft, W. S., Lucas, C. C. and Ridout, J. H. (1949). Liver damage produced by feeding alcohol or sugar and its prevention by choline. *Br. Med. J.*, **ii,** 1001
128. Pequignot, G. (1962). Die Rolle des Alkohols bei der Atiologie von Leberzirrhosen in Frankreich. *München Med. Wochenschr.*, **103,** 1464
129. Lelbach, W. K. (1967). Leberschaden bei chronischem Alkoholismus. *Acta Hepatosplen.*, **14,** 9
130. Lieber, C. S., Jones, D. P. and DeCarli, L. M. (1965). Effects of prolonged ethanol intake: production of fatty liver despite adequate diets. *J. Clin. Invest.*, **44,** 1009
131. DeCarli, L. M. and Lieber, C. S. (1967). Fatty liver in the rat after prolonged intake of ethanol with a nutritionally adequate new liquid diet. *J. Nutr.*, **91,** 331
132. Lieber, C. S. and DeCarli, L. M. (1973). Ethanol dependence and tolerance: a nutritionally controlled experimental model in the rat. *Res. Commun. Chem. Path. Pharmacol.*, **6,** 983
133. Lieber, C. S. and DeCarli, L. M. (1970). Quantitative relationship between the amount of dietary fat and the severity of the alcoholic fatty liver. *Am. J. Clin. Nutr.*, **23,** 474
134. Barak, A. J., Tuma, D. J. and Sorrell, M. F. (1973). Relationship of ethanol to choline metabolism in the liver: a review. *Am. J. Clin. Nutr.*, **26,** 1234
135. Mendenhall, C. L. and Wilson, N. L. (1973). Observations on the relationship of hepatic choline uptake to ethanolic fatty liver in the rat. *Can. J. Biochem.*, **51,** 1010
136. Hoffbauer, F. W. and Zaki, F. G. (1965). Choline deficiency in baboon and rat compared. *Arch. Pathol.*, **79,** 364
137. Olson, R. E. (1964). Nutrition and alcoholism. In M. G. Wohl and R. S. Goodhart, eds. *Modern Nutrition in Health and Disease.* Philadelphia: Lea and Febiger
138. Rubin, E. and Lieber, C. S. (1968). Alcohol-induced hepatic injury in non-alcoholic volunteers. *N. Engl. J. Med.*, **278,** 869
139. Ashworth, C. T., Wrightsman, F. and Buttram, V. (1961). Hepatic lipids. *Arch. Pathol.*, **72,** 620
140. Edreira, J. G., Hirsch, R. L. and Kennedy, J. A. (1974). Production of fatty liver with dietary ethanol despite orotic acid supplementation. *Q. J. Stud. Alc.*, **35,** 20
141. French, S. W. (1966). Effect of acute and chronic ethanol ingestion on rat liver ATP. *Proc. Soc. Exp. Biol. Med.*, **121,** 681
142. Walker, J. E. C. and Gordon, E. R. (1970). Biochemical aspects associated with an ethanol-induced fatty liver. *Biochem. J.*, **119,** 511
143. Bernstein, J., Videla, L. and Israel, Y. (1973). Metabolic alterations produced in the liver by chronic ethanol administration. II. Changes related to energetic parameters of the cell. *Biochem. J.*, **134,** 515
144. Shull, K. H., Oler, A. and Lombardi, B. (1972). Hepatic adenosine triphosphate levels during acute choline deficiency in the rat. *Proc. Soc. Exp. Biol. Med.*, **140,** 575
145. Corredor, C., Mansbach, C. and Bressler, R. (1967). Carnitine depletion in the choline-deficient state. *Biochim. Biophys. Acta,* **144,** 366

146. Kondrup, J. and Grunnet, N. (1973). The effect of acute and prolonged ethanol treatment on the contents of coenzyme A, carnitine and their derivatives in rat liver. *Biochem. J.*, **132**, 373
147. Oler, A. and Lombardi, B. (1970). Further studies on a defect in the intracellular transport and secretion of proteins by the liver of choline-deficient rats. *J. Biol. Chem.*, **245**, 1282
148. Ruebner, B. H., Moore, J., Rutherford, R. B., Seligman, A. M. and Zuidema, G. D. (1969). Nutritional cirrhosis in rhesus monkeys: electron microscopy and histochemistry. *Exp. Molec. Pathol.*, **11**, 53
149. Di Luzio, N. R. (1958). Effect of acute ethanol intoxication on liver and plasma lipid fractions of the rat. *Am. J. Physiol.*, **194**, 53
150. Lieber, C. S. and DeCarli, L. M. (1966). Study of agents for the prevention of the fatty liver produced by prolonged alcohol intake. *Gastroenterology*, **50**, 316
151. Takeuchi, J., Takada, A., Hasumura, Y., Matsuda, Y. and Ikegami, F. (1972). Acute alcoholic liver injury and choline deficiency. *Meth. Achievm. Exper. Path.*, **6**, 81
152. Patek, A. J., Bowry, S. C. and Anuras, S. (1973). Alcohol and sucrose in choline deficiency cirrhosis in the rat. *Arch. Pathol.*, **96**, 377
153. Lieber, C. S., DeCarli, L. M., Gang, H., Walker, G. and Rubin, E. (1972). Hepatic effect of long-term ethanol consumption in primates. In E. I. Goldsmith and J. Moor-Jankowski, eds. *Medical Primatology*, Part III, p. 270. Basel: Karger
154. Kumar, V., Deo, M. G. and Ramalingaswami, V. (1972). Mechanism of fatty liver in protein deficiency. *Gastroenterology*, **62**, 445
155. Klatskin, G., Krehl, W. A. and Conn, H. O. (1954). The effect of alcohol on the choline requirement. I. Changes in the rat's liver following prolonged ingestion of alcohol. *J. Exp. Med.*, **100**, 605
156. Ericsson, J. L. E., Orrenius, S. and Holm, I. (1966). Alterations in canine liver cells induced by protein deficiency. Ultrastructural and biochemical observations. *Exp. Molec. Pathol.*, **5**, 329
157. Patrick, R. S., MacKay, A. M., Coward, D. G. and Whitehead, R. G. (1973). Experimental protein-energy malnutrition in baby baboons. *Br. J. Nutr.* **30**, 171
158. Lane, B. P. and Lieber, C. S. (1966). Ultrastructural alterations in human hepatocytes following ingestion of ethanol with adequate diets. *Am. J. Pathol.*, **49**, 593
159. Holt, L. E., Snyderman, S. E., Norton, P. M. and Roitman, R. (1968). In J. H. Leathem, ed. *Protein Nutrition and Free Amino Acid Patterns*. New Brunswick, N.J.: Rutgers, Univ. Press
160. Shaw, S. and Lieber, C. S. (1975). Plasma amino acids in alcoholic liver injury: contrast with protein malnutrition. *Clin. Res.*, **23**, 459A
161. Moxley, R. T., Pozefsky, T. and Lockwood, D. H. (1974). Protein nutrition and liver disease after jejunoileal bypass for morbid obesity. *N. Engl. J. Med.*, **290**, 921
162. Zinneman, H. H., Seal, U. S. and Doe, R. P. (1969). Plasma and urinary amino acids in Laennec's cirrhosis. *Am. J. Dig. Dis.*, **14**, 118
163. Ning, M., Lowenstein, L. M. and Davidson, C. S. (1967). Serum amino acid concentrations in alcoholic hepatitis. *J. Lab. Clin. Med.*, **70**, 554
164. Siegel, F. L., Roach, M. K. and Pomeroy, L. R. (1964). Plasma amino acid patterns in alcoholism: the effects of ethanol loading. *Proc. Nat. Acad. Sci. USA*, **51**, 605
165. Shaw, S. and Lieber, C. S. (1976). Characteristic plasma amino acid abnormalities in the alcoholic: respective roles of alcoholism, nutrition and liver injury. *Clin. Res.*, **24**, 291
166. Finkelstein, J. D., Cello, J. P. and Kyle, W. E. (1974). Ethanol-induced changes in methionine metabolism in rat liver. *Biochem. Biophys. Res. Commun.*, **61**, 475
167. Baraona, E., Leo, M., Borowsky, S. A. and Lieber, C. S. (1975). Alcoholic hepatomegaly: accumulation of protein in the liver. *Science*, **190**, 794
168. Baraona, E., Leo, M. A., Borowsky, S. A. and Lieber, C. S. (1975). Hepatic accumulation of export proteins after chronic ethanol consumption. *Gastroenterology*, **69**, 806

169. Lamy, J., Lamy, J., Aron, E. and Weill, J. (1974). Profil biologique des premières étapes de la cirrhose alcoolique: IgA, transferrine, haptoglobine, orosomucoide et α_1-antitrypsine. *Pathol.-Biol.*, **Mai 22,** 401

170. Dajani, R. M. and Kouyoumjian, C. (1967). A probable direct role of ethanol in the pathogenesis of fat infiltration in the rat. *J. Nutr.*, **91,** 535

171. Madsen, N. P. (1969). Reduced serum very low-density lipoprotein levels after acute ethanol administration. *Biochem. Pharmacol,* **18,** 261

172. Koga, S. and Hirayama, C. (1968). Disturbed release of lipoprotein from ethanol-induced fatty liver. *Experientia,* **24,** 438

173. Mookerjea, S. and Chow, A. (1969). Impairment of glycoprotein synthesis in acute ethanol intoxication in rats. *Biochim. Biophys. Acta,* **184,** 83

174. Marzo, A., Ghirardi, P. and Sardini, D. (1970). Serum lipids and total fatty acids in chronic alcoholic liver disease at different stages of cell damage. *Heft. Unfallheilk,* **48,** 949

175. Cachera, R., Lamotte, M. and Lamotte-Barrillon, S. (1950). Étude clinique, biologique et histologique des stéatoses du foie chez les alcooliques. *Sem. Hôp., Paris,* **26,** 3497

176. Papadopoulos, N. M. and Charles, M. A. (1970). Serum lipoprotein patterns in liver disease. *Proc. Soc. Exp. Biol. Med.*, **134,** 797

177. Lieber, C. S. and DeCarli, L. M. (1974). An experimental model of alcohol feeding and liver injury in the baboon. *J. Med. Primatol.*, **3,** 153

178. Borowsky, S. A., Perlow, W., Baraona, E. and Lieber, C. S. (1976). Disappearance of alcoholic hyperlipemia as a sign of advancing liver damage. *Gastroenterology,* **70,** 978

179. Rubin, E. and Lieber, C. S. (1967). Early fine structural changes in the human liver induced by alcohol. *Gastroenterology,* **52,** 1

180. Kuriyama, K., Sze, P. T. and Rauscher, G. E. (1971). Effects of acute and chronic ethanol administration on ribosomal protein synthesis in mouse brain and liver. *Life Sci.*, **10,** 181

181. Jeejeebhoy, K. N., Ho, J., Greenberg, G. R., Phillips, M. J., Bruce-Robertson, A. and Sodtke, U. (1975). Albumin, fibrinogen and transferrin synthesis in isolated rat hepatocyte suspensions. *Biochem. J.*, **146,** 141

182. Nadkarni, G.-S. D. (1974). Effect of acute ethanol administration of rat plasma protein synthesis. *Biochem. Pharmacol.*, **23,** 389

183. Rothschild, M., Oratz, M., Mongelli, J. and Schreiber, S. (1971). Alcohol-induced depression of albumin synthesis: reversal by tryptophan. *J. Clin. Invest.*, **50,** 1812

184. Jeejeebhoy, K. N., Phillips, M. J., Bruce-Robertson, A., Ho, J. and Sodtke, U. (1972). The acute effect of ethanol on albumin, fibrinogen and transferrin synthesis in the rat. *Biochem. J.*, **126,** 1111

185. Kirsch, R. E., Frith, L. O'C., Stead, R. H. and Saunders, S. J. (1973). Effect of alcohol on albumin synthesis by the isolated perfused rat liver. *Am. J. Clin. Nutr.*, **26,** 1191

186. Oratz, M. and Rothschild, M. A. (1975). The influence of alcohol and altered nutrition on albumin synthesis. In M. A. Rothschild, M. Oratz and S. S. Schreiber, eds. *Alcohol and Abnormal Protein Biosynthesis,* p. 343. New York: Pergamon Press

187. Perin, A., Scalabrino, G., Sessa, A. and Arnaboldi, A. (1974). *In vitro* inhibition of protein synthesis in rat liver as a consequence of ethanol metabolism. *Biochim. Biophys. Acta,* **366,** 101

188. Freinkel, N., Cohen, A. K. and Arky, R. A. (1965). Alcohol hypoglycemia: II. A postulated mechanism of action based on experiments with rat liver slices. *J. Clin. Endocrinol. Metab.*, **25,** 76

189. Chambers, J. W., Georg, R. H. and Bass, A. D. (1966). The effect of ethanol on the uptake of α-aminoisobutyric acid by the isolated perfused rat liver. *Life Sci.*, **5,** 2293

190. Chambers, J. W. and Piccirillo, V. J. (1973). Effects of ethanol on amino-acid uptake and utilization by the liver and other organs of rats. *Q. J. Stud. Alc.*, **34,** 707

191. Renis, M., Giovinc, A. and Bertolino, A. (1975). Protein synthesis in mitochondrial and microsomal fractions from rat brain and liver after acute or chronic ethanol administration. *Life Sci.*, **16,** 1447

192. Banks, W. L., Kline, E. S. and Higgins, E. S. (1970). Hepatic composition and metabolism after ethanol consumption in rats fed liquid purified diets. *J. Nutr.*, **100,** 581
193. Morland, J. (1975). Incorporation of labelled amino acids into liver protein after acute ethanol administration. *Biochem. Pharmacol.*, **24,** 439
194. Svoboda, D. J. and Manning, R. T. (1964). Chronic alcoholism with fatty metamorphosis of the liver. Mitochondrial alterations in hepatic cells. *Am. J. Pathol.*, **44,** 645
195. Konttinen, A., Hartel, G. and Louhija, A. (1970). Multiple serum enzyme analyses in chronic alcoholics. *Acta Med. Scand.*, **188,** 257
196. Kiessling, K. H. and Pilstrom, L. (1971). Ethanol and the human liver structural and metabolic changes in liver mitochondria. *Cytobiology,* **4,** 339
197. Rubin, E., Beattie, D: S. and Lieber, C. S. (1970). Effects of ethanol on the biogenesis of mitochondrial membranes and associated mitochondrial functions. *Lab. Invest.*, **23,** 620
198. Oudea, M. C., Launay, A. N., Queneherve, S. and Oudea, P. (1970). The hepatic lesions produced in the rat by chronic alcoholic intoxication. Histological, ultrastructural and biochemical observations. *Rev. Eur. Études Clin. Biol.*, **15,** 748
199. Videla, L. and Israel, Y. (1970). Factors that modify the metabolism of ethanol in rat liver and adaptive changes produced by its chronic administration. *Biochem. J.*, **118,** 275
200. Hasumura, Y., Teschke, R. and Lieber, C. S. (1975). Acetaldehyde oxidation by hepatic mitochondria: its decrease after chronic ethanol consumption. *Science,* **189,** 727
201. Kiessling, K.-H. and Pilstrom, L. (1968). Effect of ethanol on rat liver. V. Morphological and functional changes after prolonged consumption of various alcoholic beverages. *Q. J. Stud. Alc.*, **29,** 819
202. Rubin, E., Beattie, D. S., Toth, A. and Lieber, C. S. (1972). Structural and functional effects of ethanol on hepatic mitochondria. *Fed. Proc.*, **31,** 131
203. Gordon, E. R. (1973). Mitochondrial functions in an ethanol-induced fatty liver. *J. Biol. Chem.*, **248,** 8271
204. Kiessling, K.-H. (1968). Effect of ethanol on rat liver. VI. A possible correlation between α-glycerophosphate oxidase activity and mitochondrial size in male and female rats fed ethanol. *Acta Pharmacol.*, **26,** 245
205. Pilstrom, L. and Kiessling, K.-H. (1972). A possible localization of α-glycerophosphate dehydrogenase to the inner boundary membrane of mitochondria in livers from rats fed with ethanol. *Histochemie,* **32,** 329
206. Cederbaum, A. I., Lieber, C. S. and Rubin, E. (1974). Effects of chronic ethanol treatment on mitochondrial functions. *Arch. Biochem. Biophys.*, **165,** 560
207. Lefevre, A., Adler, H. and Lieber, C. S. (1970). Effect of ethanol on ketone metabolism. *J. Clin. Invest.*, **49,** 1775
208. Jenkins, D. W., Eckel, R. W. and Craig, J. W. (1971). Alcoholic ketoacidosis. *J. Am. Med. Ass.*, **217,** 177
209. Levy, L. J., Duga, J., Girgis, M. and Gordon, E. E. (1973). Ketoacidosis associated with alcoholism in nondiabetic subjects. *Ann. Intern. Med.*, **78,** 213
210. Cederbaum, A. I., Lieber, C. S., Beattie, D. S. and Rubin, E. (1975). Effect of chronic ethanol ingestion on fatty acid oxidation by hepatic mitochondria. *J. Biol. Chem.*, **250,** 5122
211. Cederbaum, A. I., Lieber, C. S. and Rubin, E. (1974). The effect of acetaldehyde on mitochondrial function. *Arch. Biochem. Biophys.*, **161,** 26
212. Majchrowicz, E. and Mendelson, J. H. (1970). Blood concentrations of acetaldehyde and ethanol in chronic alcoholics. *Science,* **168,** 1100
213. Truitt, E. B. (1971). Blood acetaldehyde levels after alcohol consumption by alcoholic and non-alcoholic subjects. In M. K. Roach, W. M. McIsaac and P. J. Creaven, eds. *Biological Aspects of Alcohol,* p. 212. Austin and London: University of Texas Press
214. Freund, G. (1971). Alcohol, barbiturate, and bromide withdrawal syndrome in mice. In *Recent Advances in Studies of Alcoholism,* U.S. Dept. of Health, Education and Welfare,

Health Services and Mental Health Administration, National Institute of Mental Health, National Institute on Alcohol Abuse and Alcoholism, p. 453. Washington, D.C.: U.S. Government Printing Office.

215. Rubenstein, J. A., Collins, M. A. and Tabakoff, B. (1975). Inhibition of liver aldehyde dehydrogenase by pyrogallol and related compounds. *Experientia,* **31,** 414

216. Collins, M. A., Gordon, R., Bidgeli, M. G. and Rubenstein, J. A. (1974). Pyrogallol potentiates acetaldehyde blood levels during ethanol oxidation in rats. *Chem.–Biol. Interactions,* **8,** 127

217. Hedlund, S. G. and Kiessling, K.-H. (1969). The physiological mechanism involved in hangover. I. The oxidation of some lower aliphatic fusel alcohols and aldehydes in rat liver and their effect on the mitochondrial oxidation of various substrates. *Acta Pharmacol. Toxicol.,* **27,** 381

218. Di Luzio, N. R. (1962). Comparative study of the effect of alcoholic beverages on the development of the acute ethanol-induced fatty liver. *Q. J. Stud. Alc.,* **23,** 557

219. Jordo, L. and Olsson, R. (1975). Effect of long-term administration of different hard liquors and red wine on the rat liver. *Acta Pathol. Microbiol. Scand.,* **83,** 345

220. Walker, F., Elmslie, W., Fraser, R. A., Snape, P. E. and Watt, G. C. M. (1974). Cytotoxic effect of alcohol on liver cells and fibroblasts *in vitro. Scot. Med. J.,* **19,** 125

221. Goldberg, D. M. and Watts, C. (1965). Serum enzyme changes as evidence of liver reaction to oral alcohol. *Gastroenterology,* **49,** 256

222. Figueroa, R. B. and Klotz, A. P. (1962). Alterations of alcohol dehydrogenase and other hepatic enzymes following oral alcohol intoxication. *Am. J. Clin. Nutr.,* **11,** 235

223. Rollason, J. G., Pincherle, G. and Robinson, D. (1972). Serum gamma glutamyl transpeptidase in relation to alcohol consumption. *Clin. Chim. Acta,* **39,** 75

224. Rosalki, S. B. and Rau, D. (1972). Serum γ-glutamyltranspeptidase activity in alcoholism. *Clin. Chim. Acta,* **39,** 41

225. Lamy, J., Baglin, M.-C., Aron, E. and Weill, J. (1975). Diminution de la γ-glutamyltranspeptidase sérique des cirrhotiques à la suite du sevrage. *Clin. Chim. Acta,* **60,** 97

226. Lamy, J., Baglin, M.-C., Ferrant, J.-P. and Weill, J. (1975). Emploi de la mesure de la glutamyltranspeptidase sérique pour controler le succès des cures de des intoxication antialcoolique. *Clin. Chim. Acta,* **60,** 103

227. Lum, G. and Gambino, S. R. (1972). Serum gamma-glutamyl transpeptidase activity as an indicator of disease of liver, pancreas, or bone. *Clin. Chem.,* **18,** 358

228. Mendelson, J. H., Stein, S. and McGuire, M. T. (1966). Comparative psychophysiological studies of alcoholic and nonalcoholic subjects undergoing experimentally induced ethanol intoxication. *Psychosom. Med.,* **28,** 1

229. Henley, K. S., Wiggins, H., Hirschowitz, B. and Pollard, H. M. (1958). The effect of oral ethanol on glutamic pyruvic and glutamic oxalacetic transaminase activity in the rat liver. *Q. J. Stud. Alc.,* **19,** 54

230. Sardesai, V. M. and Provido, H. S. (1972). The effect of ethyl alcohol on rat liver tryptophan oxygenase. *Life Sci.,* **11,** 1023.

231. Badawy, A. A.-B. and Evans, M. (1972). Alcohol addiction, porphyria and mental disorders. *Lancet,* **ii,** 374

232. Morland, J., Christoffersen, T., Osnes, J. B., Seglen, P. O. and Jervell, K. F. (1972). An effect of ethanol administration on tryptophan oxygenase in the perfused rat liver. *Biochem. Pharmacol.,* **21,** 1849

233. Gorman, R. E. and Bitensky, M. W. (1970). Selective activation by short-chain alcohols of glucagon-responsive adenyl cyclase in liver. *Endocrinology,* **87,** 1075

234. Ammon, H. P. T., Estler, C. J. and Heim, F. (1969). Inactivation of coenzyme A by ethanol. I. Acetaldehyde as mediator of the inactivation of coenzyme A following the administration of ethanol *in vivo. Biochem. Pharmacol.,* **18,** 29

235. Bode, C., Stahler, E., Kono, H. and Goebell, H. (1970). Effects of ethanol on free coenzyme A. Free carnitine and their fatty acid esters in rat liver. *Biochim. Biophys. Acta,* **210,** 448
236. Breen, K. J., Shaw, J., Levinson, J. D. and Schenker, S. (1971). The acute effect of alcohol on hepatic coenzyme A and acetyl CoA concentrations. *Proc. Soc. Exp. Biol. Med.,* **138,** 1096
237. Paraf, A., Renault, G., Rautureau, J., Fabia, F. and Damour-Lebard, J. (1975). Modification immunitaires et infections dans les cirrhoses alcooliques. *Sem. Hôp. Paris,* **51,** 811
238. Zinneman, M. D. (1975). Autoimmune phenomena in alcoholic cirrhosis. *Dig. Dis.,* **20,** 337
239. Berenyi, M. R., Straus, B. and Cruz, D. (1974). *In vitro* and *in vivo* studies of cellular immunity in alcoholic cirrhosis. *Am. J. Dig. Dis.,* **19,** 199
240. Berenyi, M. R., Straus, B. and Avila, L. (1975). T rosettes in alcoholic cirrhosis of the liver. *J. Am. Med. Ass.,* **232,** 44
241. Lundy, J., Raaf, J. H., Deakins, S., Wanebo, H. J., Jacobs, D. A., Lee, T., Jacobowitz, D., Spear, C. and Oettgen, H. F. (1975). The acute and chronic effects of alcohol on the human immune system. *Surg. Gynecol. Obstet.,* **141,** 212
242. Bernstein, I. M., Webster, K. H., Williams, R. C. and Strickland, R. G. (1974). Reduction in circulating T lymphocytes in alcoholic liver disease. *Lancet,* **ii,** 488
243. Sorrell, M. F. and Leevy, C. M. (1972). Lymphocyte transformation and alcoholic liver injury. *Gastroenterology,* **63,** 1020
244. Pettigrew, N. M., Goudie, R. B., Russell, R. I. and Chaudhuri, A. K. R. (1972). Evidence for a role of hepatitis virus B in chronic alcoholic liver disease. *Lancet,* **ii,** 724
245. Tennenbaum, J. L., Ruppert, R. D., St. Pierre, R. L. and Greenberger, N. J. (1969). The effect of chronic alcohol administration on the immune responsiveness of rats. *J. Allergy,* **44,** 272
246. Mihas, A. A., Bull, D. M. and Davidson, C. S. (1975). Cell-mediated immunity to liver in patients with alcoholic hepatitis. *Lancet,* **i,** 951
247. Zetterman, R. K., Chen, T. and Leevy, C. M. (1974). Role of altered lymphocyte function in alcoholic liver disease. *Gastroenterology,* **67,** 837
248. Paronetto, F. and Lieber, C. S. (1976). Alcoholic liver injury in baboons: cytotoxicity of lymphocytes. *Clin. Res.,* **24,** 434
249. Tisman, G. and Herbert, V. (1973). *In vitro* myelosuppression and immunosuppression by ethanol. *J. Clin. Invest.,* **52,** 1410
250. McLaren, D. S., Faris, R. and Zekain, B. (1968). The liver during recovery from protein-calorie malnutrition. *J. Trop. Med. Hyg.,* **71,** 271
251. Lieber, C. S., DeCarli, L. M. and Rubin, E. (1975). Sequential production of fatty liver, hepatitis and cirrhosis in sub-human primates fed ethanol with adequate diets. *Proc. Nat. Acad. Sci. USA,* **72,** 437
252. MacSween, R. N. M. (1973). Mallory's (alcoholic) hyaline in primary biliary cirrhosis. *J. Clin. Pathol.,* **26,** 340
253. Gerber, M. A., Orr, W., Denk, H., Schaffner, F. and Popper, H. (1973). Hepatocellular hyalin in cholestasis and cirrhosis: its diagnostic significance. *Gastroenterology,* **64,** 89
254. Monroe, S., French, S. W. and Zamboni, L. (1973). Mallory bodies in a case of primary biliary cirrhosis. *Am. J. Clin. Patho.,* **59,** 254
255. Keeley, A. F., Iseri, O. A. and Gottlieb, L. S. (1972). Ultrastructure of hyaline cytoplasmic inclusions in a human hepatoma: relationship to Mallory's alcoholic hyalin. *Gastroenterology,* **62,** 280
256. Roy, S., Ramalingaswami, V. and Nayak, N. C. (1971). An ultrastructural study of the liver in Indian childhood cirrhosis with particular reference to the structure of alcoholic hyaline. *Gut,* **12,** 693
257. Denk, H., Gschnait, F. and Wolff, K. (1975). Hepatocellular hyalin (Mallory bodies) in long term griseofulvin-treated mice: a new experimental model for the study of hyalin formation. *Lab. Invest.,* **32,** 773

258. Kojima, K. (1975). Alcoholic hyalin-like bodies found in the pancreatic acinar cells and nerve cells of the brain. *Acta Pathol. Jap.*, **25,** 281
259. Lischner, M. W., Alexander, J. F. and Galambos, J. T. (1971). Natural history of alcoholic hepatitis. I. The acute disease, *Am. J. Dig. Dis.*, **16,** 481
260. Harinasuta, U. and Zimmerman, H. J. (1971). Alcoholic steatonecrosis. I. Relationship between severity of hepatic disease and presence of Mallory bodies in the liver. *Gastroenterology,* **60,** 1036
261. Biava, C. (1964). Mallory alcoholic hyalin: a heretofore unique lesion of hepatocellular ergastoplasm. *Lab. Invest.*, **13,** 301
262. Flax, M. H. and Tisdale, W. A. (1964). An electron microscopic study of alcoholic hyalin. *Am. J. Pathol.*, **44,** 441
263. Smuckler, E. A. (1968). The ultrastructure of human alcoholic hyaline. *Am. J. Clin. Pathol.*, **49,** 790
264. Iseri, O. A. and Gottlieb, L. S. (1971). Alcoholic hyalin and megamitochondria as separate and distinct entities in liver disease associated with alcoholism. *Gastroenterology,* **60,** 1027
265. Wiggers, K. D., French, S. W., French, B. A. and Carr, B. N. (1973). The ultrastructure of Mallory body filaments. *Lab. Invest.*, **29,** 652
266. Yokoo, H., Minick, O. T., Batti, F. and Kent, G. (1972). Morphologic variants of alcoholic hyalin. *Am. J. Pathol.*, **69,** 25
267. Ma, M. H. (1972). Ultrastructural pathologic findings of the human hepatocyte I. Alcoholic liver disease. *Arch. Pathol.*, **94,** 554
268. Horvath, E., Kovacs, K. and Ross, R. C. (1973). Subcellular features of alcoholic liver lesion: alcoholic hyalin. *J. Pathol.*, **110,** 245
269. French, S. W. and Davies, P. L. (1975). The Mallory body in the pathogenesis of alcoholic liver disease. In J. M. Khanna, Y. Israel and H. Kalant, eds. *Alcoholic Liver Pathology,* p. 113. Toronto: Addiction Research Foundation
270. Edmondson, H. A. (1958). Tumors of the liver and intrahepatic bile ducts. In *Atlas of Tumor Pathology,* Armed Forces Institute of Pathology, Section VII, Fascicle 25, p. 49, Washington, D.C.
271. Lieber, C. S., Zimmon, D., Kessler, R. and DeCarli, L. M. (1976). Portal hypertension in experimental alcoholic liver injury. *Clin. Res.*, **24,** 478
272. Patrick, R. S. (1973). Alcohol as a stimulus to hepatic fibrogenesis. *J. Alcoholism,* **8,** 13
273. McGee, J. O'D., Patrick, R. S., Rodger, M. C. and Luty, C. M. (1974). Collagen proline hydroxylase activity and ^{35}S sulphate uptake in human liver biopsies. *Gut,* **15,** 260
274. Resnick, R. H., Cerda, J. C., Boitnott, J., Aron, J. and Iber, F. L. (1973). Urinary hydroxyproline excretion in hepatic disorders. *Am. J. Gastroenterol.*, **60,** 576
275. Lelbach, W. K. (1975). Cirrhosis in the alcoholic and its relation to the volume of alcohol abuse. *N.Y. Acad. Sci.*, **252,** 85
276. Wilgram, G. F. (1959). Experimental Laennec type of cirrhosis in monkeys. *Ann. Intern. Med.*, **51,** 1134
277. Bhuyan, U. N., Nayak, N. C., Deo, M. G., Ramalingaswami, V. (1965). Effect of dietary protein on carbon tetrachloride-induced hepatic fibrogenesis in albino rats. *Lab. Invest.*, **14,** 184
278. Bhuyan, U. N., Deo, M. G., Ramalingaswami, V. and Nayak, N. C. (1972). Fibroplasia in experimental protein deficiency: a study of fibroblastic growth and of collagen formation and resorption in the rat. *J. Pathol.*, **108,** 191
279. Kyösola, K. and Salorinne, Y. (1975). Liver biopsy and liver function tests in 28 consecutive long-term alcoholics. *Ann. Clin. Res.*, **7,** 80
280. Patek, A. J., Toth, I. G., Saunders, M. G., Castro, G. A. M. and Engel, J. J. (1975). Alcohol and dietary factors in cirrhosis. *Arch. Intern. Med.*, **135,** 1053
281. Sorrel, M. F., Baker, H., Barabk, A. J. and Frank, O. (1974). Release by ethanol of vitamins into rat liver perfusates. *Am. J. Clin. Nutr.*, **27,** 743

282. Di Luzio, N. R. (1966). A mechanism of the acute ethanol-induced fatty liver and the modification of liver injury by antioxidants. *Lab. Invest.*, **15**, 50
283. Hartman, A. D., Di Luzio, N. R. (1968). Inhibition of the chronic ethanol-induced fatty liver by antioxidant administration. *Proc. Soc. Exp. Biol. Med.*, **127**, 270
284. Spritz, N. and Lieber, C. S. (1966). Decrease of ethanol-induced fatty liver by ethyl *α-p*-chlorophenoxyisobutyrate. *Proc. Soc. Exp. Biol. Med.*, **121**, 147
285. Brown, D. F. (1966). The effect of ethyl *α-p*-chlorophenoxyisobutyrate on ethanol-induced hepatic steatosis in the rat. *Metabolism*, **15**, 868
286. Adams, L. L., Webb, W. W. and Fallon, H. J. (1971). Inhibition of hepatic triglyceride formation by clofibrate, *J. Clin. Invest.*, **50**, 2339
287. Kahonen, M. T., Ylikahri, R. H. and Hassinen, I. (1972). Studies on the mechanism of inhibition of acute alcoholic fatty liver by clofibrate. *Metabolism*, **21**, 1021
288. Vincenzi, L., Meldolesi, J., Morini, M. T. and Bassan, P. (1967). Protective effect of phenobarbital and SKF 525a on the acute ethanol-induced fatty liver. *Biochem. Pharmacol.*, **16**, 2431
289. Koff, R. S., Carter, E. A., Lui, S. and Isselbacher, K. J. (1970). Prevention of the ethanol-induced fatty liver in the rat by phenobarbital. *Gastroenterology*, **59**, 50
290. Baker, H., Luisada-Opper, A., Sorrel, M. F., Thomson, A. D. and Frank, O. (1973). Inhibition by nicotinic acid of hepatic steatosis and alcohol dehydrogenase in ethanol-treated rats. *Exp. Molec. Pathol.*, **19**, 106
291. Wooles, W. R. and Weymouth, R. J. (1968). Prevention of the ethanol-induced fatty liver by chlorcyclizine-induced maintenance of hepatic lipid oxidation. *Lab. Invest.*, **18**, 709
292. Lansford, E. M., Hill, I. and Shive, W. (1962). Effects of asparagine and other related nutritional supplements upon alcohol-induced rat liver triglyceride elevation. *J. Nutr.*, **78**, 219
293. Chew, B. K., Alexander, N. M., Scheig, R. and Klatskin, G. (1968). Fatty liver, adenosine triphosphate and asparagine. *Biochem. Pharmacol.*, **17**, 2463
294. Lieber, C. S. (1966). Hepatic and metabolic effects of alcohol. *Gastroenterology*, **50**, 119
295. Estler, C.-J. and Ammon, H. P. T. (1967). The influence of beta-adrenergic blockade on the ethanol-induced derangement of lipid transport (1). *Arch. Intern. Pharmacodyn.*, **166**, No. 2
296. Ammon, H. P. T. and Zeller, W. (1965). Der Einfluss von *α*-pyridylcarbinol auf die durch Alcohol erzeugte Fettleber der Ratte. *Arzneim. Forsch.*, **15**, 1369
297. Radomski, M. W. and Wood, J. D. (1964). The lipotropic action of cold. I. The influence of cold and choline deficiency on liver lipids of rats at different intake of dietary methionine. *Can. J. Physiol. Pharmacol.*, **42**, 769
298. L'Huillier, J. R., Roudier, R. and Thuillier, J. (1967). Évidence histologique de l'efficacité et de l'innocuité de l'oxygene hyperbare dans le traitement de l'intoxication ethylique experimentale. *Med. Pharmacol. Exp.*, **16**, 513
299. Hyams, D. E. and Isselbacher, K. J. (1964). Prevention of fatty liver by administration of adenosine triphosphate. *Nature* (*London*), **204**, 1196
300. Marchetti, M., Ottani, V., Zanetti, P. and Puddu, P. (1968). Aspects of lipid metabolism in ethanol-induced fatty liver. *J. Nutr.*, **95**, 607
301. Koff, R. S. and Fitts, J. J. (1972). Chlorpromazine inhibition of ethanol metabolism without prevention of fatty liver. *Biochem. Med.*, **6**, 77
302. Bustos, G. O., Kalant, H., Khanna, J. M. and Loth, J. (1970). Pyrazole and induction of fatty liver by a single dose of ethanol. *Science*, **168**, 1598
303. Morgan, J. C. and Di Luzio, N. R. (1970). Inhibition of the acute ethanol-induced fatty liver by pyrazole. *Proc. Soc. Exp. Biol. Med.*, **134**, 462
304. Blomstrand, R. and Forsell, L. (1971). Prevention of the acute ethanol-induced fatty liver by 4-methypyrazole. *Life Sci.*, **10**, 523
305. Nordmann, R., Ribière, C., Rouach, H. and Nordmann, J. (1972). Paradoxical effects of pyrazole on acute ethanol-induced fatty liver. *Rev. Eur. Étud. Clin. Biol.*, **17**, 592

306. Domanski, R., Rifenberick, D., Stearns, F., Scorpio, R. M. and Narrod, S. A. (1971). Ethanol-induced fatty liver in rats: effects of pyrazole and glucose. *Proc. Soc. Exp. Biol. Med.*, **138,** 18
307. Prancan, A. V. and Nakano, J. (1972). Effect of pyrazole on conversion of ethanol and acetate in lipids in rat liver. *Res. Commun. Chem. Pathol. Pharmacol.*, **4,** 181
308. Kalant, H., Khanna, J. M. and Bustos, G. O. (1972). Effect of pyrazole on the induction of fatty liver by chronic administration of ethanol. *Biochem. Pharmacol.*, **21,** 811
309. Lieber, C. S., Rubin, E., DeCarli, L. M., Misra, P. S. and Gang, H. (1970). Effects of pyrazole on hepatic function and structure. *Lab. Invest.*, **22,** 615
310. Bizzi, A., Tacconi, M. T., Veneroni, E. and Garattini, S. (1966). Triglyceride accumulation in liver. *Nature (London)*, **209,** 1025
311. Fenster, L. F. (1966). The nonefficacy of short-term anabolic steroid therapy in alcoholic liver disease. *Ann. Intern. Med.*, **65,** 738
312. Jabbari, M. and Leevy, C. M. (1967). Protein anabolism and fatty liver of the alcoholic. *Medicine*, **46,** 131
313. Mendenhall, C. L. (1968). Anabolic steroid therapy as an adjunct to diet in alcoholic hepatic steatosis. *Am. J. Dig. Dis.*, **13,** 783
314. Porter, H. P., Simon, F. R., Pope, C. E., Volwiler, W. and Fenster, L. F. (1971). Corticosteroid therapy in severe alcoholic hepatitis. *N. Engl. J. Med.*, **284,** 1350
315. Reynolds, T. B. and Edmondson, H. A. (1971). Alcoholic hepatitis. *Ann. Intern. Med.*, **74,** 440
316. Campra, J. L., Hamlin, E. M., Kirshbaum, R. J., Olivier, M., Redeker, A. G. and Reynolds, T. B. (1973). Prednisone therapy of acute alcoholic hepatitis (Report of a controlled trial). *Ann. Intern. Med.*, **79,** 625
317. Helman, R. A., Temko, M. H., Nye, S. W. and Fallon, H. J. (1971). Alcoholic hepatitis. *Ann. Intern. Med.*, **74,** 311
318. Lesesne, H. R., Bozynski, E. and Fallon, H. J. (1974). Treatment of alcoholic hepatitis with encephalopathy: comparison of prednisolone with caloric supplements. *Gastroenterology*, **67,** 808
319. Resnick, R. H., Boitnott, J., Iber, F. L., Makopour, H. and Cerda, J. J. (1974). Preliminary observations of d-pencillamine therapy in acute alcoholic liver disease. *Digestion*, **11,** 257
320. Lieber, C. S. (1967). Chronic alcoholic hepatic injury in experimental animals and man: biochemical pathways and nutritional factors. *Fed. Proc.*, **26,** 1443
321. Lieber, C. S. (1975). Alcohol and malnutrition in the pathogenesis of liver disease. *J. Am. Med. Ass.*, **233,** 1077

3
Metabolic Effects of Alcohol on the Intestine

E. BARAONA and J. LINDENBAUM

3.1 INTRODUCTION 82
3.2 CLINICAL FEATURES 82
3.3 EVIDENCE OF MALABSORPTION 82
3.4 DIRECT EFFECTS OF ETHANOL IN THE INTESTINE 84
3.4.1 *Acute administration of ethanol* 84
3.4.1.1 Studies in man 84
3.4.1.2 Studies in animals 84
3.4.2 *Chronic administration of ethanol while maintaining adequate nutrition* 86
3.4.2.1 Studies in man 86
3.4.2.2 Studies in animals 88
3.5 MECHANISMS OF THE EFFECTS OF ETHANOL ON THE SMALL INTESTINE 89
3.5.1 *Effects of ethanol on gastric emptying* 89
3.5.2 *Effects of ethanol on small intestinal motility* 90
3.5.3 *Effects of ethanol on biliary and pancreatic secretions* 90
3.5.4 *Metabolic effects of ethanol on mucosal epithelial cells* 91
3.5.4.1 Acute metabolic effects 91
3.5.4.2 Chronic metabolic effects 97
3.5.5 *Structural effects of ethanol on the intestinal epithelia* 99
3.5.5.1 Acute effects 99
3.5.5.2 Chronic effects 99
3.5.6 *Effects of ethanol on splanchnic circulation of blood and lymph* 103
3.5.7 *Conclusions* 105
3.6 OTHER FACTORS AFFECTING INTESTINAL ABSORPTION IN ALCOHOLICS 106
3.6.1 *Nutritional deficiency states* 106
3.6.2 *Pancreatic disease* 108
3.6.3 *Cirrhosis* 108
3.7 SUMMARY 109
References 110

3.1 INTRODUCTION

Diarrhea and weight loss are frequent manifestations of alcoholism. Alterations in the intestinal absorption of nutrients have long been suspected in alcoholics. The presence of malabsorption was first documented in patients with alcoholic cirrhosis[1,2]. Impaired fat absorption in these patients was attributed to the chronic hepatic and pancreatic complications of alcoholism rather than to ethanol ingestion itself. It subsequently became apparent[3] that malabsorption could also occur in alcoholics without cirrhosis or pancreatitis. In the largest reported series, impairment of intestinal absorption has been found in approximately 50 % of hospitalized alcoholics with[4–8] and without[9–11] cirrhosis.

3.2 CLINICAL FEATURES

In a series of 29 hospitalized chronic alcoholics who were drinking heavily up to the time of admission, complaints of weakness and weight loss were present in 31 %, and vague abdominal pain in 24 %[9]. Similar figures for the incidence of diarrhea in chronic alcoholics have been reported by others[8,12]. These symptoms usually clear after a period of alcohol withdrawal and ingestion of hospital diet.

A close correlation between the presence of intestinal symptoms and impairment of absorptive function, however, has not been apparent[9,11]. Another source of intestinal symptoms could be food intolerance due to incomplete intestinal digestion. This has been recently shown with respect to some disaccharides, mainly lactose[13]. Because of a striking reduction in lactase activity in alcoholics, lactose administration resulted in an increased incidence of diarrhea, cramps and distension[13].

3.3 EVIDENCE OF MALABSORPTION

Steatorrhea has been reported in 35 % to 56 % of alcoholics who have been drinking until a few days prior to testing[9,11]. The steatorrhea has usually been mild, though in a few patients a fecal fat excretion greater than 15 g a day has been noted[9–11]. Low serum carotene[10] and vitamin A levels[14] have also been reported, though these may have been more likely caused by decreased dietary intake of vegetables and impaired hepatic synthesis of retinol-binding protein[14] than by malabsorption.

Evidence of impaired absorption of other substances has frequently been found. The urinary excretion of d-xylose after oral administration was abnormally low in 16 % to 76 % of alcoholics[3,9,11]. Malabsorption of water-soluble vitamins such as thiamine[15,16], folic acid[17] and vitamin B_{12}[9,18] has been demonstrated. A high incidence of elevated fecal excretion of nitrogen[9] has also been reported. Sodium and water transport, as studied during jejunal perfusion, was also found to be impaired[19–21]. There has been a poor correlation between evidence of malabsorption of one substance with that of another[9,11]; this has been particularly true for xylose and fat, suggesting that different mechanisms may account for the impaired assimilation of these substances.

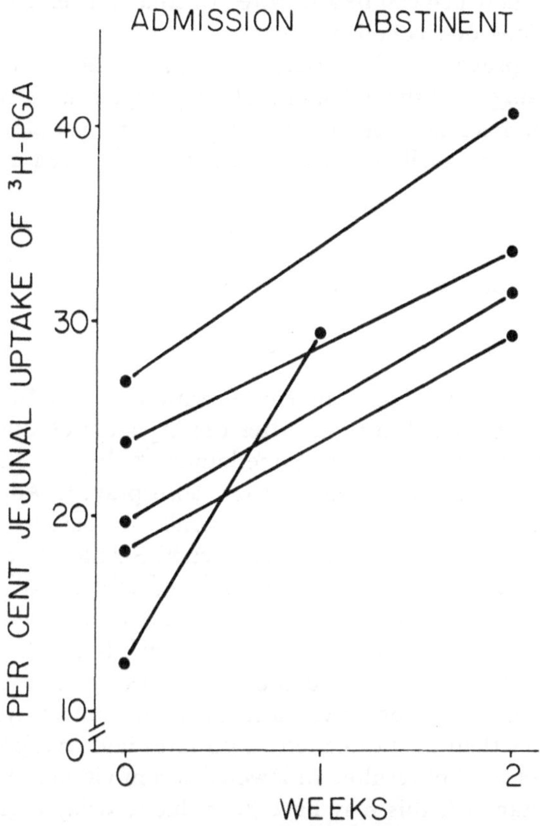

Figure 3.1 Improvement of jejunal uptake of [^{3}H]pteroylglutamic acid in five patients who were treated with abstinence and a hospital diet after admission to hospital. Four patients were restudied after 2 weeks and one after 1 week (from Halsted *et al.*[20])

The abnormalities in absorptive function usually return to normal within a few weeks of hospitalization (Figure 3.1), during which time alcohol has been withdrawn, and nutritional status and hepatic and pancreatic function have often improved. Malabsorption of fat may persist, however, especially in patients with severe hepatic or pancreatic disease, and, in a minority of malnourished patients, xylose absorption may not improve for many weeks[9,22].

3.4 DIRECT EFFECTS OF ETHANOL ON THE INTESTINE

Malabsorption in alcoholics cannot be attributed to a single cause. The direct effects of ethanol ingestion as well as other disorders associated with alcoholism appear to contribute to its pathogenesis. Among the latter alterations, malnutrition, pancreatic insufficiency and cirrhosis of the liver are important causes of malabsorption in alcoholics. Therefore we will attempt to separate the effects which can be attributed to ethanol itself from those due to other complications of alcoholism.

The rapid improvement in absorptive capacity observed after alcohol withdrawal has suggested that ethanol itself may impair intestinal functions. A number of experimental observations in man and animals indicate that ethanol affects the small intestine even in the absence of associated malnutrition.

3.4.1 Acute administration of ethanol

3.4.1.1 Studies in man

Jejunal perfusion with ethanol in concentration of 2 g/100 ml, which is reached in the upper small intestine after the ingestion of a moderate dose[23], interfered with the absorption of L-methionine[24] (Figure 3.2), but had no significant effects on sodium and water absorption[25]. Administration of ethanol in doses of 1.5 g/kg/b.w., either orally or parenterally, decreased thiamine absorption in four of twelve subjects[16]. Smaller doses, administered orally, had no effect on the absorption of calcium[26], folic acid[17], and ferrous or haemoglobin iron[27] in human volunteers. Single doses of alcohol were reported to increase the absorption of ferric iron[27]. Since this effect was not seen in three of four achlorhydric subjects, it was postulated that ethanol enhanced ferric iron absorption via stimulation of gastric hydrochloric acid production rather than by a direct effect on intestinal transport[27]. The acute administration of alcohol resulted in lowered serum vitamin A levels 4 h after a dose of the vitamin[28]; this may have been due to delayed gastric emptying rather than to an effect on intestinal absorption. It must be pointed out that the experimental doses of ethanol given to human volunteers have usually been much lower than those spontaneously consumed by alcoholics. Most of the absorptive capacity of the intestine will remain unaffected by the administration of a dose of ethanol which is rapidly absorbed in the upper portion of the gastrointestinal tract.

3.4.1.2 Studies in animals

In rats, the acute administration of ethanol (2.5 g/kg/b.w.) decreased the absorption of an actively transported amino acid, L-phenylalanine, but not that of the passively absorbed isomer, D-phenylalanine[29]. Absorption was judged from the blood levels achieved after intragastric administration; therefore, the possibility that ethanol could have affected amino acid metabolism was not ruled out. The previous administration of an intragastric ethanol dose (3.2 g/kg) to rats was reported to reduce the ability of isolated duodenal loops (with intact circulation) to absorb ferrous iron[30]; a smaller dose of ethanol was

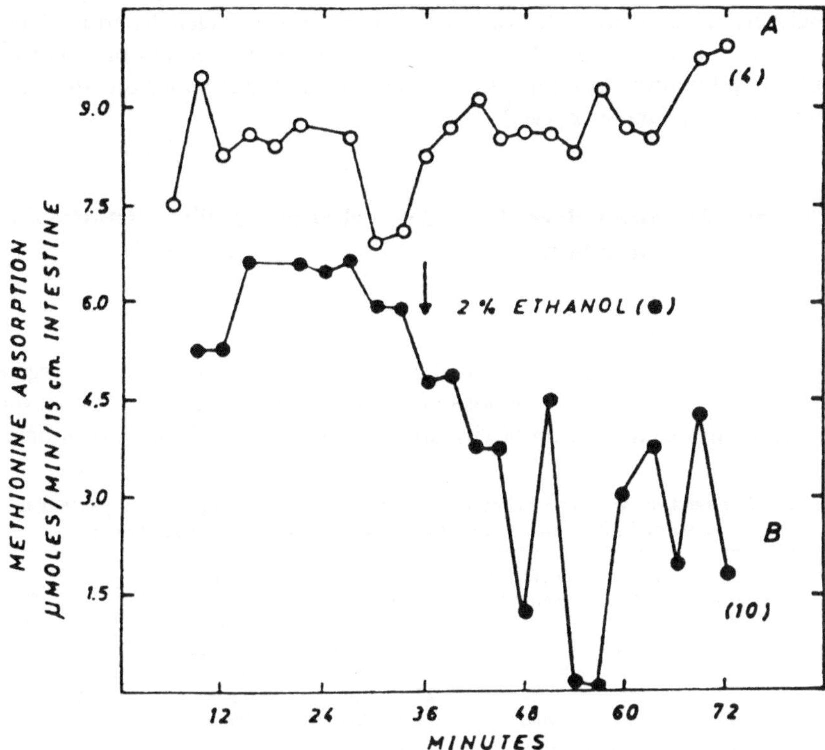

Figure 3.2 Methionine absorption in perfusion studies of human small intestine. The points represent the average for four subjects in curve A and ten in curve B. The arrow shows the time at which alcohol was added to the perfusion fluid. No alcohol was added throughout the experiment to the subjects in curve A (from Israel *et al.*[24])

reported to have no effect on iron absorption[31]. After a very large single dose (7.5 g/kg), which caused gross intestinal lesions, inhibition of calcium transport was reported[32]. Acute alcohol administration to rats inhibited the active transport of thiamine at low concentrations, but did not affect the passive diffusion of the vitamin at high concentrations[33].

In vitro, ethanol inhibited the active transport of D-glucose[34] and L-amino acids[29,34] by everted sacs of small intestine. Minimal effects were observed at ethanol concentrations as low as 0.5 g/100 ml; marked changes were found at concentrations of 2–3 g/100 ml. At the highest concentration (3 g/100 ml) there was tissue damage and increased permeability to passively transported substances[34]. The addition of ethanol *in vitro* was also found to depress the uptake of trace elements by chick duodenal segments[35].

In contrast, single doses of ethanol have been reported to enhance the absorption of some substances. Fat absorption was increased after a single dose of alcohol in rats[36]. When a lipid emulsion, containing fatty acids, monoglycerides, and bile salts was administered intraduodenally to rats, the addition of ethanol (2.5 g/100 ml) markedly increased the output of lipid into the intestinal lymph[36]. Alcohol has also been reported to enhance the intestinal transport of manganese in rats[37].

3.4.2 Chronic administration of ethanol while maintaining adequate nutrition

3.4.2.1 Studies in man

Experimental administration of alcohol in man has resulted in divergent results. Ethanol ingestion for periods of several weeks along with a nutritious diet resulted in malabsorption of vitamin B_{12} in six of eight human volunteers

Table 3.1 Per cent urinary excretion of Co-57 vitamin B_{12} during control periods and ethanol administration in human volunteers (from Lindenbaum and Lieber[39])

Subject	*% Urinary Co-57 B_{12} excretion* Control (pre- and/or post-ethanol) 24 h	*Control 48 h*	*Ethanol 24 h*	*Ethanol 48 h*	*Number of days on ethanol when tested*	*Maximum ethanol dose % total caloric intake*
1	42.4	51.4	27.4	33.0	13	46
	40.7*	50.6	11.9	20.6	26	
2	12.1	16.2	5.9		21	60
	12.1*	16.8	6.7	11.0	31	
	11.2*	17.5				
3	17.0	21.0	13.1	17.4	21	60
4	10.5	15.4	5.9	10.2	34	66
5	18.3	18.8	3.1	3.9	21	46
	14.7*	19.4	6.1†	7.9	28	
6	20.9	30.0	14.5	22.7	23	46
	15.4	25.3	10.2	10.5	37	
7	10.2	14.4	17.3	23.1	25	46
			17.8	25.5	33	
8	7.4	10.6	8.8	11.0	25	46

* Post-ethanol period, 8–22 days after cessation of alcohol administration
† 57Co-B_{12} given with 9 g pancreatin (Viokase)

(Table 3.1)[38,39]. The coadministration of intrinsic factor or pancreatin with cyanocobalamin did not correct the absorptive defect, suggesting interference with ileal function[38,39]. In the same subjects, however, serum and urinary xylose levels (Figure 3.3) after an oral dose were increased during ethanol administration as compared to control periods; alcohol did not appear to affect the clearance or urinary excretion of intravenously administered xylose[39]. Fat

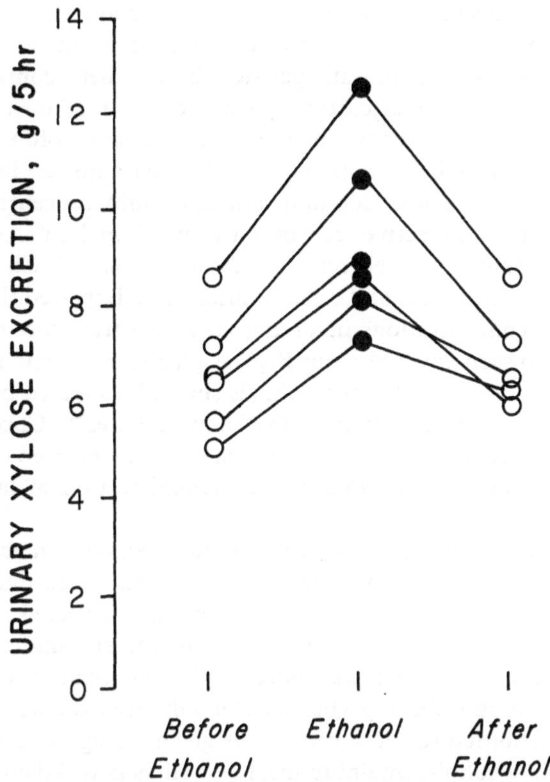

Figure 3.3 Urinary xylose excretion after an oral 25 g dose in six subjects after several weeks on ethanol and nutritious diet as compared to pre- and post-ethanol control periods (from Lindenbaum and Lieber[39])

absorption also appeared to improve or show no change during chronic ethanol ingestion[39] and the absorption of a large dose of folic acid was unaffected[40].

Other investigators have reported that 2–3 weeks of alcohol administration along with a nutritious diet did not cause xylose or fat malabsorption[11,20]. The uptake of small doses of folic acid in jejunal perfusion studies was unchanged or improved in five, and depressed in two, of seven patients given ethanol along with hospital diet for 2 weeks[20]. Sodium and water absorption was impaired by a 2-week period of alcohol feeding in four human volunteers[25] and after 26 days in another subject[21].

3.4.2.2 *Studies in animals*

The administration of ethanol (20 g/100 ml in the drinking water) to rats for 3 weeks resulted in decreased absorption of intraduodenally administered xylose[41]. An inhibitory effect of chronic ethanol feeding on carbohydrate absorption was demonstrated in rats pair-fed liquid diets containing either ethanol or, in controls, isocaloric carbohydrate for 25 to 39 days[42]. Decreased mucosal uptake of xylose, 2-deoxyglucose, and glucose was found in isolated jejunal loops with intact blood supply in alcohol-fed animals; impairment of glucose absorption was seen at 200 mM, but not 2 mM concentrations of the sugar, suggesting that the active transport was not impaired[42]. Alternatively, these alterations could reflect a decreased absorptive area[43]. Chronic ethanol feeding with adequate protein and vitamin intake also impaired the absorption of vitamin B_{12} at concentrations involving an active transport mechanism[44]. The effect was also seen when vitamin B_{12} was placed in intestinal loops along with rat intrinsic factor. Alcohol-fed animals showed decreased binding of the B_{12}-intrinsic factor complex by intestinal homogenates[44]. Chronic ethanol feeding also interfered with active calcium transport by everted duodenal sacs of rats[45] and this was not restored by the administration of large doses of vitamin D[46].

Chronic alcohol feeding was found to have no effect on iron absorption[30,31]. In rats fed alcohol chronically, there were no increased fecal losses of nitrogen[47,48]. Fat absorption also appeared to be little affected in rats by the chronic administration of ethanol. In contrast to the stimulatory effect of a single dose of ethanol on the transport of dietary lipid into the lymph, previous chronic ethanol feeding abolished or inhibited the acute effect of a single dose[36]. Ethanol-fed rats absorbed lipids given intragastrically[49] or intraduodenally[36] in an alcohol-containing meal as well as pair-fed controls. When rats chronically fed alcohol were then given a meal containing no ethanol, the animals showed a slight decrease in fat absorption compared to their pair-fed controls[36]. However, steatorrhea did not occur in rats chronically fed alcohol[48]. Chronic ethanol feeding, with or without restriction of protein intake, had no effect on the uptake of folic acid by perfused rat jejunum[49a].

In conclusion, ethanol administration markedly depresses the transport of some substances and stimulates or has little or no effect on that of others (Table 3.2). The reasons for the different effects of ethanol on small bowel function, depending upon the substance tested, the mode of administration or the animal species studied, are not yet understood. It has been suggested that in *man* alcohol impairs the absorption of actively transported nutrients, but has no effect (or even an enhancing one) on passive diffusion processes[39]. In

Table 3.2 Effects of experimental alcohol administration on intestinal absorption in the absence of nutritional deficiency

Substance	*Single ethanol doses*		*Chronic ethanol administration*	
	Rats	*Humans*	*Rats*	*Humans*
Glucose	↓	NS	↓	0
Xylose	NS	↓	↓	0 or ↑
L-Amino acids	↓	↓	NS	NS
D-Phenylalanine	0	NS	NS	NS
Iron	0 or ↓	0 or ↑	0	NS
Calcium	0 or ↓	0	↓	NS
Sodium, water	NS	0	NS	↓
Manganese	↑	NS	NS	NS
Thiamine	↓	0 or ↓	NS	NS
Folic acid	NS	0	0	0
Vitamin B_{12}	NS	NS	↓	↓
Fat	↑	NS	0	0 or ↑
Nitrogen	NS	NS	0	NS

NS = not studied ↑ = increased ↓ = decreased 0 = unchanged

the *rat*, as mentioned above, a differential effect of acute ethanol administration on the active and passive transport of nutrients was demonstrated. However, chronic ethanol feeding in rats may interfere with passive transport as well, perhaps as a consequence of a reduced absorptive area[43].

3.5 MECHANISMS OF THE EFFECTS OF ETHANOL ON THE SMALL INTESTINE

Only a limited amount has been learned about the mechanisms underlying the effects of ethanol on intestinal absorption, and mostly in the rat model. Alcohol could modify intestinal absorption by acting on processes preceding the actual absorption of nutrients, by affecting the absorptive capacity of individual villus epithelial cells, or the number of cells present, or by modifying the blood or lymphatic circulation of the small bowel.

3.5.1 Effects of ethanol on gastric emptying

In early studies the rate of gastric emptying was studied after administration of alcoholic beverages[50–52]. Such beverages contain ethanol in concentrations which modify gastric emptying, but they also contain congeners which may possibly affect the rate of gastric emptying. The effects of ethanol itself on gastric emptying are concentration-dependent. A concentration of approximately 8–10 g/100 ml (such as those found in wines) is needed to demonstrate significant changes in gastric emptying[53,54]. Concentrations of ethanol of this order of magnitude have been reported to accelerate[54,55] as well as delay[53] gastric emptying. Greater concentrations (such as those found in common spirits) inhibit gastric emptying[54,56]. This inhibitor effect may be mediated by hyperosmolarity[57] or by irritative actions of ethanol on gastric mucosa[53]. In addition, a central nervous system mechanism has been proposed for the inhibition of gastric emptying produced by intoxicating doses of ethanol given intravenously[58] or intraperitoneally[59].

3.5.2 Effects of ethanol on small intestinal motility

In electromanometric and cineradiological studies in normal human subjects, intravenously administered ethanol caused a significant increase in motility in the second part of the duodenum[60]. Increases in pressure and in the number of waves, were followed by decreased activity with a slow return to normality. More recently, the effects of ethanol on motility in the human jejunum and ileum have been measured after oral and intravenous administration[61]. Ethanol given by either route decreased type I (impending) waves in the jejunum and increased type III (propulsive) waves, more strikingly in the ileum. This pattern of motility should result in accelerated transit through the small intestine and possibly may contribute to the diarrhea seen in alcoholics[61]. It has been observed that alterations in gastric or intestinal motor function could account for the changes in xylose absorption noted in humans chronically fed alcohol[39].

3.5.3 Effects of ethanol on biliary and pancreatic secretions

Ethanol was reported to exert a dual effect on bile secretion in the rat. After acute administration, when blood concentrations were high (over 50 mg/100 ml), bile secretion was depressed; this effect was observed both in bile fistula rats[62,63] and in isolated perfused liver preparations[63,64]. By contrast, chronic ethanol feeding increased the flow of bile and the secretion of both bile salts and the non bile salt dependent fraction of bile[63]. This increased bile salt secretion probably reflects an increased bile salt pool rather than increased synthesis since bile salt turnover has been shown to be decreased by chronic ethanol feeding[65].

The acute administration of ethanol stimulates pancreatic secretion both in man and animals[66], but this effect is suppressed by gastrectomy[67], suggesting that it is mediated by stimulation of gastric acid secretion. If the gastric acid–duodenal secretin mechanism is eliminated, ethanol has a direct inhibitory effect on pancreatic secretion of fluid, bicarbonate concentration and output of enzymes in the dog[68]. The effects of ethanol in the intact individual are complex, depending on the magnitude of the direct and indirect effects[69–71]. In dogs who have been fed alcohol chronically, acute ethanol administration has been reported to stimulate pancreatic secretion[72]. Chronic ethanol administration in rats has been found to cause either an increase or a decrease in enzyme synthesis, depending on the protein and fat content of the diet[72]. The theory that alcohol causes pancreatitis by stimulating increased secretion as well as obstructing the main pancreatic duct by increasing pressure at the sphincter of Oddi has not been widely accepted[72,73]. It has been proposed that chronic alcohol ingestion in man may cause the precipitation of enzyme proteins in the smaller pancreatic ducts which results in obstruction and pancreatitis[72].

The effects of experimental chronic ethanol ingestion on pancreatic function in man have not been extensively studied. The administration of 256 g of alcohol daily (along with 105 g of protein) to alcoholic patients for 2 weeks did not prevent improvement of previously depressed pancreatic function as measured by secretin tests[11].

3.5.4 Metabolic effects of ethanol on mucosal epithelial cells

3.5.4.1 Acute metabolic effects

The cellular effects produced by ethanol are generally due either to direct effects of this substance or to metabolic imbalances secondary to its oxidation. The small intestine possesses some alcohol dehydrogenase (ADH) activity[74,75] and it is able to oxidize ethanol to CO_2[76]. However the magnitude of this oxidation is small. The predominant role of the liver in ethanol oxidation is well documented[77–80]. It has been reported that the capacity of intestinal slices to produce CO_2 from ethanol is about two-thirds that of liver slices. However, in these experiments the capacity of the liver to oxidize ethanol was greatly underestimated: the production of CO_2 only reflects a minimal fraction of the ethanol oxidized because most of the acetate resulting from hepatic ethanol oxidation does not complete its oxidation to CO_2 in the liver, but is released into the blood and oxidized by extrahepatic tissues[81].

In support of the possibility that some effects of ethanol could be linked to its oxidation by the small intestine, pyrazole (a known inhibitor of alcohol dehydrogenase) has been reported to prevent stimulatory effects of ethanol on intestinal triglyceride synthesis[82] and transport of manganese[37]. The effects of pyrazole on the intestine are not well known. In the liver, however, this substance not only inhibits ADH activity, but also depresses a variety of other enzymes and produces striking structural alterations[83]. Animals given a single injection of pyrazole or fed a pyrazole-containing diet for 28 days exhibited a 70 % increase in small intestinal ATP content without concomitant alterations in hepatic ATP[84]. This suggests that pyrazole exerts effects on the intestine which are not linked to inhibition of ethanol oxidation. The effects of ethanol on triglyceride synthesis and manganese transport have been observed at ethanol concentrations of 2.6 and 3 g/100 ml, respectively. Because of its low K_m, alcohol dehydrogenase should be fully saturated at ethanol concentrations of about 10 mg/100 ml. Therefore, the effects secondary to the metabolic imbalances produced by the oxidation of ethanol through this pathway should be

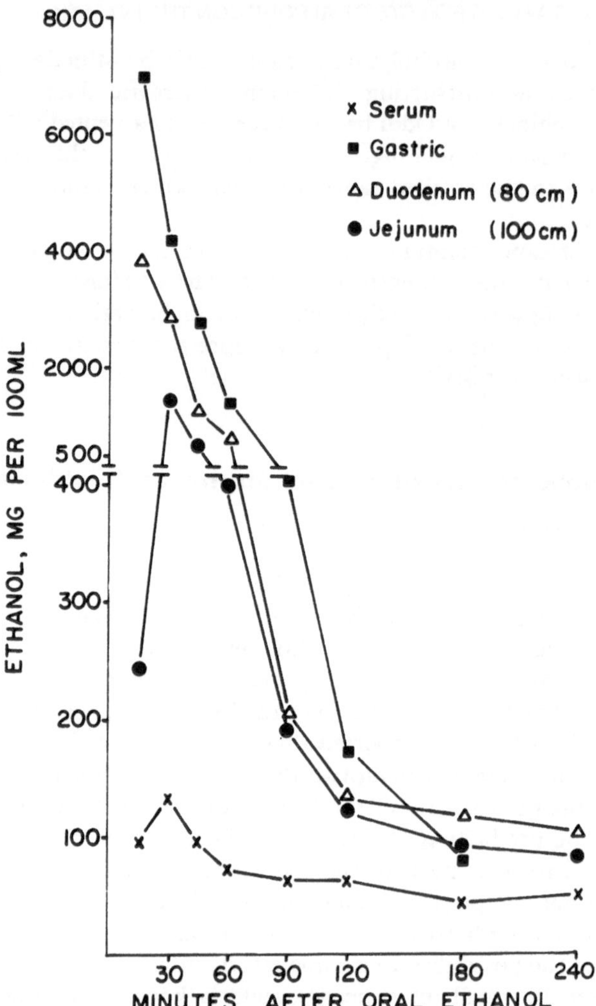

Figure 3.4 Concentrations of ethanol in the serum, and in the gastric, duodenal and proximal jejunal contents of an alcoholic patient at timed intervals after the acute oral ingestion of ethanol, 0.8 g/kg b.w. (Numbers in parentheses refer to distance from the teeth to each aspiration port.) From Halsted *et al.*[23]

apparent at this low ethanol concentration. A system for ethanol oxidation of much higher K_m, the microsomal ethanol oxidizing system (MEOS) has been described in the liver[85], but it has not been found in the intestine. An *in vitro* concentration of ethanol (125 mg/100 ml) sufficient to saturate both oxidative systems failed to demonstrate significant effects on intestinal lipid metabolism[86].

The oral or intragastric administration of ethanol in concentrations similar to those of alcoholic beverages produces in the lumen of the small intestine ethanol concentrations much greater than those necessary to saturate all

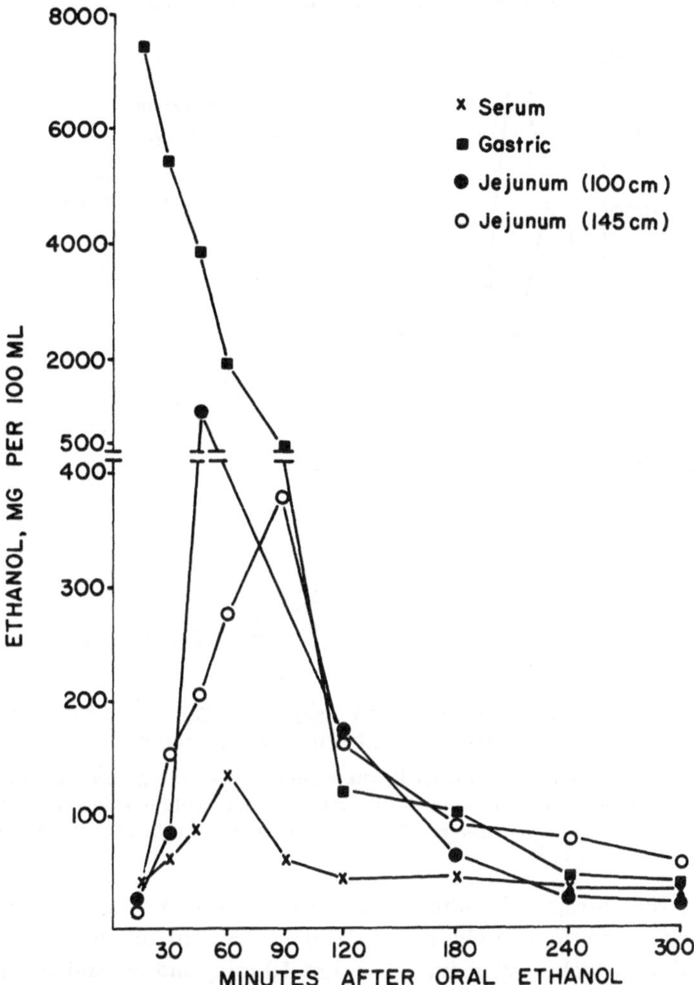

Figure 3.5 Concentrations of ethanol in the serum, and in the gastric, proximal jejunal and midjejunal contents of an alcoholic patient at timed intervals after the acute oral ingestion of ethanol. Conditions similar to those of Figure 3.4 (from Halsted *et al.*[23]).

known ethanol oxidizing systems. After oral ingestion by three human subjects of 0.8 g of ethanol per kg/b.w. (a dose which results in blood concentrations of 100–150 mg/100 ml), in a concentration of 25 g/100 ml (less than that in most spirits), the highest ethanol concentrations in the lumen of the gastrointestinal tract were observed within the first hour[23] (Figures 3.4, 3.5 and 3.6). At this time, ethanol concentrations reached a maximum between 7–8 g/100 ml in the stomach, 4 g/100 ml in the duodenum and between 1–4 g/100 ml in the upper jejunum. The concentrations in the duodenum and upper jejunum remained greater than 400 mg/100 ml for more than 1 h. Ileal ethanol concentrations were lower and paralleled those in the serum[23].

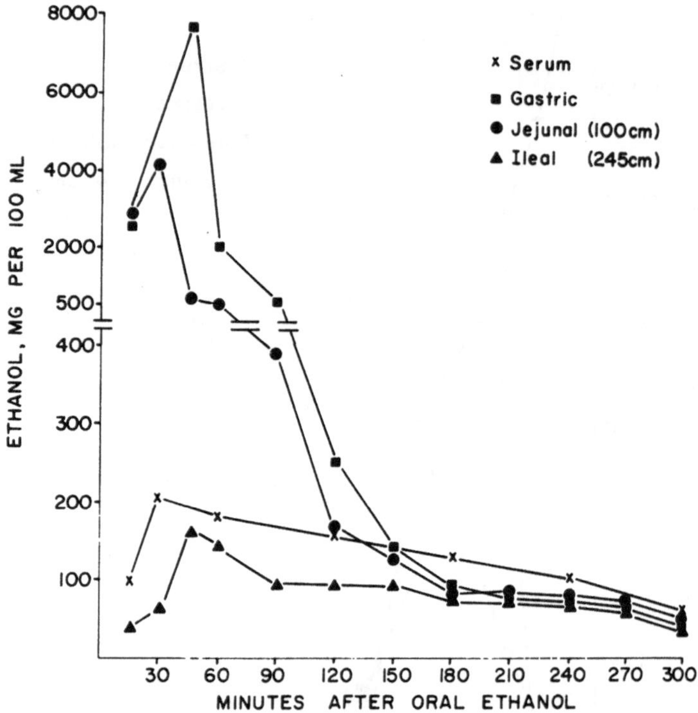

Figure 3.6 Concentrations of ethanol in the serum, and in the gastric, jejunal and ileal contents of an alcoholic patient at timed intervals after the acute oral ingestion of ethanol, 0.8 g/kg b.w. (Numbers in parentheses refer to the distance from the teeth to each aspiration port). From Halsted *et al.*[23]

In rats, the intragastric administration of an ethanol dose which led to blood levels of approximately 150 mg/100 ml resulted in intestinal luminal concentrations which were maximal within 10 min, and dependent upon the concentration of ethanol administered[43]. After ethanol was given in a concentration of 35 g/100 ml (similar to common spirits), a concentration of about 3 g/100 ml was found in the upper jejunum whereas an equal dose administered at a concentration of 5 g/100 ml (similar to that of beers) led to intraluminal concentrations which averaged 1.2 g/100 ml[43]. After administration of an intermediate concentration (20 g/100 ml) to the rat, the jejunal concentration peak occurred at 10 min and averaged 1.75 g/100 ml (range: 2.70–0.98)[29]. Thus, the upper small intestine, both in man and rat, is exposed during ethanol ingestion to local concentrations much greater than those encountered in other tissues even during severe intoxication. The next highest ethanol concentrations are found in the portal blood[87] and in the mesenteric lymph[49]. The ethanol concentration in the mixed (portal and arterial) hepatic blood is probably reflected in the bile, resulting in an enterohepatic circulation of ethanol[87].

Single doses of ethanol have been shown to affect predominantly the absorption of nutrients which require an active transport mechanism. The active absorption of glucose and amino acids depends upon sodium transport. In concentrations attainable in the small intestine, ethanol inhibits the ($Na^+ + K^+$)-activated ATPase activity of brain and other tissues[88]. A fully operative sodium transport system depends upon this activity. Therefore, it has been postulated that ethanol impairs intestinal transport via inhibition of this enzyme[29,33,34]. The inhibition of intestinal thiamine transport was reported to be at the exit of the vitamin from the cell rather than at the uptake from the gut lumen[33]. A similar effect on thiamine transport was found with ouabain, a known inhibitor of ATPase[33]. It has not yet been demonstrated that acute or chronic ethanol administration affects this enzyme in the small bowel.

Though ATPase inhibition may well be a site of ethanol action, the cellular alterations produced by ethanol at the concentrations achieved in the intestine are more generalized. Concentrations of ethanol of 1.6–3.2 g/100 ml have been shown to inhibit oxygen consumption both in isolated epithelial cells[89] and intestinal slices[29]. Much stronger inhibition of oxygen consumption, however, was produced by a dose of cyanide that inhibited active amino acid transport to the degree seen with ethanol[29]. It was therefore argued that the effect of alcohol on amino acid transport was not due to direct interference with oxidative metabolism[29]. Jejunal slices obtained from rats given an acute dose of alcohol prior to sacrifice also showed a depressed oxygen consumption even when incubated without ethanol[43]. In addition, previous administration of an ethanol dose *in vivo* diminished the ability of the slices to survive *in vitro*[43], suggesting a more diffuse and permanent alteration of the cell.

Intestinal ATP content has also been found decreased after acute and chronic ethanol administration and after *in vitro* incubation with ethanol (2.6 g/100 ml)[84]. These effects of ethanol were not prevented by pyrazole[84]. The administration of a moderate dose of alcohol to normal volunteer subjects decreased the activity of jejunal glycolytic (hexokinase, fructose-1-phosphate aldolase and fructose-1,6-diphosphate aldolase) and gluconeogenetic (fructose-1,6-diphosphatase) enzymes within 24 h[90]. On the other hand, ethanol increased the activity of pyruvate kinase. Folic acid, which is a potent stimulator of jejunal glycolytic enzymes, reversed the inhibitory action of ethanol. Conversely, the response of these activities to folate administration was decreased by the concomitant administration of ethanol (producing a 42–45 % increase in the glycolytic activities and no change in the gluconeogenetic activity instead of the 1.6–2-fold increase seen after folate alone). Folate and ethanol exerted a synergistic stimulation of pyruvate kinase activity[90]. It is not clear whether folic acid actually antagonized a reversible inhibitory effect of ethanol or acted on cell populations which remain unaffected by ethanol.

As in many other tissues, fatty acids are the preferred fuel for the small intestine[91]. In rats, intraduodenal infusion of a solution containing ethanol (3.4 g/100 ml) for 15 hours decreased the oxidation of intravenously injected

[^{14}C]palmitate to water-soluble metabolites (including $^{14}CO_2$) in the small intestine[92]. This effect was attributed to ethanol oxidation by the intestine. In *in vitro* studies, however, the incorporation of palmitate label into $^{14}CO_2$ was inhibited by ethanol in concentrations of 2.5 g/100 ml or greater, but was unaffected by concentrations of 0.5 and 1 g/100 ml, suggesting that this effect is not linked to ethanol oxidation[86] (Table 3.3). Total CO_2 production was also decreased, which excludes the possibility that the inhibition of the labelling could be accounted for by isotopic dilution of the acetylCoA pool by the acetate resulting from the oxidation of ethanol. In addition, the intragastric administration of ethanol (3 g/kg/b.w.) to rats prior to sacrifice reduced the ability of jejunal (but not ileal) slices to oxidize fatty acids even in the absence of ethanol in the media[86]. These findings suggest a more permanent inability of the ethanol-exposed intestine to perform a variety of biochemical reactions.

Table 3.3 Effects of ethanol on palmitate oxidation and esterification by intestinal slices* (from Baraona *et al.*[86])

Ethanol concentration	*[^{14}C]palmitate disappearance* (dpm/mg tissue)	*$^{14}CO_2$ production* (dpm/mg tissue)	*[^{14}C]triglyceride production* (dpm/mg tissue)	*[^{14}C]ethylpalmitate production†* (dpm/mg tissue)
0	1679 ± 98	246 ± 17	343 ± 46	0
0.5	1543 ± 50	202 ± 15	263 ± 34	91 ± 81
1.0	1466 ± 105	220 ± 20	98 ± 10‡	15 ± 81
2.5	1500 ± 128	88 ± 10‡	82 ± 14‡	433 ± 116‡
5.0	1808 ± 101	34 ± 4‡	44 ± 9‡	551 ± 120‡

* Jejunal slices obtained from seven chow-fed rats (fasted overnight), were incubated in Krebs–Ringer phosphate medium containing a micellar solution of [^{14}C]palmitate, mono-oleate and taurocholate for 30 min, with and without ethanol. Each value represents the mean ± SE

† Identification based on chromatographic characteristics and labelling with [^{14}C]ethanol

‡ $P < 0.01$, paired comparisons with slices incubated without ethanol

The *in vitro* activity of intestinal adenyl cyclase, an enzyme involved in the formation of cyclic AMP was increased by ethanol in concentrations much higher than those attainable *in vivo*[93]. The acute perfusion of ethanol in concentrations of 1–8 g/100 ml was reported to have no effect on jejunal cAMP levels in man[28].

A point of controversy concerns the effects of ethanol on intestinal triglyceride synthesis. Intestinal slices incubated with ethanol (2.5–2.6 g/100 ml) were reported to have a 30 % increase in triglyceride synthesis by some investigators[82] and a 76 % decrease by others[86]. In both studies the incorporation of [^{14}C]palmitate into triglyceride fractions isolated by thin-layer chromatography was measured, but in the second study[86] a much higher concentration of fatty acid was used. Under the latter conditions, the incorporation of labelled palmitate into intestinal triglycerides was progressively inhibited by ethanol concentrations from 1–5 g/100 ml while an increasing amount of the fatty acid label was incorporated into a lipid band, adjacent to that of triglycerides, which was readily visible at high concentrations of both ethanol and fatty acids[86] (Table 3.3). This lipid fraction incorporated not only fatty acids but also equimolar amounts of labelled ethanol and was identified as ethylpalmitate by gas liquid chromatography and by the splitting off of ethanol during saponification[86]. The increased esterification of fatty acids with ethanol disappeared in boiled slices[86], suggesting that ethylpalmitate formation requires some enzymatic system either in the intestinal cells or in the contaminating luminal contents[94]. Contamination of triglycerides with ethyl fatty acid esters could account for as much as a 50 % increase in apparent triglyceride synthesis in the presence of high ethanol concentrations.

There are also divergent results in studies in which the ability of the ethanol-exposed intestine to synthesize triglycerides has been assessed in the absence of significant amounts of ethanol in the preparation. It has been reported that microsomes obtained from intestinal slices incubated for 1 h in a medium containing ethanol (2.6 g/100 ml), have an increased ability to convert [^{14}C]palmitate into triglyceride in a medium containing no ethanol[82]. By contrast, decreased triglyceride synthesis was found in jejunal slices obtained from rats given ethanol intragastrically 1 h prior to sacrifice and then washed and incubated without ethanol[86].

A number of studies have been performed in rats in the fasting state, 15–18 h after intragastric administration of ethanol in a high dose (7.5 g/kg/b.w.)[82,95] or after prolonged (5–15 h) jejunal perfusion with high ethanol concentrations (3.4–15 g/100 ml)[92,96,97]. Under these conditions, increased mucosal triglyceride[82,92,96] and cholesterol[95] synthesis, enhanced activities of jejunal lipid re-esterifying enzymes (microsomal acylCoA synthetase and acylCoA: monoglyceride acyltransferase)[97], and increased lymph output of cholesterol[95] and triglycerides[96] have been found after ethanol. However, in view of the rapid cell turnover of the small intestine, one wonders whether the observed effects can be attributed not only to direct actions of ethanol on intestinal lipid metabolism but also to cellular necrosis and repair as a consequence of the high ethanol concentrations[32,43,98] or to increased intraluminal content of lipids and other nutrients derived from sloughed cells.

In summary, the ingestion of alcohol results in intestinal concentrations of ethanol which are much greater than those necessary to saturate all known pathways of ethanol oxidation. The intestinal effects observed at these high concentrations are most likely due to a direct action of ethanol rather than to the metabolic disturbances associated with its local oxidation. These direct effects include inhibition of active transport and of a variety of metabolic activities, suggestive of diffuse cell damage.

3.5.4.2 Chronic metabolic effects

Striking changes in metabolic activities occur in the small intestine after chronic ethanol feeding along with nutritionally adequate diets. Intestinal slices obtained from rats which have been fed ethanol for several weeks showed increased oxygen consumption[43], increased ability to oxidize fatty acids[86] and to synthesize triglycerides[82,86] (Figure 3.7). The effects on lipid metabolism were associated with increased activity of palmitoylCoA synthetase in the mucosal homogenates of ethanol-fed rats[86]. This suggests that these rats may develop an increased intestinal capacity to form acylCoA esters, a step which is necessary for both fatty acid oxidation and triglyceride synthesis. These metabolic changes are opposite to those found 1 h after acute ethanol administration and similar to some of the changes observed 16–18 h after administration of a high ethanol dose. The mechanisms underlying these increased metabolic activities are unknown.

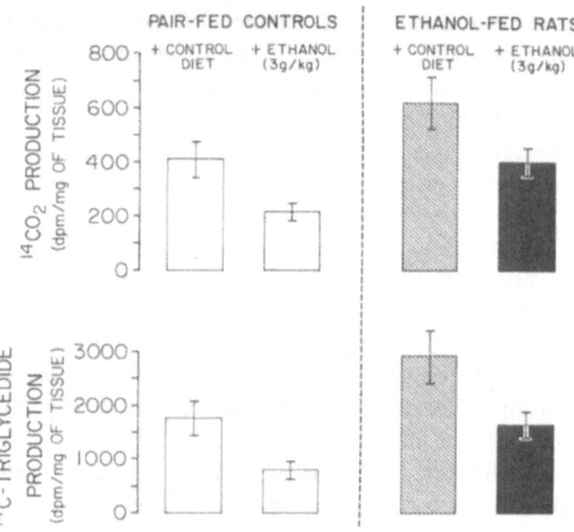

Figure 3.7 Effects of acute and chronic ethanol pretreatment on jejunal oxidation of palmitate and triglyceride synthesis *in vitro*. Intestinal slices were obtained from seven groups of four rats 1 h after intragastric administration of a single dose of diet containing either ethanol (3 g/kg/b.w.) or isocaloric carbohydrate. The slices were incubated in Krebs–Ringer phosphate medium containing a micellar solution of [^{14}C]palmitate, mono-oleate and taurocholate for 30 min. Two rats of each group were previously fed an ethanol-containing diet for 3–4 weeks, and two were fed similar amounts of control diet. Each value represents the mean ± SEM of seven determinations

The chronic metabolic changes are not, however, associated with enhanced absorptive function; frequently the opposite relationship has been found. Fat absorption in ethanol-fed rats was either unaffected or slightly depressed depending upon whether an acute dose of ethanol was given before the test[36]. Chronic ethanol feeding impaired the absorption of carbohydrate[42] and vitamin B_{12}[44] in rats. The intrinsic factor-mediated vitamin B_{12} uptake by intestinal homogenates was also impaired in these rats[44]. Duodenal calcium transport in everted sacs from ethanol-fed rats was also inhibited[46]. Duodenal calcium-binding activity was not depressed[46].

3.5.5 Structural effects of ethanol on the intestinal epithelia

3.5.5.1 Acute effects

In addition to this wide spectrum of metabolic alterations, the concentrations of ethanol to which the upper small intestine is exposed during drinking produce structural alterations of the rat small intestine both *in vivo*[43,98] and *in vitro*[32,34]. Intragastric administration of ethanol, in concentrations similar to those of common alcoholic beverages, produced haemorrhagic erosions of rat jejunal villi[32,43] (Figure 3.8 A–C). These alterations were seen within 10 min, were well defined at 1 h and were less apparent or had even disappeared at 4 and 16 h[43]. The intensity of the lesions was maximal proximally, decreased toward the ileum, and was proportional to the concentration of ethanol administered (Figure 3.9)[43]. *In vitro,* similar alterations were apparent with ethanol concentrations as low as 1.5 g/100 ml[32]. The morphological lesions and the inhibitory effects of ethanol on calcium absorption and fatty acid oxidation have been reproduced by urea[43,86] or mannitol[32,86] in hyperosmolar concentrations comparable to those of ethanol. It has been postulated that the caustic effects of these ethanol concentrations are due, at least in part, to hypertonicity. Even in the almost total absence of microscopic lesions, the chronic administration of liquid diets containing only 5 g ethanol/100 ml decreased jejunal lactase and thymidine kinase activities and irreversibly depressed intestinal oxygen consumption[43]. These findings suggest that acute ethanol administration, even in the absence of gross lesions, affects the integrity and survival of intestinal epithelial cells.

Similar gastric lesions and similar ethanol concentrations in the intestinal lumen are observed in man and rat after ethanol ingestion, but there was no clear documentation of ethanol-induced intestinal lesions in man: duodenal biopsies from alcoholic patients (within 15 h of alcohol withdrawal) failed to demonstrate duodenitis[99]. More recently, however, haemorrhage of duodenal villus tips has been produced in alcoholic volunteers by ingestion of ethanol in doses (1 g/kg b.w.) and concentrations (35 g/100 ml) which they commonly ingested[100].

3.5.5.2 Chronic effects

Chronic ethanol feeding with nutritionally adequate diets in man and in the rat produces ultrastructural abnormalities of the intestinal epithelial cells[101]. These alterations include mitochondrial abnormalities and dilatation of the endoplasmic reticulum and cisternae of the Golgi apparatus. Biopsies from human subjects also showed focal cytoplasmic degradation. These changes were found in villus and crypt cells both in the jejunum and in the ileum. There were no gross histological alterations[101]. However, quantitative studies in the jejunum of the rat showed fewer cells per villi and slightly decreased

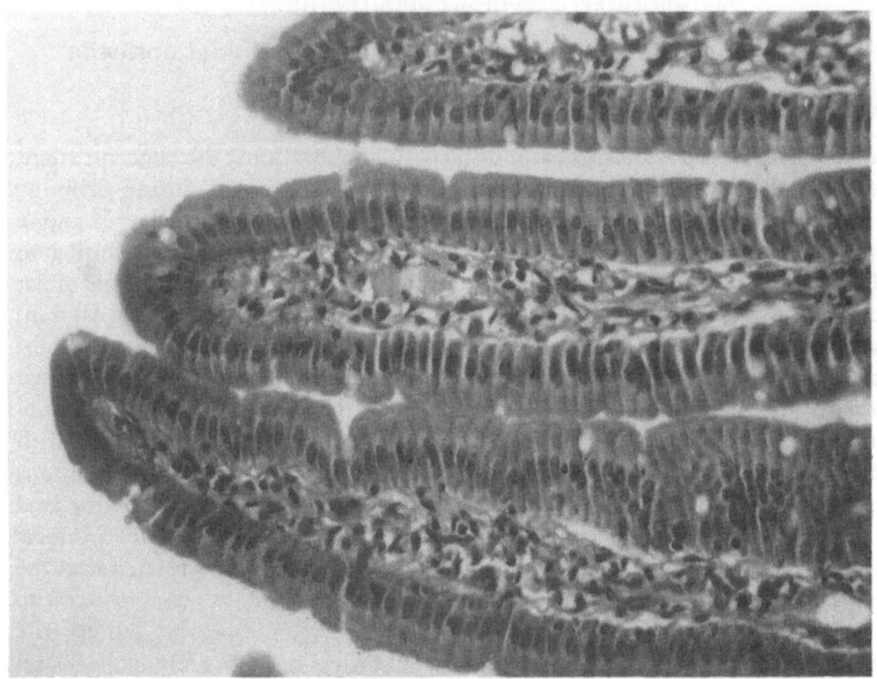

Figure 3.8A

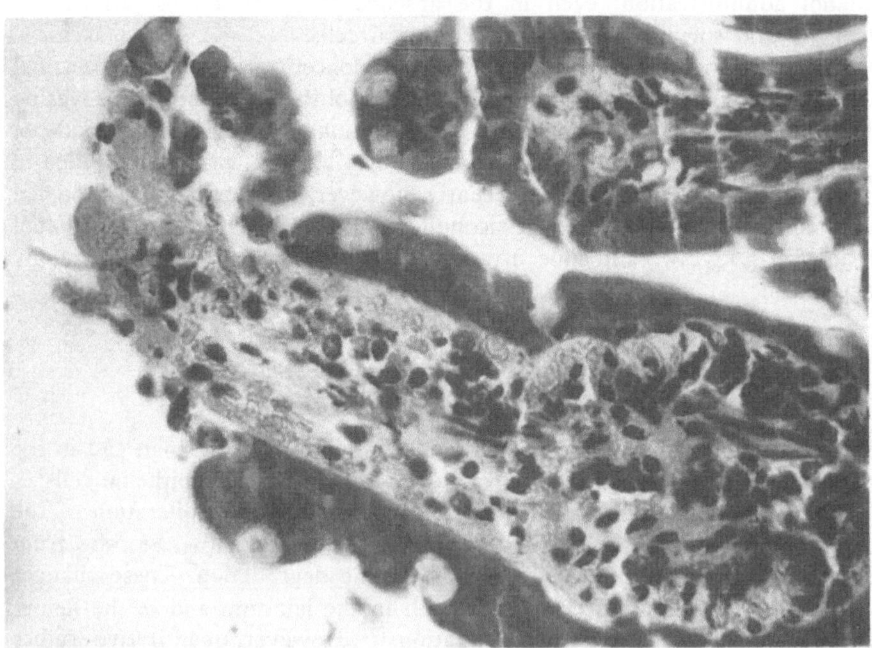

Figure 3.8B

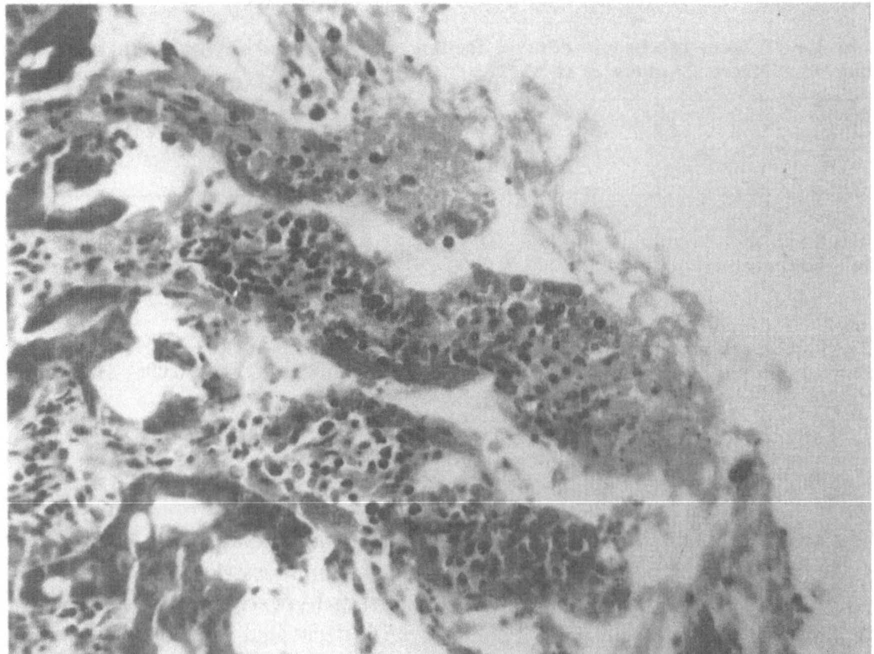

Figure 3.8C Microscopic appearances of rat jejunal villi 1 h after intragastric administration of saline or ethanol solutions; A: Normal appearances from a control rat after intubation with saline (H and E, × 100); B: Typical changes seen after ethanol administration with epithelial cell loss mainly affecting the villus tips and with haemorrhage in the corium (H and E, × 200); C: Gross damage of villi in an area of confluent haemorrhage after ethanol administration (H and E, × 100). From Baraona *et al.*[43]

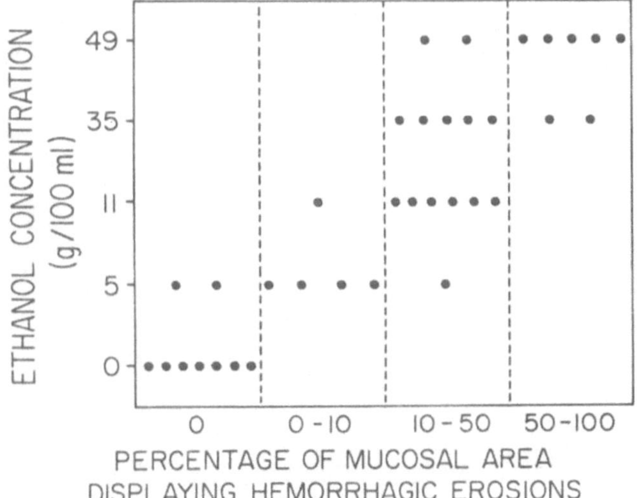

Figure 3.9 Effect of varying the concentration of ethanol administered intragastrically (in a dose of 3 g/kg) on the severity of damage in the proximal 20 cm of rat small intestine. Each animal is represented by a dot (from Baraona *et al.*[43])

Table 3.4 Effects of chronic ethanol feeding on villus and crypt length and cell population *(from Baraona *et al.*[43])

	Villus		*Crypt*	
	Length (mm)	*Number of cells*†	*Length* (mm)	*Number of cells*†
Jejunum				
Rats fed ethanol chronically	0.449 ± 0.017	92.4 ± 2.3	0.185 ± 0.014	41.4 ± 1.7
Pair-fed controls	0.600 ± 0.022	120.8 ± 2.5	0.159 ± 0.007	32.1 ± 0.7
P	<0.001	<0.01	NS‡	<0.01
Ileum				
Rats fed ethanol chronically	0.285 ± 0.010	78.0 ± 2.8	0.155 ± 0.009	43.4 ± 1.5
Pair-fed controls	0.291 ± 0.020	83.6 ± 1.8	0.138 ± 0.006	33.8 ± 0.5
P	NS	NS	NS	<0.01

*Means ± SE of determinations in twelve pairs of rats fed liquid diets containing either ethanol or isocaloric carbohydrate
†Average number of epithelial cell nuclei visualized on one side of longitudinal sections of villi and crypts
‡NS, not significant

villus height after ethanol feeding compared to pair-fed controls[43] (Table 3.4). On the other hand, the number of crypt cells and mitoses were greater in the alcohol-fed rats, mainly in the ileum, suggesting hyperregenerative activity. The shortened jejunal villi were associated with decreased activity of enzymes which are typical of mature villus cells, such as lactase, sucrase and alkaline phosphatase, whereas the morphological changes in the crypt were associated with increased activity of thymidine kinase (an enzyme typical of proliferating crypt cells) and increased incorporation of tritiated thymidine into desoxyribonucleic acid (DNA)[43]. Thus, chronic ethanol feeding not only altered cell ultrastructure but also the relative numbers of crypt and villus cells, at least in the rat[43]. There is no documented evidence that similar changes in intestinal cell populations are produced by ethanol in man. Decreases in villus height[102]

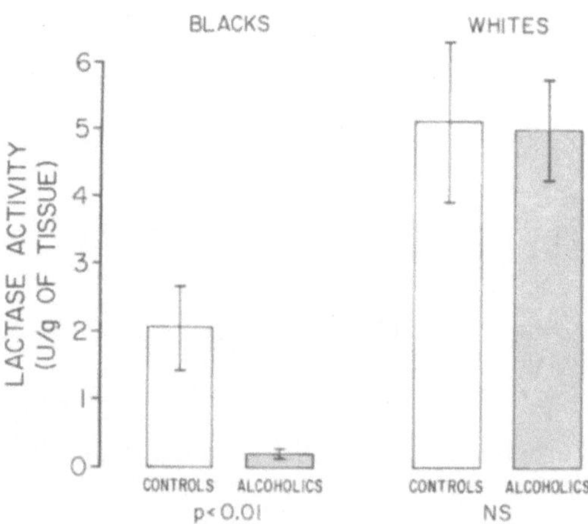

Figure 3.10 Comparison of jejunal lactase activity between controls and alcoholics from two racial populations: American blacks and whites of Northern European origin

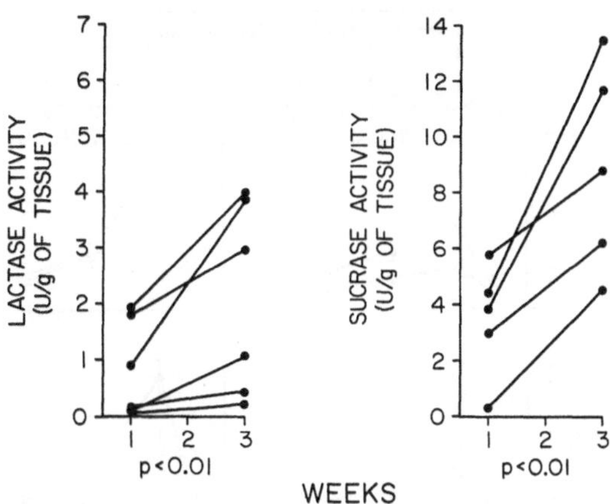

Figure 3.11 Jejunal lactase and sucrase activities in successive biopsies done after 1 and 3 weeks of ethanol abstinence in six male alcoholics (from Perlow *et al.*, unpublished data)

and disaccharidase activity[103] of mucosal biopsy specimens have been found in alcoholics, but the relative importance of alcohol ingestion and nutritional deficiency states, such as folate depletion, in the genesis of these abnormalities was not determined. Recently, in a group of well-nourished alcoholics, disaccharidase activity was generally found to be less than in non-alcoholics, but striking racial differences in the effect of alcoholism on lactase activity were described[13] (Figure 3.10). In a human population of Northern European origin (with genetically determined high levels of lactase), significant differences were not noted between alcoholics and non-alcoholics. However, in American blacks (whose lactase levels are comparable to the majority of the world population[104]), the activity of this enzyme was strikingly lower in alcoholics than in non-alcoholics, with virtual disappearance of lactase in the small intestine of some alcoholics and a higher incidence of lactose intolerance[13]. Disaccharidase activities recovered during alcohol abstinence (Figure 3.11).

3.5.6 Effects of ethanol on splanchnic circulation of blood and lymph

Ethanol is a well-recognized peripheral vasodilator. It also affects the splanchnic circulation. In man, hepatic blood flow has been found to be increased after infusion of relatively small doses of ethanol[105,106]. Other authors failed to demonstrate this effect with similar[107] or smaller doses[81]. The increased hepatic blood flow was associated with decreased splanchnic vascular resistance and increased cardiac output[106]. The increased circulation could facilitate the passive diffusion of some substances: increased intestinal blood flow after experimental and therapeutic portocaval shunt was associated with increased absorption of d-xylose[108]. The absorption of actively transported nutrients is unaffected unless extreme circulatory changes are produced[109,110].

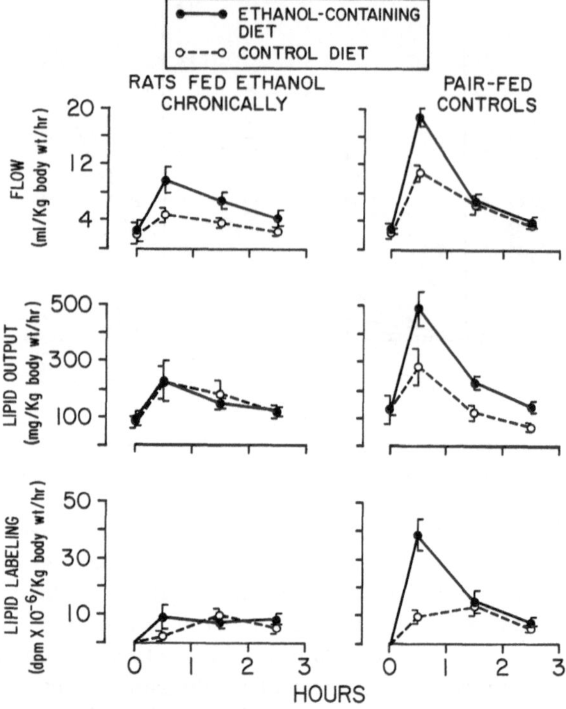

Figure 3.12 Time-course of intestinal lymph changes after intragastric administration of single doses of diets containing either ethanol (3 g/kg/b.w.) (solid lines) or isocaloric carbohydrate (broken lines) to rats pretreated for 3 to 4 weeks with either alcohol-containing or control diets. Dietary lipids were labelled with (carboxyl-^{14}C)tripalmitin (from Baraona and Lieber[36])

Mesenteric lymph formation varies with changes in the splanchnic circulation[111]. Recently, it has been shown that ethanol markedly increased the flow of intestinal lymph in rats, most strikingly in animals not previously fed ethanol[36] (Figure 3.12). This effect was smaller or disappeared in rats fed ethanol for several weeks. The lymphagogue effect of ethanol was associated with an increased output of both dietary lipids and plasma proteins into the lymph. The administration of ethanol without exogenous lipids produced a rapid increase in the lymph flow at a time when there were no changes in lymph lipid output[36] (Figure 3.13), indicating that the lymphagogue effect does not depend on increased fat transport. The alternative possibility that the lymphagogue action of ethanol could enhance the transport of dietary lipids is supported by reports that other lymphagogue agents (neostigmine[36] and overload of water[36,112]) also increased dietary lipid transport into the lymph. All these lymphagogue effects, as well as that of fat itself[113,114], are associated with the outpouring of proteins from the plasma into the lymph. It has been suggested that plasma apolipoproteins originating in the liver may be necessary for the assembly of lymph lipoproteins[115].

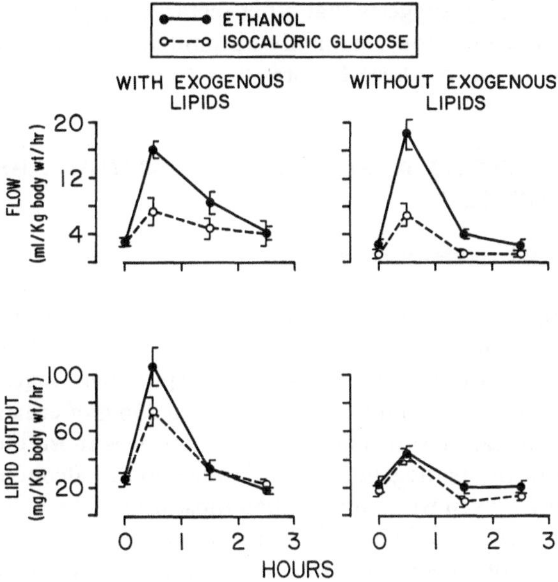

Figure 3.13 Intestinal lymph changes after intraduodenal administration of either ethanol (0.75 g/kg) (solid lines) or isocaloric glucose (broken lines), with (left) and without (right) emulsions containing palmitate, mono-oleate, and taurocholate (from Baraona and Lieber[36])

3.5.7 Conclusions

The acute and chronic administration of ethanol to man and animals affects the absorption of various nutrients in the absence of nutritional deficiency. The high ethanol concentrations to which the upper small intestine is exposed during drinking have deleterious effects on the function, structure, and survival of intestinal epithelial cells in the rat. Prolonged ethanol consumption in the rat results in decreased numbers of villus cells, increased regenerative activity in crypts, and a decreased mature villus cell/proliferating crypt cell ratio. These structural changes are associated with impaired intestinal transport of some substances, but not others (see Table 3.1). On the other hand, fat absorption may even be enhanced, probably as a consequence of the lymphagogue effects of ethanol.

The relevance of the findings in the rat model to the effects of alcohol in man is uncertain. In both species, experimental chronic ethanol administration depresses vitamin B_{12} absorption, and causes ultrastructural changes in mucosal cells; in both species, fat absorption is unchanged or stimulated by alcohol. In contrast, chronic alcohol feeding produces opposite effects on carbohydrate absorption in the two species (see Table 3.2).

While ethanol alone clearly has some deleterious effects on intestinal absorption and ultrastructure in man, the failure to induce xylose or fat malabsorption by chronic alcohol administration in human subjects in the absence of nutritional deficiency suggests that other factors may play a major etiological role in the malabsorption commonly encountered in alcoholics. We turn now to a consideration of those factors.

3.6 OTHER FACTORS AFFECTING INTESTINAL ABSORPTION IN ALCOHOLICS

3.6.1 Nutritional deficiency states

Malabsorption in alcoholics is usually associated with a history of inadequate diet, but less commonly with gross signs of malnutrition[9–11]. Since absorptive function usually improved after admission to hospital with ingestion of a normal diet despite the daily administration of 134 to 256 g of ethanol[11,20], it was concluded that clinical or subclinical malnutrition was more important than ethanol toxicity in the pathogenesis of malabsorption in alcoholics. However, the doses of ethanol given were smaller than those often taken by patients with malabsorption prior to admission[9,10]. In addition, a possible synergism between the effects of alcohol ingestion and malnutrition on gut function was not excluded in these studies. Such a synergism has been well documented in the pathogenesis of alcohol-induced megaloblastic and sideroblastic anaemias (see Chapter 8).

Multiple nutritional deficiency states occur in chronic alcoholics. Of these, at least folate and protein deficiency, and perhaps others, may adversely affect absorptive function.

Depletion of body stores of either folic acid or vitamin B_{12} severe enough to cause megaloblastic anaemia in man is associated with macrocytosis of jejunal epithelial cells, decreased mitotic activity in crypt cells, and reduction in villus height. The changes revert to normal after vitamin therapy[102,116–118]. Reversible impairment of the absorption of xylose and cyanocobalamin is also frequently associated with deficiency of B_{12} or folate (Figure 3.14)[18,119,120]. Decreased intestinal absorption secondary to folate deficiency has been documented in both alcoholics and non-alcoholic patients[18,119].

In alcoholic patients, a strong association has been noted between xylose and folic acid malabsorption and evidence of folate deficiency[21,22]. In perfusion studies, decreased intestinal uptake of tritiated folic acid in binge-drinking alcoholics strongly correlated with serum folate levels[21]. In a series of 71 alcoholics studied within a day of admission to hospital, 29 had folate deficiency severe enough to cause haematological abnormalities, and 42 were hematologically normal. The incidence of xylose malabsorption in the two groups was 79 % and 5 %, respectively; of B_{12} malabsorption, 29 % and 0 %, respectively[22]. There was no correlation between malabsorption and hypoalbuminaemia in these patients. While the possible role of associated deficiency of other nutrients cannot be excluded, the findings suggest that folic acid deficiency is a major cause of impaired intestinal function in

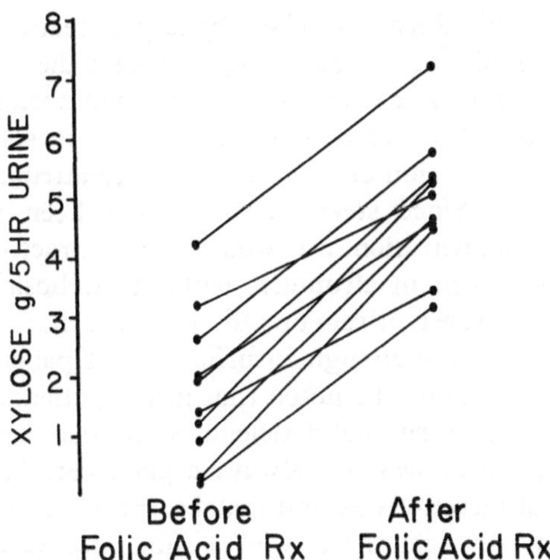

Figure 3.14 Urinary xylose excretion after a 25 g oral dose in ten patients with folate-deficiency megaloblastic anaemia studied before and after 1–2 weeks of therapy with folic acid. In seven patients folate deficiency was associated with alcoholism, in two with poor diet and chronic infection, and in one, with oral contraceptive therapy (from Lindenbaum *et al.*, unpublished data)

alcoholic patients. This notion is further supported by recent studies[21,25]. Two subjects developed malabsorption of folic acid, xylose, and glucose after 5 weeks on 200 g of ethanol daily plus a diet selectively deficient in folate. Absorption of these substances returned to normal after 2 weeks on hospital diet and folate supplements even though ethanol was continued at the same dosage level[21]. While the simultaneous alteration of diet and folate status renders interpretation of these experiments slightly ambiguous, the findings are consistent with the idea that folate deficiency was the major factor in the malabsorption state. Less striking abnormalities in absorptive function were produced in single subjects by ethanol with a nutritious diet, or by the folate deficient diet alone, suggesting that alcohol and folate deficiency act synergistically to depress jejunal function. Other experimental studies[25] provide support for this hypothesis. Alcohol ingestion by human volunteers for 2 weeks as 36 % of caloric intake produced more striking abnormalities of sodium and water transport in jejunal perfusion studies when a folate-deficient diet was given with ethanol[25].

The possibility that protein malnutrition also plays an important role in malabsorption in alcoholics is less well established. Clinically severe protein malnutrition is a well-recognized cause of functional and structural alterations of the small intestine in children[121,122]. Similar changes have been observed in adults in tropical countries with severe protein malnutrition[123]. In addition tc the small intestinal changes, profound dietary protein deficiency produces pancreatic acinar atrophy and fibrosis and reduces pancreatic exocrine secretion in rats[124] and man[125,126]. Recovery of exocrine pancreatic function in adult man occurs with the administration of high protein diets[126].

In a group of alcoholic patients, most of whom had normal serum albumin concentrations, abnormalities of pancreatic response to secretin stimulation which improved after ingestion of hospital diet were attributed to subclinical protein malnutrition[11]. Since steatorrhea has not been produced by experimental ethanol administration, this would be an attractive explanation for the fat malabsorption seen in alcoholics without cirrhosis or clinically apparent pancreatitis. However, it remains to be shown that subclinical protein malnutrition causes a severe enough insufficiency of pancreatic function to result in steatorrhea. It should be noted that in the patients of the study discussed above[11], multiple nutritional deficiency states may have been corrected simultaneously; also, there was not always a good correlation between the presence of abnormal secretin tests and malabsorption of fat and xylose. The possible roles of clinically apparent as well as subclinical protein malnutrition in the abnormalities of pancreatic and intestinal function common in alcoholics require further study. The effects on gastrointestinal function of other deficiency states frequently encountered in alcoholics, such as depletion of thiamine, pyridoxal phosphate, magnesium, and phosphorus, have yet to be explored.

3.6.2 Pancreatic disease

Clinically apparent acute and chronic pancreatitis occurs frequently in alcoholic patients. In addition, abnormalities in pancreatic exocrine function are commonly found in alcoholics with no history suggestive of pancreatic disease[11]. Pancreatic insufficiency undoubtedly accounts for the presence of fat and nitrogen malabsorption in some alcoholics. In addition, vitamin B_{12} malabsorption, which may be corrected by the administration of pancreatic extracts during the performance of the Schilling test, may occur in as many as 40 % of patients with alcoholic pancreatitis[127].

3.6.3 Cirrhosis

Steatorrhea has been found in approximately 50 % of patients with cirrhosis with and without associated alcoholism[4,7,8,128]. The malabsorption observed in cirrhotics appears to affect exclusively the assimilation of lipids and lipid-soluble vitamins. Urinary excretion and blood levels of xylose after oral administration may be abnormal in some patients with cirrhosis[4,128–130], probably due either to alterations in renal excretion[131,132] or to loss of xylose into ascitic fluid[132]. Studies of intraluminally perfused substances in cirrhotics showed that while triolein was poorly absorbed, intestinal uptake of d-xylose, glucose, electrolytes and water was normal[133,134]. Vitamin B_{12} absorption has also been reported to be normal in alcoholics with cirrhosis[8].

Several factors may contribute to the steatorrhea in cirrhosis. The degree of portal hypertension did not correlate with the presence of steatorrhea[4]. In addition, steatorrhea was not affected by portocaval shunting[135] and experimentally induced portal hypertension had little effect on protein or fat absorption in the dog[136].

Postmortem studies have revealed a high incidence of degenerative and fibrotic changes in the pancreas of cirrhotic patients without a history of clinical pancreatitis[128,137–139]. Patients with cirrhosis, with and without a history of alcoholism, also display a variety of alterations in pancreatic secretory function. The most frequently reported changes are an increase in the volume of pancreatic secretion and a decrease in the concentration of bicarbonate in response to stimuli. The total output of bicarbonate and enzymes has been reported to be normal or decreased. The correlation between these abnormalities and the presence of steatorrhea has been poor in some series[4,5,140], but good in others[7,8]. Improvement in fat absorption has been reported in some patients after supplementation with pancreatic extract[7,8]. It is unlikely, however, that pancreatic insufficiency accounts for all cases of steatorrhea in cirrhotics. In some patients, neomycin administration has been postulated as the cause of malabsorption[8].

Hepatic cirrhosis is associated with slowed clearance of bile salts[141] and decreased bile salt excretion[142,143]. Non-alcoholic cirrhotics with steatorrhea were shown to have subnormal duodenal bile salt concentrations and significantly less incorporation of lipids into the micellar phase during intraluminal digestion than control subjects without steatorrhea[144]. Since impaired hydrolysis of triglycerides could not be demonstrated, it was postulated that steatorrhea in those patients was due to reduced bile salt excretion rather than insufficient pancreatic lipase. It is not clear, however, whether this reduced incorporation of dietary lipids into the micellar phase is sufficient to account for the steatorrhea. In addition, artificially prepared micelles (with bile salts) were found to be poorly absorbed in cirrhotics with steatorrhea[145], suggesting that a defect in mucosal transport or lymphatic hypertension[146] may also contribute to the production of lipid malabsorption.

Malabsorption of fat in cirrhotics thus appears to be due to multiple causes, which may vary with the individual patient, including pancreatic insufficiency, decreased duodenal bile salt concentrations, neomycin administration, and possibly lymphatic hypertension.

3.7 SUMMARY

Malabsorption is a common finding in alcoholics. The magnitude of this alteration is generally moderate, although in occasional patients it may contribute to malnutrition in a degree comparable to that seen in patients with sprue. Both ethanol and associated complications of alcoholism contribute to its pathogenesis. The high ethanol concentrations to which the small intestine is exposed during drinking have direct deleterious effects on epithelial cell function and survival. Prolonged ethanol feeding in rats changes the epithelial cell population, resulting in a more immature type of intestine. These structural alterations may account for the defective absorption of nutrients which require active transport mechanisms. By contrast, fat absorption is unaffected by ethanol. Nonetheless, steatorrhea is commonly present in alcoholics. Nutritional, pancreatic and hepatic complications of alcoholism are the most likely causes of the fat malabsorption. Folate deficiency also probably plays a major role in diffuse mucosal dysfunction seen in chronic alcoholics.

References

1. Gross, J. B., Comfort, M. W., Wollaeger, E. E. and Power, M. H. (1950). Total solids, fat and nitrogen in the feces: V. A study of patients with primary parenchymatous hepatic disease. *Gastroenterology*, **16**, 140
2. Fast, B. B., Wolfe, S. J., Stormont, J. M. and Davidson, C. S. (1959). Fat absorption in alcoholics with cirrhosis. *Gastroenterology*, **37**, 321
3. Small, M., Longarini, A. and Zamcheck, N. (1959). Disturbances of digestive physiology following acute drinking episodes in 'skid-row' alcoholics. *Am. J. Med.*, **27**, 575
4. Baraona, E., Orrego, H., Fernandez, O., Amenabar, E., Maldonado, E., Tag, F. and Salinas, A. (1962). Absorptive function of the small intestine in liver cirrhosis. *Am. J. Dig. Dis.*, **7**, 318
5. Van Goldsenhoven, G. E., Henke, W. J., Vacca, J. G. and Knight, W. A. (1963). Pancreatic function in cirrhosis of the liver. *Am. J. Dig. Dis.*, **8**, 160
6. Linscheer, W. G., Patterson, J. F., Moore, E. W., Clemont, R. J., Robins, S. J. and Chalmers, T. C. (1966). Medium and long-chain fat absorption in patients with cirrhosis. *J. Clin. Invest.*, **45**, 1317
7. Sun, D. C. H., Albacete, R. A. and Chen, J. K. (1967). Malabsorption studies in cirrhosis of the liver. *Arch. Intern. Med.*, **119**, 567
8. Marin, G. A., Clark, M. L. and Senior, J. R. (1969). Studies of malabsorption occurring in patients with Laennec's cirrhosis. *Gastroenterology*, **56**, 727
9. Roggin, G. M., Iber, F. L., Kater, R. M. H. and Tobon, F. (1969). Malabsorption in the chronic alcoholic. *Johns Hopkins Med. J.*, **125**, 321
10. Insunza, I. and Ugarte, G. (1970). Esteatorrea en alcoholicos con y sin cirrosis hepatica. *Rev. Med. Chile*, **98**, 669
11. Mezey, E., Jow, E., Slavin, R. E. and Tobon, F. (1970). Pancreatic function and intestinal absorption in chronic alcoholism. *Gastroenterology*, **59**, 657
12. Herbert, V., Zalusky, R. and Davidson, C. S. (1963). Correlation of folate deficiency with alcoholism and associated macrocytosis, anemia and liver disease. *Ann. Intern. Med.*, **58**, 977
13. Perlow, W., Baraona, E. and Lieber, C. S. (1975). Symptomatic intestinal disaccharidase deficiency in alcoholics. *Gastroenterology*, **68**, 935
14. Smith, F. R. and Lindenbaum, J. (1974). Human serum retinol transport in malabsorption. *Am. J. Clin. Nutr.*, **27**, 700
15. Tomasulo, P. A., Kater, R. M. H. and Iber, F. L. (1968). Impairment of thiamine absorption in alcoholism. *Am. J. Clin. Nutr.*, **21**, 1340
16. Thomson, A. D., Baker, H. and Leevy, C. M. (1970). Patterns of ^{35}S-thiamine hydrochloride absorption in the malnourished alcoholic patient. *J. Lab. Clin. Med.*, **76**, 34

17. Halsted, C. H., Criggs, R. C. and Harris, J. W. (1967). The effect of alcoholism on the absorption of folic acid (^{3}H-PGA) evaluated by plasma levels and urine excretion. *J. Lab. Clin. Med.*, **69,** 116
18. Lindenbaum, J. and Pezzimenti, J. F. (1973). Effects of B_{12} and folate deficiency on small intestinal function. *Clin. Res.*, **21,** 518
19. Krasner, N., Cochran, K. M., Thompson, C. G., Carmichael, H. A. and Russel, R. I. (1974). Effects of ethanol on small intestinal absorption. *Gut,* **15,** 831
20. Halsted, C. H., Robles, E. A. and Mezey, E. (1971). Decreased jejunal uptake of labeled folic acid (^{3}H-PGA) in alcoholic patients: Roles of alcohol and nutrition. *N. Engl. J. Med.*, **285,** 701
21. Halsted, C. H., Robles, E. A. and Mezey, E. (1973). Intestinal malabsorption in folate-deficient alcoholics. *Gastroenterology,* **64,** 526
22. Marxer, F. and Lindenbaum, J. Unpublished observations
23. Halsted, C. H., Robles, E. A. and Mezey, E. (1973). Distribution of ethanol in the human gastrointestinal tract. *Am. J. Clin. Nutr.*, **26,** 831
24. Israel, Y., Valenzuela, J. E., Salazar, I. and Ugarte, G. (1969). Alcohol and amino acid transport in the human intestine. *J. Nutr.*, **98,** 222
25. Mekhjian, H. S., May, E. S. and Sury, T. (1974). The effect of ethanol on human jejunal absorption. *Clin. Res.*, **22,** 604A
26. Verdy, M. and Caron, D. (1973). Ethanol et absorption du calcium chez l'humain. *Biol. Gastroenterol. (Paris)*, **6,** 157
27. Charlton, R. W., Jacobs, P., Seftel, H. and Bothwell, T. H., (1964). Effect of alcohol on iron absorption. *Br. Med. J.*, **ii,** 1427
28. Althausen, T. L., Uyeyama, K. and Loran, M. R. (1960). Effects of alcohol on absorption of vitamin A in normal and gastrectomized subjects. *Gastroenterology,* **38,** 942
29. Israel, Y., Salazar, I. and Rosenmann, E. (1968). Inhibitory effects of alcohol on intestinal amino acid transport *in vivo* and *in vitro*. *J. Nutr.*, **96,** 499
30. Tapper, E. J., Bushi, S., Ruppert, R. D. and Greenberger, N. J. (1968). Effect of acute and chronic ethanol treatment on the absorption of iron in rats. *Am. J. Med. Sci.*, **255,** 46
31. Murray, M. J. and Stein, N. (1965). Effect of ethanol on absorption of iron in rats. *Proc. Soc. Exp. Biol. Med.*, **120,** 816
32. Krawitt, E. L. (1974). Effect of acute ethanol administration on duodenal calcium transport. *Proc. Soc. Exp. Biol. Med.*, **146,** 406
33. Hoyumpa, A., Middleton, H., Wilson, F. and Schenker, S. (1974). Dual system of thiamine transport: Characteristics and effect of ethanol. *Gastroenterology,* **66,** 714
34. Chang, T., Lewis, J. and Glazko, A. J. (1967). Effects of ethanol and other alcohols on the transport of amino acids and glucose by everted sacs of rat small intestine. *Biochim. Biophys. Acta,* **135,** 1000
35. Hill, C. H. (1960). The effects of alcohols on absorption of trace elements. *Fed. Proc.*, **28,** 300
36. Baraona, E. and Lieber, C. S. (1975). Intestinal lymph formation and fat absorption: Stimulation by acute ethanol administration and inhibition by chronic ethanol feeding. *Gastroenterology,* **68,** 495
37. Schafer, D. F., Stephenson, D. V., Barak, A. J. and Sorrell, M. F. (1974). Effects of ethanol on the transport of manganese by small intestine of the rat. *J. Nutr.*, **104,** 101
38. Lindenbaum, J. and Lieber, C. S. (1969). Alcohol-induced malabsorption of vitamin B_{12} in man. *Nature (London)*, **224,** 806
39. Lindenbaum, J. and Lieber, C. S. (1975). Effects of chronic ethanol administration on intestinal absorption in man in the absence of nutritional deficiency. *Ann. N.Y. Acad. Sci.*, **252,** 228
40. Lindenbaum, J. and Lieber, C. S. (1971). Effects of ethanol on the blood, bone marrow and small intestine of man. In M. K. Roach, W. M. McIsaac and P. J. Creaven, eds. *Biological Aspects of Alcohol,* Vol. 3, p. 27. Austin and London: University of Texas Press

41. Small, M. D., Gershoff, S. N., Broitman, S. A., Colon, P. L., Cavanagh, R. C. and Zamcheck, N. (1960). Effect of alcohol and dietary deprivation on absorption of xylose from the rat small intestine. *Am. J. Dig. Dis.*, **5**, 801
42. Lindenbaum, J., Shea, N., Saha, J. R. and Lieber, C. S. (1972). Alcohol-induced impairment of carbohydrate (CHO) absorption. *Clin. Res.*, **20**, 459
43. Baraona, E., Pirola, R. C. and Lieber, C. S. (1974). Small intestinal damage and changes in cell population produced by ethanol ingestion in the rat. *Gastroenterology*, **66**, 226
44. Lindenbaum, J., Saha, J. R., Shea, N. and Lieber, C. S. (1973). Mechanism of alcohol-induced malabsorption of vitamin B_{12}. *Gastroenterology*, **64**, 762
45. Krawitt, E. L. (1973). Ethanol inhibits intestinal calcium absorption. *Gastroenterology*, **64**, 757
46. Krawitt, E. L. (1975). Effect of ethanol ingestion on duodenal calcium transport. *J. Lab. Clin. Med.*, **85**, 665
47. Klatskin, G. (1961). The effect of ethyl alcohol on nitrogen excretion in the rat. *Yale J. Biol. Med.*, **34**, 124
48. Rodrigo, C., Antezana, C. and Baraona, E. (1971). Fat and nitrogen balances in rats with alcohol-induced fatty liver. *J. Nutr.*, **101**, 1307
49. Baraona, E., Pirola, R. C. and Lieber, C. S. (1973). Pathogenesis of postprandial hyperlipemia in rats fed ethanol-containing diets. *J. Clin. Invest.*, **52**, 296
49a. Halsted, C. H., Bhanthumnavin, K. and Mezey, E. (1974). Jejunal uptake of tritiated folic acid in the rat studied by *in vivo* perfusion. *J. Nutr.*, **104**, 1674
50. Franzen, G. (1928). Untersuchungen über Alkohol. VII. Mitteilung: Alkoholwirkungen auf die Magenverdauung. *Arch. Exp. Pathol. Pharmakol.*, **134**, 129
51. Barlow, O. W., Beams, A. J. and Goldblatt, H. (1936). Studies on the pharmacology of ethyl alcohol. I. A comparative study of the pharmacologic effects of grain and synthetic ethyl alcohols. *J. Pharmacol. Exp. Ther.*, **56**, 117
52. Pihkanen, T. A. (1957). Neurological and physiological studies on distilled and brewed beverages. *Ann. Med. Exp. Fenn.*, **35**, Suppl. 9
53. Cooke, A. R. (1972). Ethanol and gastric function. *Gastroenterology*, **62**, 501
54. Harichaux, P. and Moline, J. (1964). Influence d'une ingestion d'ethanol à 10 p. 100 sur l'évacuation gastrique chez le rat. *C.R. Soc. Biol. (Paris)*, **158**, 1389
55. Harichaux, P., Lienard, J., Capron, J.-P., Freville, M. and Moline, J. (1971). Action de l'ethanol sur la motricité antro-pylorique. Étude expérimentale et clinique. *Therapie*, **26**, 1039
56. Barboriak, J. J. and Meade, R. C. (1970). Effect of alcohol on gastric emptying in man. *Am. J. Clin. Nutr.*, **23**, 1151
57. Iber, F. L. (1971). Alcohol and the gastrointestinal tract. *Gastroenterology*, **61**, 120
58. Greenberg, L. A., Lolli, G. and Rubin, M. (1942). The influence of intravenously administered alcohol on the emptying time of the stomach. *Q. J. Stud. Alc.*, **3**, 371
59. Tennent, D. M. (1941). The influence of alcohol on the emptying time of the stomach and the absorption of glucose. *Q. J. Stud. Alc.*, **2**, 271
60. Pirola, R. C. and Davis, A. E. (1970). Effects of intravenous alcohol on motility of the duodenum and of the sphincter of Oddi. *Aust. Ann. Med.*, **19**, 1
61. Robles, E. A., Mexey, E., Halsted, C. H. and Schuster, M. M. (1974). Effect of ethanol on motility of the small intestine. *Johns Hopkins Med. J.*, **135**, 17
62. Boyer, J. L. (1972). Effect of chronic ethanol feeding on bile formation and secretion of lipids in the rat. *Gastroenterology*, **62**, 294
63. Maddrey, W. C. and Boyer, J. L. (1973). The acute and chronic effects of ethanol administration on bile secretion in the rat. *J. Lab. Clin. Med.*, **82**, 215
64. Schapiro, R. H., Drummey, G. D., Shimizu, Y. and Isselbacher, K. J. (1964). Studies on the pathogenesis of ethanol-induced fatty liver II. Effect of ethanol on palmitate-1-^{14}C metabolism by the isolated perfused rat liver. *J. Clin. Invest.*, **43**, 1338
65. Lefevre, A. F., DeCarli, L. M. and Lieber, C. S. (1972). Effect of ethanol on cholesterol and bile acid metabolism. *J. Lipid Res.*, **13**, 48

66. Dreiling, D. A., Richman, A. and Fradkin, N. F. (1952). The role of alcohol in the etiology of pancreatitis: a study of the effect of intravenous ethyl alcohol on the external secretion of the pancreas. *Gastroenterology,* **20,** 636
67. Whalton, B., Schapiro, H. and Woodward, E. R. (1962). The effect of alcohol and histamine on pancreatic secretion. *Ann. Surg.,* **28,** 443
68. Bayer, M., Rudick, J., Lieber, C. S. and Janowitz, H. D. (1972). Inhibitory effect of ethanol on canine exocrine pancreatic secretin. *Gastroenterology,* **63,** 619
69. Mott, C. B., Sarles, H., Tiscornia, O. and Gullo, L. (1972). Inhibitory action of alcohol on human exocrine pancreatic secretion. *Am. J. Dig. Dis.,* **17,** 902
70. Tiscornia, O., Gullo, L. and Sarles, H. (1972). The inhibition of canine exocrine pancreatic secretion by intravenous ethanol. *Gastroenterology,* **62,** 866
71. Tiscornia, O. M., Gullo, L., DeBarros Mott, C., Devauz, M. A., Palasciano, G., Hage, G. and Sarles, H. (1974). The effects of intragastric ethanol administration upon canine exocrine pancreatic secretion. *Digestion,* **9,** 490
72. Sarles, H. and Tiscornia, O. (1974). Ethanol and chronic calcifying pancreatitis. *Med. Clin. N. Am.,* **58,** 1333
73. Baum, R. and Iber, F. L. (1973). Alcohol, the pancreas, pancreatic inflammation and pancreatic insufficiency. *Am. J. Clin. Nutr.,* **26,** 347
74. Spencer, R. P., Brody, K. R. and Lutters, B. M. (1964). Some effects of ethanol on the gastrointestinal tract. *Am. J. Dig. Dis.,* **9,** 599
75. Mistilis, S. P. and Garske, A. (1969). Induction of alcohol dehydrogenase in liver and gastro-intestinal tract. *Aust. Ann. Med.,* **18,** 227
76. Carter, E. A. and Isselbacher, K. J. (1971). The metabolism of ethanol to carbon dioxide by stomach and small intestinal slices. *Proc. Soc. Exp. Biol. Med.,* **138,** 817
77. Harger, R. N. and Hulpieu, H. R. (1956). The pharmacology of alcohol. In G. N. Thompson, ed. *Alcoholism.* Springfield, Ill.: Charles C. Thomas
78. Winkler, K., Lundquist, F. and Tygstrup, N. (1969). The hepatic metabolism of ethanol in patients with cirrhosis of the liver. *Scand. J. Clin. Lab. Invest.,* **23,** 59
79. Larsen, J. A. (1959). Extrahepatic metabolism of ethanol in man. *Nature (London),* **184,** 1236
80. Forsander, O., Raiha, N. and Suomalainen, H. (1960). Oxydation des Athylalkohols in isolierter Leber und isolierten Hinterkorper der Ratte. *Hoppe-Seyler's Z. Physiol. Chem.,* **318,** 1
81. Lundquist, E., Tygstrup, N., Winkler, K., Mellengaard, K. and Munch-Petersen, S. (1962). Ethanol metabolism and production of free acetate in the human liver. *J. Clin. Invest.,* **41,** 955
82. Carter, E. A., Drummey, G. D. and Isselbacher, K. J. (1971). Ethanol stimulates triglyceride synthesis by the intestine. *Science,* **174,** 1241
83. Lieber, C. S., Rubin, E., DeCarli, L. M., Misra, P. and Gang, H. (1970). Effects of pyrazole on hepatic function and structure. *Lab. Invest.,* **22,** 615
84. Carter, E. A. and Isselbacher, K. J. (1973). Effect of ethanol on intestinal adenosine triphosphate (ATP) content. *Proc. Soc. Exp. Biol. Med.,* **142,** 1171
85. Lieber, C. S. and DeCarli, L. M. (1970). Hepatic microsomal ethanol-oxidizing system. *In vitro* characteristics and adaptive properties *in vivo. J. Biol. Chem.,* **245,** 2505
86. Baraona, E., Pirola, R. C. and Lieber, C. S. (1975). Acute and chronic effects of ethanol on intestinal lipid metabolism. *Biochim. Biophys. Acta,* **388,** 19
87. Beck, I. T., Paloschi, G. B., Dinda, P. K. and Beck, M. (1974). Effects of intragastric administration of alcohol on ethanol concentrations and osmolality of pancreatic juice, bile, and portal and peripheral blood. *Gastroenterology,* **67,** 484
88. Israel, Y., Kalant, H. and Laufer, L. (1965). Effects of ethanol on Na, K, Mg-stimulated microsomal ATPase activity. *Biochem. Pharmacol.,* **14,** 1803
89. Van Tuan, T., Mitjavila, M. T. and Derache, R. (1971). Effet de l'éthanol sur la respiration des cellules épitheliales isolées de l'intestin de rat. *C.R. Soc. Biol. (Paris),* **165,** 2011

90. Greene, H. L., Stifel, F. B., Herman, R. H., Herman, Y. F. and Rosensweig, N. S. (1974). Ethanol-induced inhibition of human intestinal enzyme activities: reversal by folic acid. *Gastroenterology*, **67**, 434
91. Hülsmann, W. C. (1971). Preferential oxidation of fatty acids by rat small intestine. *FEBS Lett.* **17**, 35
92. Gangl, A. and Ockner, R. K. (1975). Intestinal metabolism of plasma free fatty acids. Intracellular compartmentation and mechanism of control. *J. Clin. Invest.*, **55**, 803
93. Greene, H. L., Herman, R. H. and Kraemer, S. (1971). Stimulation of jejunal adenyl cyclase by ethanol. *J. Lab. Clin. Med.*, **78**, 336
94. Newsome, W. H. and Rattray, J. B. M. (1965). The enzymatic esterification of ethanol with fatty acids. *Can. J. Biochem.*, **43**, 1223
95. Middleton, W. R. J., Carter, E. A., Drummey, G. D. and Isselbacher, K. J. (1971). Effect of oral ethanol administration on intestinal cholesterogenesis in the rat. *Gastroenterology*, **60**, 880
96. Mistilis, S. P. and Ockner, R. K. (1972). Effects of ethanol on endogenous lipid and lipoprotein metabolism in the small intestine. *J. Lab. Clin. Med.*, **80**, 34
97. Rodgers, J. B. and O'Brien, R. J. (1975). The effect of acute ethanol treatment on lipid-reesterifying enzymes of the rat small bowel. *Am. J. Dig. Dis.*, **20**, 354
98. Maling, H. M., Highman, B., Hunter, J. M., Butler, W. M. and Williams, M. A. (1967). Blood alcohol levels, triglyceride fatty livers, and pathologic changes in rats after single doses of alcohol. In R. P. Maickel, ed. *Biochemical Factors in Alcoholism*, p. 185. New York: Pergamon Press
99. Pirola, R. C., Bolin, T. D. and Davis, A. E. (1969). Does alcohol cause duodenitis? *Am. J. Dig. Dis.*, **14**, 239
100. Gottfried, E. B., Korsten, M. A. and Lieber, C. S. (1976). Gastritis and duodenitis induced by alcohol: an endoscopic and histologic assessment. *Gastroenterology*, **70**, 890
101. Rubin, E., Rybak, B. J., Lindenbaum, J., Gerson, C. D., Walker, G. and Lieber, C. S. (1972). Ultrastructural changes in the small intestine induced by ethanol. *Gastroenterology*, **63**, 801
102. Hermos, J. A., Adams, W. H., Liu, Y. K., Sullivan, L. W. and Trier, J. S. (1972). Mucosa of the small intestine in folate-deficient alcoholics. *Ann. Intern. Med.*, **76**, 957
103. Madzarovova-Nohejlova, J. (1971). Activité des disaccharidases intestinales chez l'adulte et chez le buveur chronique de bière de Pilsen. *Biol. Gastro-Enterol.*, **4**, 325
104. Bayless, T. M., Paige, D. M. and Ferry, G. D. (1971). Lactose intolerance and milk-drinking habits. *Gastroenterology*, **60**, 605
105. Mendeloff, A. I., Kramer, P., Ingelfinger, F. J. and Bradley, S. E. (1949). Studies with bromsulfalein. II. Factors altering its disappearance from the blood after a single intravenous injection. *Gastroenterology*, **13**, 222
106. Stein, S. W., Lieber, C. S., Leevy, C. M., Cherrick, G. R. and Abelmann, W. H. (1963). The effect of ethanol upon systemic and hepatic blood flow in man *Am. J. Clin. Nutr.*, **13**, 68
107. Castenfors, H., Hultman, E. and Josephson, B. (1960). Effect of intravenous infusions of ethyl alcohol on estimated hepatic blood flow in man. *J. Clin. Invest.*, **39**, 776
108. Price, J. B., McCullough, W., Peterson, L., Britton, R. C. and Voorhees, A. B. (1967). Effects of portal systemic shunting on intestinal absorption in the dog and in man. *Surg. Gyn. Obstet.*, **125**, 305
109. Varro, V., Jung, I., Szarvas, F., Csernay, L., Savay, G. and Okros, J. (1967). The effect of vasoactive substances on the circulation and glucose absorption of an isolated jejunal loop in dog. *Am. J. Dig. Dis.*, **12**, 46
110. Bynum, T. E. and Jacobson, E. D. (1971). Blood flow and gastrointestinal function. *Gastroenterology*, **60**, 325
111. Yoffey, J. M. and Courtice, F. C. (1956). Lymphatics. In *Lymph and Lymphoid Tissue*. Cambridge, Mass.: Harvard University Press

112. Shepherd, P. and Simmonds, W. J. (1959). Some conditions affecting the maintenance of a steady lymphatic absorption of fat. *Aust. J. Exp. Biol.*, **37**, 1
113. Borgström, B. and Laurell, C. B. (1953). Studies on lymph and lymph-proteins during absorption of fat and saline by rats. *Acta Physiol. Scand.*, **29**, 264
114. Simmonds, W. J. (1955). Some observations on the increase in thoracic duct lymph flow during intestinal absorption of fat and saline by rats. *Acta Physiol. Scand.*, **29**, 264
115. Windmueller, H. G., Herbert, P. N. and Levy, R. I. (1973). Biosynthesis of lymph and plasma lipoprotein apoproteins by isolated perfused rat liver and intestine. *J. Lipid Res.*, **14**, 215
116. Foroozan, P. and Trier, J. S. (1967). Mucosa of the small intestine in pernicious anemia. *N. Engl. J. Med.*, **277**, 553
117. Bianchi, A., Chipman, D. W., Dreskin, A. and Rosensweig, N. S. (1970). Nutritional folic acid deficiency with megaloblastic changes in the small-bowel epithelium. *N. Engl. J. Med.*, **282**, 859
118. Weinstein, W. M., Tytgat, G. N., Eichner, E. R., Pierce, H. T., Hillman, R. S. and Saunders, D. R. (1974). The small intestinal mucosa in human folic acid (FA) deficiency. *Clin. Res.*, **22**, 738
119. Hift, W. and Adams, E. B. (1963). Malabsorption of vitamin B_{12} in megaloblastic anemia among Africans and Indians in Durban. *Trans. Roy. Soc. Trop. Med. Hyg.*, **57**, 445
120. Lindenbaum, J., Pezzimenti, J. F. and Shea, N. (1974). Small intestinal function in vitamin B_{12} deficiency. *Ann. Intern. Med.*, **80**, 326
121. James, W. P. T. (1968). Intestinal absorption in protein–calorie malnutrition. *Lancet*, **i**, 333
122. Brunser, O., Reid, A., Monckeberg, F., Maccioni, A. and Contreras, I. (1968). Jejunal mucosa in infant malnutrition. *Am. J. Clin. Nutr.*, **21**, 976
123. Mayoral, L. G., Tripathy, K., Garcia, F. T., Klahr, S., Bolanos, O. and Ghitis, J. (1967). Malabsorption in the tropics: a second look. *Am. J. Clin. Nutr.*, **20**, 866
124. Lemire, S. and Iber, F. L. (1967). Pancreatic secretion in rats with protein malnutrition. *Johns Hopkins Med. J.*, **120**, 21
125. Davies, J. N. P. (1948). The essential pathology of kwashiorkor. *Lancet*, **i**, 317
126. Tandon, B. N., Banks, P. A., George, P. K., Sama, S. K., Ramachandran, K. and Gandhi, P. C. (1970). Recovery of exocrine pancreatic function in adult protein–calorie malnutrition. *Gastroenterology*, **58**, 358
127. Toskes, P. P., Hansell, J., Cerda, J. and Deren, J. J. (1971). Vitamin B_{12} malabsorption in chronic pancreatic insufficiency: studies suggesting the presence of a pancreatic 'intrinsic factor'. *N. Engl. J. Med.*, **284**, 627
128. Losowsky, M. S. and Walker, B. E. (1969). Liver disease and malabsorption. *Gastroenterology*, **56**, 589
129. Benson, J. A., Culver, P. J., Ragland, S., Jones, C. M., Drummey, G. D. and Bougas, E. (1957). The d-xylose absorption test in malabsorption syndromes. *N. Engl. J. Med.*, **256**, 335
130. Shamma'a, N. H. and Ghazanfar, S. A. S. (1960). D-xylose test in enteric fever, cirrhosis, and malabsorptive states. *Br. Med. J.*, **ii**, 836
131. Fishberg, E. H. and Friedfeld, L. (1932). The excretion of xylose as an index of damaged renal function. *J. Clin. Invest.*, **11**, 501
132. Marin, G. A., Clark, M. L. and Senior, J. R. (1968). Distribution of d-xylose in sequestered fluid resulting in false-positive tests for malabsorption. *Ann. Intern. Med.*, **69**, 1155
133. Oberhauser, E., Orrego Matte, H., Salinas, A. and Baraona, E. (1962). Further studies on intestinal absorption in liver cirrhosis, using an intraintestinal reference substance (polyethylene glycol). *Am. J. Dig. Dis.*, **7**, 699
134. Talley, R. B., Schedl, H. P. and Clifton, J. A. (1964). Small intestinal glucose, electrolyte and water absorption in cirrhosis. *Gastroenterology*, **47**, 382

135. Fisher, B., Lee, S., Fedor, E. J. and Levine, M. (1968). Intestinal absorption and nitrogen balance following portocaval shunt. *Ann. Surg.*, **167,** 41
136. Enquist, I. F., Golding, M. R., Aiello, R. G., Fierst, S. M. and Solomon, N. A. (1965). The effect of portal hypertension on intestinal absorption. *Surg. Gyn. Obstet.*, **120,** 87
137. Weiner, H. A. and Tennant, R. (1938). A statistical study of acute hemorrhagic pancreatitis (hemorrhagic necrosis of pancreas). *Am. J. Med. Sci.*, **196,** 167
138. Sobel, H. J. and Waye, J. D. (1963). Pancreatic changes in various types of cirrhosis in alcoholics. *Gastroenterology*, **45,** 341
139. Stinson, J. C., Baggenstoss, A. H. and Morlock, C. G. (1952). Pancreatic lesions associated with cirrhosis of the liver. *Am. J. Clin. Path.*, **22,** 117
140. Gross, J. B., Comfort, M. W., Wollaeger, E. E. and Power, M. H. (1950). External pancreatic function in primary parenchymatous hepatic disease as measured by analysis of duodenal contents before and after stimulation with secretin. *Gastroenterology*, **16,** 151
141. Blum, M. and Spritz, N. (1966). The metabolism of intravenously injected isotopic cholic acid in Laennec's cirrhosis. *J. Clin. Invest.*, **45,** 187
142. Vlahcevic, Z. R., Buhac, I., Farrar, J. T., Cooper Bell, C., and Swell, L. (1971). Bile acid metabolism in patients with cirrhosis. I. Kinetic aspects of cholic acid metabolism. *Gastroenterology*, **60,** 491
143. Vlahcevic, Z. R., Juttijudata, P., Bell, C. C. and Swell, L. (1972). Bile acid metabolism in patients with cirrhosis. II. Cholic and chenodeoxycholic acid metabolism. *Gastroenterology*, **62,** 1174
144. Badley, B. W. D., Murphy, G. M., Bouchier, I. A. D. and Sherlock, S. (1970). Diminished micellar phase lipid in patients with chronic nonalcoholic liver disease and steatorrhea. *Gastroenterology*, **58,** 781
145. Malagelada, J. R., Owe, P. and Linscheer, W. G. (1974). Impaired absorption of micellar long-chain fatty acid in patients with alcoholic cirrhosis. *Am. J. Dig. Dis.*, **19,** 1016
146. Dumont, A. E. and Mulholland, J. H. (1962). Alterations of thoracic duct lymph flow in hepatic cirrhosis: significance of portal hypertension. *Ann. Surg.*, **156,** 668

4
The Effect of Alcohol on the Heart

R. J. BING and H. TILLMANNS

4.1 HISTORICAL CONSIDERATIONS	117
4.2 CLINICAL FEATURES	119
4.3 THE ACUTE EFFECT OF ALCOHOL ON CORONARY FLOW AND MYOCARDIAL PERFORMANCE	121
4.3.1 *Chronic haemodynamic changes induced by alcohol*	123
4.4 THE ACUTE EFFECT OF ALCOHOL ON CARDIAC METABOLISM	124
4.5 CORRELATION OF FUNCTION WITH STRUCTURE	128
4.6 SUMMARY	129
4.6.1 *Clinical studies*	129
4.6.2 *Haemodynamics*	130
4.6.3 *Effects of ethanol on cardiac metabolism*	130
References	130

4.1 HISTORICAL CONSIDERATIONS

Most of the early publications dealing with the effect of alcohol on the heart make little distinction between the action of ethanol and that of nutritional factors; however, the effect of alcohol in general on the heart was recognized as early as 1855 by Wood[1], in 1861 by Friedreich[2], and in 1873 by Walshe[3]. Walshe described a localized form of cirrhosis occurring in the myocardial wall and in the Trabeculae carneae in the absence of impaired coronary circulation. One of the most original papers in this field was that of Bollinger, who introduced the term 'Munich beer heart' in describing cardiac dilatation and hypertrophy secondary to chronic alcoholism[4]. The paper was presented

Original work was sponsored by the United States Public Health Service #RO1 AA 00304-02, The Margaret W. and Herbert Hoover, Jr. Foundation, The Kenneth and Eileen L. Norris Foundation and the Council for Tobacco Research, U.S.A., Inc.

at a meeting of the Medical Society of Munich in February, 1884; in it, Bollinger mentioned that cardiac hypertrophy was more common in Munich than anywhere else, quoting statistics from the pathological laboratory of the University of Munich. Among 1000 autopsies he discovered 46 cases (4.6 %) of cardiac hypertrophy as a cause of death. Bollinger stated that this could only be explained by invoking the effect of habitual excess in beer drinking. He was foresighted enough to state that: 'With excessive habitual use of beer, one has to take into account the direct effect of alcohol on the heart, and to a much lesser degree, a large volume of fluid ingested'. Most of those patients were in the age group 31–40 years, and most of these individuals were overweight. Bollinger determined that the amount of beer consumed *per capita* in Munich in 1882 was 432 *l*/y, whereas the overall beer consumption in Germany was 'only' 88 *l per capita*. Bollinger concludes that this idiopathic hypertrophy cannot be explained by either myocarditis or rheumatic carditis, but represents a toxic, functional hypertrophy induced by habitual beer and alcohol consumption. In 1895, Aufrecht noted alcoholic myocarditis associated with liver disease and albuminuria[5]. He mentions that 'alcoholism leads to diminished cardiac contractility with cardiac dilatation and subsequent cardiac hypertrophy'.

However, the term 'alcoholic heart disease' was first used in 1902 by John MacKenzie in his monograph *The Study of the Pulse*[6]. In the second edition of his book *Diseases of the Heart* published in 1910, he mentions that 'the heart may be only slightly enlarged, or there may be great dilatation, usually accompanied by enlargement of the liver, and tenderness of the tissues covering it'[7]. He adds that with abstinence from alcohol these cases quickly recover, but with 'continuance of the habit all these characters of the heart failure supervene'. In the index MacKenzie lists this condition as 'alcoholic heart'.

In 1906, Graham Steell noted the similarity of alcoholic heart disease to beri-beri heart disease[8]; since then, until quite recently, the effect of alcohol and of nutritional factors are usually discussed together as it was felt by most clinicians that the effects of alcohol were primarily the result of nutritional deficiencies. The first complete description of beri-beri heart disease was presented in 1929 by Aalsmer and Wenckebach, who described the chronic and the acute form (shoshin beri-beri); their patients were orientals, and there was no ingestion of alcohol[9]. Keefer in 1930 mentioned that beri-beri was caused by a deficiency in thiamine with secondary changes in heart muscle[10]. No connection to ethanol was mentioned in his report, primarily since his patients were also orientals who refrained from alcohol. Laubry in 1930 introduced the phrase 'myocardie' in describing heart disease occurring in alcoholic patients[11]. In 1937, Weiss and Wilkins described occidental beri-beri heart disease and mentioned its connection to alcoholism[12]. In their analyses of 900 patients suffering from various types of nutritional deficiencies, a great number were afflicted with chronic alcoholism with or without polyneuritis. It is likely that the relation to alcoholism was made by these authors because they studied occidentals, whereas Wenckebach's and Keefer's patients were mostly oriental. Blankenhorn in 1946 reported on twelve alcoholic patients with heart disease who showed a poor response to thiamine[13].

In 1957, Brigdon recognized the high incidence of alcoholism in patients with non-coronary myocardial disease and later differentiated isolated alcoholic cardiomyopathy from nutritional heart disease on the basis of haemodynamic observations[14]. Evans in 1959 described electrocardiographic changes supposedly characteristic for alcoholic heart disease and also stressed the association between cardiomyopathy and excessive alcoholic intake[15]. Robin and Goldschlager in 1970 clearly separated alcoholic cardiomyopathy from beri-beri heart disease[16].

4.2 CLINICAL FEATURES

Several comprehensive articles have been published on the clinical features of alcoholic cardiomyopathy[17–19,20–23]. Most of these articles stress that the clinical symptoms of alcoholic cardiomyopathy are usually indistinguishable from those of other cardiomyopathies. Alcoholic cardiomyopathy however does not exclude the possibility of involvement of the coronary arteries, leading to advanced congestive failure. The history usually discloses heavy alcohol intake and more than often irregular meals of poor nutritional quality. Physical examination reveals tachycardia, shortness of breath persisting for many months or years, orthopnea and paroxysmal nocturnal dyspnea[18]. Third heart sounds are frequently heard, and the pulmonic component of the second sound may be intensified. Frequently, a murmur of mitral regurgitation is audible. The pulse pressure may be narrow due to increased diastolic pressure[18]. The presence of pulmonary emboli is not infrequent in alcoholic cardiomyopathy; often the diagnosis is made easier by the finding of neurological deficits manifested by sensory disturbances in the lower extremities and absent deep reflexes. The chest x-ray is usually non-specific and shows cardiac enlargements.

Much has been written about the electrocardiogram in alcoholic cardiomyopathy, but it is generally agreed that changes are not characteristic. Sinus tachycardia with ST and T changes, conduction defects and atopic rhythms are not uncommon. Demakis, in a recent paper, uses the following diagnostic criteria for alcoholic cardiomyopathy[23]: (1) congestive cardiac failure in patients under 50 years old; (2) no evidence of the usual causes of heart disease; and (3) presence of alcoholism. This is presumed to be present when the patient has consumed more than 227 ml of whisky or gin, or 1.1 *l* of wine or 2.2 *l* of beer daily over the last 5 years. As Demakis states, most patients with alcoholic cardiomyopathy consume far more alcohol than these amounts. Most of them are heavy, daily drinkers.

The natural course of alcoholic cardiomyopathy as described by Demakis and co-workers is greatly influenced by continued inebriety or by the advent of sobriety[23]. The objective signs usually consist of cardiomegaly, rales, edema, hepatomegaly, third and fourth heart sounds, and a cardiac murmur. The electrocardiogram shows primarily left ventricular hypertrophy, with abnormal T waves, normal or low voltage QRS with abnormal T waves, and some type of conduction disturbances. Atrial fibrillation, premature ventricular or atrial beats are rare.

Sobriety leads to a marked improvement in the functional classification. On the other hand, in patients who do not improve, but become stationary, cardiomegaly and the abnormal electrocardiogram persist, but no further episodes of chronic congestive heart failure are encountered. In the third group of patients in whom deterioration is the rule, heart size continues to increase; there are recurrent episodes of cardiac failure and pulmonary emboli. The mortality in this group is 80 % within the first 3 years of observation. Of patients who continue to drink heavily during the follow-up period, only four, that is 10 % of the whole population, improve. Individuals with the shortest duration of symptoms prior to the initiation of therapy had the best prognosis. Abstinence from alcohol is the most important therapeutic consideration. Whether prolonged bed rest, as recommended by MacDonald and his co-workers, is beneficial, is not certain[24].

Asokan, Frank and Witham have described alcoholic cardiomyopathy without cardiomegaly[25]. Apparently this occurred primarily in the early stages. Despite the absence of cardiomegaly, early haemodynamic findings were present such as elevated left ventricular end-diastolic pressure, low cardiac output, and depressed myocardial contractility. It is therefore likely that true functional cardiac impairment can exist in these patients prior to the development of abnormal clinical parameters. This is in line with the observations of Regan and co-workers in patients with long-standing alcoholism, who show no obvious failure but in whom stress tests or ingestion of alcohol cause marked haemodynamic changes which are absent in patients not exposed to alcohol[26]. Left ventricular function curves showed that, as left ventricular end-diastolic pressure increased following administration of angiotensin, stroke work failed to rise proportionally.

A peculiar form of alcoholic cardiomyopathy has been described in 1964 which has been termed 'cobalt-beer cardiomyopathy'. Epidemics of this condition have occurred in Quebec[27], Omaha[28], and Minneapolis[29] as well as in Belgium[30]. Two unique features are polycythaemia and pericardial effusion. In Quebec, where the disease was first discovered, Morin and Coté believed that the condition was due to the drinking of large quantities of beer which contained from 0.5 to 1.5 parts/million of cobalt[31]. The Omaha group recognized that severe lactate acidosis was probably responsible for the high mortality[28]. Haemodynamic changes consisted of a severe depression of myocardial contractility and reduction in coronary flow. The mortality of this condition is high.

As Alexander states, it has been difficult to explain the cardiotoxic effect of 10–15 mg of cobalt per day, when patients with pernicious anaemia take from 50–100 mg/d and tolerate this dose without developing cardiotoxicity[29]. It is possible that diminished protein intake can aggravate the condition. Furthermore, cobalt and iron compete for the same absorption sites, and the presence of iron in the preparation probably reduces the amount of cobalt absorbed[29]. Finally, anaemic patients preferably eat a well-balanced diet free of alcohol, two factors which protect the heart from the cardiotoxic effect of cobalt.

The toxic effects of cobalt are probably due to its blockage of the oxidation of pyruvate to acetylCoA and of α-ketoglutarate to succinylCoA. Thiamine pyrophosphate is required as a co-factor.

4.3 THE ACUTE EFFECT OF ALCOHOL ON CORONARY FLOW AND MYOCARDIAL PERFORMANCE

In 1971, Mendoza and his co-workers reported their work on coronary flow and referred to the work of others on the effect of alcohol on coronary flow[31]. The effect of alcohol on the coronary circulation is controversial; some workers found an increase in coronary flow[32–34], others a diminution[35–38], while a third group found no change[34,39–42]. Mendoza and his co-workers found in anaesthetized dogs and in man, that after an intravenous infusion of alcohol resulting in blood concentration of 50 mg/%, there was a consistent but not significant increase in coronary flow as measured with coincidence counting, using ^{81}Rb; at the same time coronary vascular resistance slightly declined[31]. In contrast, at a higher dose with consequently higher blood concentrations of ethanol, a significant increase in coronary flow was noted together with a fall in coronary vascular resistance. With alcohol blood levels of about 200 mg/%, the coronary blood flow increased approximately 60 % and the coronary vascular resistance (mmHg/cc/min) declined. These results indicate that the response of the coronary circulation to alcohol is largely dependent on the ethanol blood concentration.

In 1972, using non-coincidence counting with ^{86}Rb, Gould and his associates studied the response of the coronary circulation in patients with and without coronary heart disease, after the ingestion of 90 ml of Canadian Club whisky[43]. Unfortunately, no data are available on the blood ethanol level. They concluded that coronary flow increased significantly in patients with coronary artery disease. They explained the lack of effect of alcohol on the coronary blood flow in the normal group by minimal alterations in myocardial oxygen consumption. In the group suffering from coronary heart disease, an increase in left ventricular end-diastolic pressure, a fall in the stroke work index and an increase in peripheral resistance were recorded[44]. They postulated that the rise in the left ventricular end-diastolic pressure is associated with an increase in left ventricular end-diastolic volume, leading to an augmentation of the myocardial oxygen requirements and consequently to an increase in coronary blood flow. Their studies, however, were carried out with ^{86}Rb, a non $\beta+$ emitter. Consequently, the accidental counts are so high that it must have been difficult to separate the radioactivity of the heart from that of surrounding structures. Furthermore, no data are available on the extraction ratio of rubidium by the heart and of the body under these conditions; inequality of these ratios can lead to considerable error.

It should be reiterated at this point that the measurement of *total* coronary blood flow permits little insight into the presence of inhomogenous perfusion[45]. This is particularly the case in the heart muscle of patients with coronary artery disease where 'coronary steal' may shunt blood away from underperfused areas of the coronary circulation[46]. Thus, a decrease in resistance at the precapillary level of non-occluded or normal vessels could result in a decrease in blood flow to muscle supplied by the artery through collaterals. In line with the observations of Bing[47] and of Knoebel[48] and their associates, alcohol should, in patients with coronary heart disease, lead to a diminution rather than an increase in coronary flow; coronary vasodilators such as dipyridamole and isoproterenol lead to a proportionally greater increase in coronary flow in patients without coronary artery disease as compared to individuals suffering from restricted coronary circulation.

The effect of ethanol on myocardial performance is less controversial. Most workers discovered depression of myocardial contractility in intact dogs and isolated heart preparations[34,35,49–51]. Working on patients and anaesthetized animals, Mendoza and co-workers found no evidence of myocardial depression at blood ethanol levels of less than 50 mg/%[31]. However, in dogs the intravenous infusion of alcohol resulting in blood levels of approximately 200 mg/% led to a significant diminution in velocity of left ventricular contraction. Depression of myocardial contractility has also been reported among others, by Lochner[34], Sulzer[35], Haggard[49], Wakim[50], and Loomis[51]. Using strain gauge analysis, Newman and Valicenti also found (in anaesthetized open-chest dog) depression of ventricular contraction, concluding that this chamber operates under increased load produced by infusion of alcohol[53]. Using human volunteers, Riff and co-workers discovered that the ingestion of 85 ml of whisky leading to alcohol levels of from 85 to 140 mg/% produces an increase in cardiac output which was primarily accounted for by an increase in heart rate[53]. The arterial pressure was unchanged and left ventricular contractility remained unimpaired.

These results are in disagreement with those of Ahmed and Regan who found that the ingestion of 170 ml of 43 % alcohol resulted in depression of myocardial contractility, as indicated by prolongation of the pre-ejection period (PEP), isovolumic left ventricular contraction time (IVT), and an increase in the PEP/left ventricular ejection (LVET) ratio (PEP/LVET)[54]. They conclude that alcohol in non-intoxicating doses elicits a depression of cardiovascular function in normal unhabituated subjects. In general, blood alcohol levels in the individual of this series ranged from approximately 50 to 120 mg/%. In 1973, Horwitz found in conscious dogs that intravenous infusion of ethanol to blood levels ranging from 120 to 311 mg/% resulted in an increase in left ventricular end-diastolic pressure and diameter and a fall in left ventricular dp/dt_{max}, following pharmacological autonomic denervation with propranolol and atropine[55]. The authors conclude that the effects of alcohol infusion on the myocardium are direct and not mediated through autonomic mechanisms.

Using non-invasive methods, other workers studied the effect of one or two cocktails in normal man[56]. After ingestion of 113 ml of Canadian whisky, pre-ejection period, isometric contraction time and the PEP/LVET ratio were prolonged, demonstrating impaired cardiac function in normal subjects. However, there appeared to be no corrections made for heart rate[56]. Wendt and co-workers found no significant haemodynamic changes in their patients 30 min after ingestion of 170 ml of vodka[57].

4.3.1 Chronic haemodynamic changes induced by alcohol

The changes induced in animals and men by prolonged periods of ethanol administration do not differ from those observed in other types of cardiomyopathy. However, since alcohol affects other organs, primarily the liver, haemodynamic changes depend on the absence or presence of hepatic disease. For example, Wendt and co-workers found differences between patients with and without hepatic involvement[58]. Alcoholic patients without overt evidence of heart disease were able to respond to exercise more effectively than patients with myocardial involvement. Mean blood pressure was low at rest in patients with cardiomyopathy but rose normally under the stress of exercise. In patients with liver disease, some elevation of mean blood pressure at rest and during exercise was found, reflecting the increased systolic and widened pulse pressures encountered clinically in this group. Abelmann and co-workers also found that alcoholics have normal cardiac output, arterial blood pressure and peripheral vascular resistance at rest[59]. In cirrhotic patients, all of whom had ascites, the cardiac index was elevated.

In experiments on rats exposed to ethanol, Maines and co-workers discovered progressive cardiovascular changes manifested by depression in myocardial contraction[60]. This was accompanied by a decrease in aortic blood pressure and heart rate and a marked tendency toward cardiac arrhythmias. The myocardial depression occurred only in the alcohol-intoxicated group regardless of whether these animals received adequate nutrition. Vitamin supplements did not protect against myocardial depression. Spodick and co-workers, using systolic time intervals to measure myocardial contractility in chronic alcoholics without clinical signs of cardiac damage, found reduced left ventricular ejection time (LVET) and an increase in the PEP/LVET ratio, indicating depressed myocardial contractility[61]. In order to evaluate properly changes in myocardial contractility on the basis of non-invasive techniques, it should be recalled that systolic time intervals only reflect major alterations in myocardial contractility. It is therefore surprising that in patients in whom no clinical signs of cardiac damage were evident, these non-invasive methods demonstrated such obvious degrees of damage[62]. Using invasive techniques, Gould and co-workers demonstrated elevated left ventricular end-diastolic pressure and mean pulmonary artery pressure as well as a fall in stroke index on exercise in patients with normal cardiovascular findings and minimal or no liver disease[63].

Diminished left ventricular function was also present in alcoholics with fatty liver but without clinical evidence of cardiac or nutritional disease[26]. Using angiotensin afterload, a 3-fold rise of left ventricular end-diastolic pressure in this group was found. The stroke volume and stroke work response in the non-cardiac alcoholic was significantly less than in controls. Ventricular function curves differed significantly from normal individuals. In normal individuals, a small rise of left ventricular end-diastolic pressure was associated with a significant stroke output and stroke work increment. In contrast, in alcoholics without clinical evidence of cardiac disease, a nearly 3-fold rise of ventricular end-diastolic pressure was found, but only a minimal stroke output and stroke work increment was present. Regan and his co-workers concluded that the cumulative effects of repeated ingestion of alcohol in intoxicating doses can produce diminished left ventricular function before any clinical evidence of cardiac abnormality occurs[26].

These findings further demonstrate that haemodynamic disturbances are present in chronic alcoholics prior to any clinical manifestation of heart disease. Pachinger and co-workers also measured the effect of angiotensin afterload in dogs exposed to alcohol for 14 weeks[64]. They found that during angiotensin infusion, the maximal rate of rise of left ventricular pressure (dp/dt_{max}) declined in animals exposed to alcohol. It increased slightly in the control group. However, these changes were not statistically significant. Only minimal changes in cardiac contractility were present in conjunction with marked mitochondrial dysfunction. It was suggested that myocardial contractility might not be dependent on the integrity of mitochondrial function alone, an opinion which was supported by recent observations that both calcium binding and uptake of mitochondria and sarcoplasmic reticulum are severely reduced in dogs exposed to alcohol for a comparable period of time, even though cardiac contractility remained essentially unimpaired[65].

4.4 THE ACUTE EFFECTS OF ALCOHOL ON CARDIAC METABOLISM

The changes induced by ethanol on cardiac metabolism and function result from its toxic action on the myocardial cell. The dynamic, metabolic and morphological consequences induced by this agent are indistinguishable from other cardiomyopathies. But, in alcoholic cardiomyopathy, the cause as well as the effect of the disease are known. Thus the whole chain of events in the disease process can be followed step by step.

Another general result of ethanol is that the metabolic effects on the heart muscle and on cells of other organs are similar, if not identical. In this chapter no special mention will be made of the work on the effect of alcohol on competitive action with hydrogen acceptors as outlined in the chapter on the effects of alcohol on the liver by Lieber and DeCarli (Chapter 2)[66]. However, although the toxic effects of ethanol on the cell are common for all cells, its action on any specific organ depends on the specific function of that organ.

The measurable metabolic effects of alcohol on the heart depend on the different techniques used. Using catheterization of the human heart, Wendt and his co-workers found as main changes a 'leakage' of enzymes from the heart muscle into the coronary vein blood. Isocitrate dehydrogenase was primarily affected: this enzyme leaked into coronary vein blood in chronic alcoholic patients prior to the administration of ethanol.[58]. This was interpreted as indicating changes in intramitochondrial metabolic pathways or altered membrane permeability or both. Regan and co-workers obtained similar results for potassium and phosphate which were present in coronary vein blood in increased concentrations, even before there was a significant rise in their arterial concentrations[38]. Later this was followed by the appearance of transaminase in the coronary vein blood.

These alterations, together with the electronmicroscopic findings, suggest definite alterations in mitochondrial function. This supposition was confirmed by Pachinger and his co-workers who studied mitochondrial respiration as well as the activity of the intramitochondrial enzyme, isocitrate dehydrogenase (ICDH) by means of biopsy specimens and material obtained at autopsy from dogs maintained on alcohol for a period of 14 weeks[64]. In the group exposed to alcohol, diminution in respiratory function of myocardial mitochondria was detected. These alterations occurred regardless of the substrate used. Thus, mitochondrial QO_2 and the respiratory control indices were markedly diminished. The ADP/O ratio showed no change. Significant diminution in the NAD–ICDH occurred in animals exposed to alcohol as compared with the control.

The metabolic defect not only extends to respiratory function of mitochondrial and some of the intramitochondrial enzymes, but also to calcium binding and uptake of sarcoplasmic reticulum and mitochondria of dogs exposed to alcohol for a period of 6 months[65]. The results suggest that ethanol causes severe damage to the sarcoplasmic reticulum and thus to excitation–contraction coupling.

Excitation–contraction coupling and relaxation in heart muscle are considered as interactions between myofibrillar protein, actin and myosin, and an energy-dependent calcium movement[67]. In general, an action potential on the depolarizing heart muscle cell travels along the transverse sarcotubular system, releases calcium from the sarcoplasmic reticulum (SR), which then results in muscular contraction. As the intracellular free Ca^{2+} is taken up by the sarcoplasmic reticulum, through ATP-dependent mechanisms, relaxation occurs[68]. The main role of the sarcoplasmic reticulum is therefore consistent with that of Ca^{2+} pumping, the Ca^{2+} being pumped out of the membrane of the SR granules in order to permit Ca^{2+} combination with contractile elements of the muscle; during relaxation, the Ca^{2+} returns to the SR granule. Thus there occurs a rapid binding and subsequent release or a rapid accumulation with no release. The former process occurs in the absence of inorganic phosphate or oxalate; the latter in the presence of either oxalate or phosphate. The accumulation of Ca^{2+} in the presence of either oxalate or phosphate is the result of movement of Ca^{2+} ions across the vesicular grana with subsequent precipitation to calcium phosphate or calcium oxalate within the vesicle[69]. The accumulation process in the absence of precipitating ions is referred to as binding, and the accumulation in the presence of a precipitating anion is referred to as uptake[70]. Apparently the binding process in the absence of oxalate is of primary significance, as shown by Ebashi[71]. There are two proposed mechanisms for intracellular Ca^{2+}: (1) The active transport hypothesis, which is based on the stoichiometry of ATP splitting and Ca^{2+} uptake; and (2) the two-stage binding and active transport process as suggested by Ebashi[71]. The latter suggested that the first step in Ca^{2+} uptake involves ATP-induced change of the membrane before any splitting of ATP occurs.

The sequence of events involving Ca^{2+} in the myocardial cell can thus be summarized: depolarization of the surface cell membrane is transmitted to the cell interior via the tubular system of the sarcotubular reticulum[67,72]. The potential change across the SR membrane causes the release of bound Ca^{2+} to the myofilaments, and this Ca^{2+} initiates and sustains contraction. Ca^{2+} release ceases as membrane repolarization commences, and relaxation is accomplished by the active return of Ca^{2+} to the SR.

We are convinced that damage to contractile proteins is of equal importance in the effect of ethanol on the heart. Ca^{2+} is primarily attached to the regulatory protein troponin-A. The evidence available indicates that this regulatory system is in part associated with actin in the I-filaments where, in a manner not yet understood, it regulates the ATPase activity of the myosin and its response to the intracellular Ca^{2+}. Now troponin has been shown to consist of at least three different distinct proteins[67,73].

The presence in actomyosin of tropomyosin and troponin under conditions of high Ca^{2+}, where the primary interaction between actin and myosin is taking place, appears to enhance the rates of both ATP hydrolysis and the physiochemical changes associated with contraction[73]. When Ca^{2+} concentration is reduced, the tropomyosin–troponin complex effects a marked inhibition of the primary interaction between actin and myosin.

Ca^{2+}, in affecting excitation–contraction coupling, acts to reverse the inhibition of the primary interaction between actin and myosin by a tropomyosin–troponin complex. Tropomyosin and troponin in the absence of Ca^{2+} act as a repressor while Ca^{2+} serves as a depressor.

The process concerned with excitation–contraction has been discussed in detail because its mechanism is of fundamental importance to the understanding of myocardial failure in general, and of the action of ethanol on the heart muscle in particular. Although ethanol injures the mitochondria, it affects excitation–contraction coupling mechanisms and contractile proteins as well.

As mentioned above, Bing and his associates showed that the administration of alcohol for a period of 6 months causes marked depression of calcium binding and uptake in the presence of succinate-linked oxidation in both mitochondria and sarcotubular reticulum[65]. Disturbed respiratory function of the mitochondria could be a contributory factor since Ca^{2+} binding and uptake by these structures depend partially on the rate of substrate oxidation and on energy-dependent processes. Deficient ability of mitochondria to take up Ca^{2+} has also been recently found by Sordahl *et al.* in failing hearts of rabbits[74].

It is therefore surprising that animals exposed to ethanol for this prolonged period of time, with daily blood levels as high as 200 mg/% a day, show no marked changes in cardiac contractility[65]. Two possible reasons may explain this: In the first place, the changes in calcium transport may not be as severe as those found after myocardial infarction or in other cardiomyopathies[74–79]. More likely, in both acute myocardial ischaemia and in the hereditary cardiomyopathy of the hamster, the contractile elements themselves are morphologically involved and the mitochondrial lesions are only part of the general process of myocardial reaction[65]. As mentioned above, the effect of ethanol on the contractile elements of the heart is of decisive importance. It has been shown that when alcohol is being administered to the experimental animal for longer periods (several years), structural changes in contractile elements appear. These morphological changes in contractile elements of the heart muscle will be described in a subsequent section.

The fact must be stressed that disturbances in contractility are not present unless the contractile elements themselves are affected. Alcohol therefore affects cardiac metabolism by a multipronged attack upon many subcellular structures. It appears to be a multifocal poison which manifests itself clinically as a result of this diverse action. Metabolic changes induced in heart muscle are also concerned with alterations in myocardial lipid metabolism. Regan discovered that when alcohol was acutely administered to dogs, the heart muscle accumulated triglycerides, and myocardial extraction of free fatty acids diminished[38]. Marciniak confirmed these findings in dogs subjected to chronic alcohol administration[80]. In 1969, Regan found similar changes in patients with liver disease, but without clinical evidence of cardiac dysfunction[26]; myocardial extraction of triglycerides was enhanced and myocardial free fatty acid uptake was reduced. It is doubtful, however, whether these disturbances in lipid metabolism of the heart muscle are responsible for clinical manifestations of advanced alcoholic cardiomyopathy.

Kako and co-workers further investigated the changes in fatty acid composition of myocardial triglycerides following a single administration of ethanol to rabbits[81]. They concluded that acute administration of ethanol to rabbits depresses fatty acid oxidation and augments their esterification to myocardial triglycerides. They are of the opinion that depressed fatty acid oxidation and enhanced esterification are a manifestation of the derangement of the mitochondrial function.

One additional effect of alcohol on the heart may be of interest. It deals with its effect on myocardial protein synthesis[82]. The work implicates acetaldehyde in the deficiency in myocardial protein synthesis induced by ethanol. The conclusions are based on the discovery that alcohol does not interfere with protein synthesis until levels lethal to the intact animal are reached. However, acetaldehyde produces marked positive inotropic and chronotropic effects and inhibits protein synthesis despite its marked stimulatory effect. The authors speculate that the metabolic effects of ethanol may be partially the result of acetaldehyde which may play a role in production of the cardiomyopathy after prolonged exposure by interfering with myocardial protein synthesis.

4.5 CORRELATION OF FUNCTION WITH STRUCTURE

The biochemical changes are the primary lesions which are later transformed into structural damage. From the previous comments, the following structures should be particularly involved: mitochondria, sarcoplasmic reticulum (SR), and in later stages of the disease, contractile proteins. Demonstration of structural changes in the contractile elements are of particular interest since this furnishes an explanation of the decline in myocardial contractility found in the later stages of chronic alcohol ingestion.

The evidence is overwhelming that all of these structures are affected in alcoholic cardiomyopathy. Bulloch also demonstrated that on the basis of structural changes no distinction can be made between idiopathic and alcoholic cardiomyopathy[83]. Thus, combined loss of contractile elements and of sarcoplasmic reticulum are the common ultrastructural abnormalities in both idiopathic and alcoholic cardiomyopathy. They are indistinguishable in those two groups. The biochemical and physiological equivalents of these structural changes have already been dwelled upon. The structural changes in sarcoplasmic reticulum express themselves biochemically as diminished calcium uptake and binding. The mitochondrial alterations are reflected in their diminished respiratory function and loss of mitochondrial enzymes. The changes in contractile proteins resulting in loss of contractile function occur after the changes in sarcotubular reticulum and mitochondrial structure have been present for some time.

The changes in SR are not restricted to the heart muscle alone. Lindbaugh and Lieber reported dilated endoplasmic reticulum as a major ultrastructural abnormality in the intestinal mucosa of patients with alcohol-induced malabsorption of vitamin B_{12}[84].

Most authors agree on the electron and light microscopic changes in heart muscle of animals and patients exposed to alcohol. Hibbs and co-workers also mention swelling of sarcoplasmic reticulum[85]; mitochondrial changes were even more pronounced than those described by Bulloch[83]. Degeneration of myofibrils is usually preceded by pronounced mitochondrial injury; the presence of numerous lipid droplets throughout the myocardium is also seen, even in areas in which no other alterations are demonstrable[85]. It is likely that these lipid droplets represent accumulation of triglycerides. In mice exposed from 4 to 10 weeks to ethanol, the ultrastructural alterations are identical. Alterations in intercalated discs are also present[86]. Alexander stressed the increased number of mitochondria found in hearts of patients exposed to alcohol for several years[87].

The biochemical lesion in cobalt-beer cardiomyopathy has been described already. Reference was made to the possible biochemical action of cobalt in blocking of oxidation of pyruvate to acetylCoA and α-ketoglutarate to succinylCoA[20]. The structural and subcellular changes in this condition have been described by Morin and Côté[22]. They described myocardial degeneration without inflammatory cell infiltration as the most consistent lesion. Myocardial degeneration was characterized by a decrease of acidophilic material inside the cell. Electronmicroscopic examination revealed that the cellular membrane was intact and pinocytosis was still active in several areas. There were also changes in mitochondria, accumulation of lipid droplets, but no depletion of glycogen. The characteristic picture of cobalt-beer cardiomyopathy is the disappearance of contractile elements in the heart muscle.

4.6 SUMMARY

The historical, clinical, biochemical, physiological, and morphological features of the effect of ethanol on the heart were discussed.

4.6.1 Clinical studies

On clinical grounds, alcoholic cardiomyopathy cannot be differentiated from other myocardial diseases unless a history of alcoholism is documented. The clinical course of the disease depends on the duration of inebriety. Abstinence from ethanol is the most important therapeutic consideration. The deleterious effect of cobalt in beer on the heart are due to the combination of this agent combined with the absence of iron and other dietary factors.

4.6.2 Haemodynamics

The effect of acute alcohol administration on the coronary circulation is controversial. In the dog, ethanol increases coronary flow and reduces coronary vascular resistance at blood alcohol concentrations exceeding 180 mg/%. At high blood ethanol levels myocardial contractility is reduced. The haemodynamic changes produced by long periods of alcohol ingestion are indistinguishable from those observed in other cardiomyopathies. The haemodynamic effects of alcohol are influenced by the presence of liver disease or overt heart disease. Diminished cardiac contractility may be present even in the absence of clinical evidence of heart disease.

4.6.3 Effects of ethanol on cardiac metabolism

These are the results of direct toxic action of alcohol on the myocardial cell. The changes induced by this agent are indistinguishable from those of other cardiomyopathies. In man, leakage of enzymes as well as of potassium and phosphate from the heart are observed. Ethanol also results in diminution of respiratory function of mitochondria and reduced activity of intra-mitochondrial isocitrate dehydrogenase. It diminishes calcium uptake and binding by the sarcoplasmic reticulum. It is also likely that it damages the contractile proteins. Alcohol results in marked changes in myocardial lipid metabolism, it depresses fatty acid oxidation and augments their esterification.

Close correlation exists between function and structural changes induced by ethanol. Alcohol affects all subcellular structures resulting in their biochemical and biophysical malfunction.

References

1. Wood, G. B. (1885). *A Treatise on the Practice of Medicine,* **2,** 168. Philadelphia: Lippincott, Grambo and Co.
2. Friedreich, N. (1861). *Handbuch der Speziellen Pathologie und Therapie,* fifth section: *Die Krankheiten des Herzens.* Erlangen: Verlag von Ferdinand Enke
3. Walshe, W. H. (1873). *Diseases of the Heart and Great Vessels,* fourth edition. London: Smith, Elder and Co.
4. Bollinger, O. (1884). Uber die Häufigkeit and Ursachen der idiopathischen Herzhypertrophie in München. *Deutsch Med. Wochenschr.,* **10,** 180
5. Aufrecht, D. (1895). Die alkoholische Myocarditis mit nachfolgender Lebererkrankung und zeitweiliger Albuminurie. *Deutsch Arch. Klin. Med.,* **54,** 615
6. Mackenzie, J. (1902). *The Study of the Pulse,* p. 237. Edinburgh and London: Y. T. Pentland
7. Mackenzie, J. (1910). *Diseases of the Heart,* second edition, p. 207. New York: Oxford Medical Publications

8. Steell, G. (1906). *Textbook on Diseases of the Heart*, p. 19. Philadelphia: P. Blakiston's Son and Co.
9. Aalsmer, W. C. and Wenckebach, K. R. (1929). Herz und Kreislauf bei der Beri-Beri Krankheit. *Wien Arch. Inn. Med.*, **16,** 193
10. Keefer, C. S. (1930). The beriberi heart. *Arch. Intern. Med.*, **45,** 1
11. Laubry, C. (1930). Les myocardies. In *Nouveau traite de pathologie interne*, 530. Paris: Gaston Doin Cie.
12. Weiss, S. and Wilkins, R. W. (1937). The nature of the cardiovascular disturbances in nutritional deficiency states (beriberi). *Ann. Intern. Med.*, **11,** 104
13. Blankenhorn, M. A., Vilter, C. F., Scheinker, I. M. and Rustin, R. S. (1946). Occidental beri-beri heart disease. *J. Am. Med. Ass.*, **131,** 717
14. Brigden, W. (1957). Uncommon myocardial diseases. The non-coronary cardiomyopathies. *Lancet*, **ii,** 1179, 1243
15. Evans, W. (1959). The electrocardiogram of alcoholic cardiomyopathy. *Br. Heart J.*, **21,** 445
16. Robin, E. and Goldschlager, N. (1970). Persistence of low cardiac output after relief of high output by thiamine in a case of alcoholic beri-beri and cardiac myopathy. *Am. Heart J.*, **80,** 103
17. Perkoff, G. T., Dioso, M. M., Bleisch, V. and Kunkerfuss, G. (1967). A spectrum of myopathy associated with alcoholism. *Ann. Intern. Med.*, **67,** 481
18. Burch, G. E. and de Pasquale, N. P. (1969). Alcoholic cardiomyopathy. *Am. J. Cardiol.*, **23,** 723
19. Gunnar, R. M., Sutton, G. C. Pietras, R. J. and Tobin, Jr., J. R. (1971). Alcoholic cardiomyopathy. Disease-a-Month, p. 1, September
20. Alexander, C. S. (1972). Nutritional heart disease. In G. E. Burch, guest editor, *Cardiomyopathy*, p. 221, *Cardiovascular Clinics*, Vol. 4, Nr. 1. Philadelphia: F. A. Davis Co.
21. Brigden, W. (1972). Alcoholic cardiomyopathy. In G. E. Burch, guest editor, *Cardiomyopathy*, p. 187, *Cardiovascular Clinics*, Vol. 4, Nr. 1. Philadelphia: F. A. Davis Co.
22. Morin, Y. and Côté, G. (1972). Toxic agents and cardiomyopathies. In G. E. Burch, guest editor, *Cardiomyopathy*, p. 245, *Cardiovascular Clinics*, Vol. 4, Nr. 1. Philadelphia: F. A. Davis Co.
23. Demakis, J. G., Proskey, A., Rahimtoola, S. H., Jamil, M., Sutton, G. C., Rosen, K. M., Gunnar, R. M. and Tobin, Jr., J. R. (1974). The natural course of alcoholic cardiomyopathy. *Ann. Intern. Med.*, **80,** 293
24. Macdonald, C. D., Burch, G. E. and Walsh, J. J. (1971). Alcoholic cardiomyopathy managed with prolonged bed rest. *Ann. Intern. Med.*, **74,** 681
25. Asokan, S. K., Frank, M. J. and Witham, A. C. (1972). Cardiomyopathy without cardiomegaly in alcoholics, *Am. Heart J.*, **84,** 13
26. Regan, T. J., Levinson, G. E. and Oldewurtel, H. A. (1969). Ventricular function in noncardiacs with fatty liver: role of ethanol in the production of cardiomyopathy. *J. Clin. Invest.*, **48,** 397
27. Morin, Y. L., Foley, A. R., Martineau, G. and Roussel, J. (1967). Quebec beer-drinkers' cardiomyopathy: forty-eight cases. *Can. Med. Ass. J.*, **97,** 881
28. McDermott, P. H., Delaney, R. L., Egan, J. D. and Sullivan, J. F. (1966). Myocardosis and cardiac failure in men. *J. Am. Med. Ass.*, **198,** 253
29. Alexander, C. S. (1972). Cobalt-beer cardiomyopathy. A clinical and pathologic study of twenty-eight cases. *Am. J. Med.*, **53,** 395
30. Kesteloot, H., Terryn, R., Bosmans, P. and Joossens, J. V. (1966). Alcoholic pericardiomyopathy. *Acta Cardiol. (Brux.)*, **21,** 34
31. Mendoza, L. C., Hellberg, K., Rickart, A., Tillich, G. and Bing, R. J. (1971). The effect of intravenous ethyl alcohol on the coronary circulation and myocardial contractility of the human and canine heart. *J. Clin. Pharmacol.*, **11,** 165

32. Lasker, N., Sherrod, T. R. and Killam, K. F. (1955). Alcohol on the coronary circulation of the dog. *J. Pharmacol. Exp. Ther.*, **113**, 414
33. Ganz, V. (1963). The acute effect of alcohol on the circulation and on the oxygen metabolism of the heart. *Am. Heart J.*, **66**, 494
34. Lochner, A., Cowley, R. and Brink, A. J. (1969). Effect of ethanol on metabolism and function of perfused rat heart. *Am. Heart J.*, **78**, 770
35. Sulzer, R. (1924). The influence of alcohol on the isolated mammalian heart. *Heart*, **11**, 141
36. Leighninger, D. S., Rueger, and Beck, C. S. (1961). Effect of pentaerythritol amyl nitrite and alcohol on arterial blood supply to ischemic myocardium. *Am. J. Cardiol.*, **7**, 533
37. Webb, W. R. and Degerli, I. U. (1965). Ethyl alcohol and the cardiovascular system. *J. Am. Med. Ass.*, **191**, 1055
38. Regan, T. J., Koroxenidis, C. B. M., Oldewurtel, H. A., Lehan, P. H. and Hellems, H. K. (1966). The acute metabolic and hemodynamic responses of the left ventricle to ethanol. *J. Clin. Invest.*, **45**, 270
39. Loeb, O. (1905). Die Wirkung des Alkohols auf das Warmblüterherz. *Arch. Exp. Pathol. Pharmakol.*, **52**, 459
40. Gilbert, N. C. and Fenn, C. K. (1929). The effect of purine base diuretics on the coronary flow. *Arch. Intern. Med.*, **44**, 118
41. Schmitthener, J. E., Hafkenschiel, J. H., Forte, I., Williams, A. J. and Riegel, C. Does alcohol increase coronary blood flow and cardiac work? *Circulation*, **18**, 778
42. Wendt, V. E., Stock, R. B., Hayden, R. O., Bruce, T. A., Gudbjarnason, S. and Bing, R. J. (1962). The hemodynamics and cardiac metabolism in cardiomyopathies. *Med. Clin. N. Am.*, **45**, 1445
43. Gould, L., Collica, C., Zahir, M. and Gomprecht, R. F. (1972). Ethyl alcohol. Effects on coronary blood flow in man. *Br. Heart J.*, **34**, 815
44. Gould, L., Jaynal, F., Zahir, M. and Gomprecht, R. F. (1972). Effects of alcohol on the systolic time intervals. *Q. J. Stud. Alc.*, **33**, 451
45. Bing, R. J. and Hellberg, K. (1972). Coronary blood flow in relation to angina pectoris. *Circulation*, **46**, 1146
46. McGregor, M. and Fam, W. M. (1966). Regulation of coronary blood flow. *Bull. N.Y. Acad. Med.*, **42**, 940
47. Cohen, A., Luebs, E. D., Zaleski, E. and Bing, R. J. (1966). A new diagnostic test for coronary disease using a coincidence counting system. *Minn. Med.*, **49**, 17
48. Knoebel, S. B., McHenry, P. L., Stein, L. and Sonel, A. (1967). Myocardial blood flow in man as measured by a coincidence counting system and a single bolus of ^{84}rubidium chloride. *Circulation*, **36**, 187
49. Haggard, H. W. (1941). Studies on the absorption, distribution and elimination of alcohol. IX. The concentration of alcohol in the blood causing primary cardiac failure. *J. Pharmacol. Exp. Ther.*, **71**, 358
50. Wakim, K. G. (1946). The effects of ethyl alcohol on the isolated heart. *Fed. Proc.*, **5**, 109
51. Loomis, T. A. (1962). Effect of alcohol on myocardial and respiratory function. The influence of modified respiratory function on the cardiac toxicity of alcohol. *Q. J. Stud. Alc.*, **13**, 461
52. Newman, W. H. and Valicenti, J. F., Jr. (1971). Ventricular function following acute alcohol administration: a strain-gauge analysis of depressed ventricular dynamics. *Am. Heart J.*, **81**, 61
53. Riff, D. P., Jain, A. C. and Doyle, J. T. (1969). Acute hemodynamic effects of ethanol on normal human volunteers. *Am. Heart J.*, **78**, 592
54. Ahmed, S. S., Levinson, G. E. and Regan, T. J. (1973). Depression of myocardial contractility with low doses of ethanol in normal man. *Circulation*, **48**, 378
55. Horwitz, L. D. and Atkins, J. M. (1974). Acute effects of ethanol on left ventricular performance. *Circulation*, **49**, 124

56. Gould, L., Reddy, R., Goswami, K., Venkataraman, K. and Gombrecht, R. F. (1973). Cardiac effects of two cocktails in normal man. *Chest,* **63,** 943
57. Wendt, V. E., Ajlumi, R., Bruce, T. A., Prasad, A. S. and Bing, R. J. (1966). Acute effects of alcohol on the human myocardium. *Am. J. Cardiol.,* **17,** 804
58. Wendt, V. E., Wu, C., Balcon, R., Doty, G. and Bing, R. J. (1965). Hemodynamic and metabolic effects of chronic alcoholism in man. *Am. J. Cardiol.,* **15,** 175
59. Abelmann, W. H., Kowlaksi, H. J. and McNeely, W. F. (1954). The circulation of blood in alcohol addicts. *Quart. J. Stud. Alcohol,* **15,** 1
60. Maines, J. E. and Aldringer, E. E. (1967). Myocardial depression accompanying chronic consumption of alcohol. *Am. Heart J.,* **73,** 55
61. Spodick, D. H., Pigott, V. M. and Chirife, P. (1972). Preclinical cardiac malfunction in chronic alcoholism. Comparison with matched normal controls and with alcoholic cardiomyopathy. *N. Engl. J. Med.,* **287,** 677
62. Sarma, R., Ishikawa, K., Getzen, J. H., McNair, J. D., Buggs, H., Johnson, J. L. and Bing, R. J. (1974). Comparison of the invasive and noninvasive measurement in coronary artery disease. *Cardiology,* **59,** 114
63. Gould, L., Zahir, M., Shariff, M. and DiLieto, M. (1969). Cardiac hemodynamics in alcoholic heart disease. *Ann. Intern. Med.,* **71,** 543
64. Pachinger, O. M. Tillmanns, H., Mao, J. C., Fauvel, J-M. and Bing, R. J. (1973). The effect of prolonged administration of ethanol on cardiac metabolism and performance in the dog. *J. Clin. Invest.,* **52,** 2690
65. Bing, R. J., Tillmanns, H., Fauvel, J-M., Seeler, K. and Mao, J. C. (1974). The effect of prolonged alcohol administration on calcium transport in heart muscle of the dog. *Circ. Res.,* **35,** 33
66. Lieber, C. S. and Davidson, C. S. (1962). Some metabolic effects of ethyl alcohol. *Am. J. Med.,* **33,** 319
67. Bing, R. J. and Tillmanns, H. (1974). Cardiac metabolism. In V. Puddu and A. B. Anguissola, eds. Torina, Italy. *Cardiologia d'Oggi* (*Cardiology Today*)
68. Weber, A. (1959). On the role of calcium in the activity of adenosine-5′-triphosphate hydrolysis by actomyosin. *J. Biol. Chem.,* **234,** 2764
69. Olson, R. E. (1971). Introduction. In P. Harris and L. H. Opie, eds. *Calcium and the Heart,* p. 1. London and New York: Academic Press
70. Schwartz, A. (1971). Calcium and the sarcoplasmic reticulum. In P. Harris and L. H. Opie, eds. *Calcium and the Heart,* p. 66. London and New York: Academic Press
71. Ebashi, S. and Lipmann, F. (1962). Adenosine triphosphate-linked concentration of calcium ions in a particulate fraction of rabbit muscle. *J. Cell. Biol.,* **14,** 389
72. Langer, G. A. (1968). Ion fluxes in cardiac excitation and contraction and their relation to myocardial contractility. *Physiol. Rev.,* **48,** 708
73. Katz, A. M. (1971–72). Effects of ischemia on the cardiac contractile proteins. *Cardiology,* **56,** 276
74. Sordahl, L. A., McCollum, W. B., Wood, W. G. and Schwartz, A. (1973). Mitochondria and sarcoplasmic reticulum function in cardiac hypertrophy and failure. *Am. J. Physiol.,* **224,** 497
75. Lee, K. S., Ladinsky, H. and Stucky, J. H. (1967). Decreased Ca^{2+} uptake by sarcoplasmic reticulum after coronary occlusion for 60 and 90 minutes. *Circ. Res.,* **21,** 439
76. Lindenmayer, G. E., Harigaya, S., Bajusz, E. and Schwartz, A. (1970). Oxidative phosphorylation and calcium transport of mitochondria isolated from cardiomyopathic hamster hearts. *J. Mol. Cell. Cardiol.,* **1,** 249
77. McCollum, W. B., Crow, C., Harigaya, S., Bajusz, E. and Schwartz, A. (1970). Calcium binding by cardiac relaxing system isolated from myopathic Syrian hamsters (strains 14.6, 82.62 and 40.54). *J. Mol. Cell. Cardiol.,* **1,** 445
78. Sulakhe, P. V. and Dhalla, N. S. (1970). Excitation–contraction coupling in heart. VII.

Calcium accumulation in subcellular particles in congestive heart failure. *J. Clin. Invest.*, **50,** 1019

79. Schwartz, A., Wood, J. M., Allen, J. C., Bornet, E. P., Entman, M. L., Goldstein, M. A., Sordahl, L. A. and Suzuki, M. (1973). Biochemical and morphologic correlates of cardiac ischemia. *Am. J. Cardiol.*, **32,** 46
80. Marciniak, M., Gudbjarnason, S. and Bruce, T. A. (1968). The effect of chronic alcohol administration on enzyme profile and glyceride content of heart muscle, brain, and liver. *Proc. Soc. Exp. Biol. Med.*, **128,** 1021
81. Kako, K. J., Liu, M. S. and Thornton, M. J. (1973). Changes in fatty acid composition of myocardial triglyceride following a single administration of ethanol to rabbits. *J. Mol. Cell. Cardiol.*, **5,** 473
82. Schreiber, S. S., Briden, K., Oratz, M. and Rothschild, M. A. (1972). Ethanol, acetaldehyde, and myocardial protein synthesis. *J. Clin. Invest.*, **51,** 2820
83. Bulloch, R. T., Pearce, M. B., Murphy, M. L., Jenkins, B. J. and Davis, J. L. (1972). Myocardial lesions in idiopathic and alcoholic cardiomyopathy. Study by ventricular septal biopsy. *Am. J. Cardiol.*, **29,** 15
84. Lindbaugh, J. and Lieber, C. S. (1969). Alcohol-induced malabsorption of vitamin B_{12} in man. *Nature (London)*, **224,** 806
85. Hibbs, R. G., Ferrans, V. J., Black, W. C., Weilbaecher, D. G., Walsh, J. J. and Burch, G. E. (1975). Alcoholic cardiomyopathy. An electron microscopic study. *Am. Heart J.*, **69,** 766
86. Burch, G. E., Harb, J. M., Colcolough, H. L. and Tsui, C. Y. (1971). The effect of prolonged consumption of beer, wine and ethanol on the myocardium of the mouse. *Johns Hopkins Med. J.*, **129,** 130
87. Alexander, C. S. (1966). Idiopathic heart disease. II. Electronmicroscopic examination of myocardial biopsy specimens in alcoholic heart disease. *Am. J. Med.*, **41,** 229

5
Alcohol and Skeletal Disease

P. D. SAVILLE

5.1 INTRODUCTION 135
5.2 GROWTH AND DEVELOPMENT 135
5.2.1 *Human growth* 135
5.2.2 *Animal growth* 136
5.3 BONE DENSITY CHANGES 136
5.3.1 *Mechanism for alcohol changes in bone* 139
5.3.1.1 Calcium metabolism 139
5.3.1.2 Phosphorus metabolism 139
5.3.1.3 Corticosteroid metabolism 140
5.4 NEUROPATHIC ARTHROPATHY IN ALCOHOLICS 140
5.5 NON-TRAUMATIC OSTEONECROSIS (ASEPTIC NECROSIS, AVASCULAR NECROSIS OF BONE) 141
5.5.1 *Pathology* 142
5.5.2 *Radiographic changes* 142
5.5.3 *Etiology* 143
5.5.4 *Diagnosis* 144
5.6 SUMMARY 144
References 146

5.1 INTRODUCTION

Chronic alcohol ingestion may affect the skeletal system in several ways: (a) growth and development; (b) decreases in bone density with increased susceptibility to fractures; (c) Charcot feet; (d) osteonecrosis (avascular necrosis, aseptic necrosis of bone).

5.2 GROWTH AND DEVELOPMENT

5.2.1 Human growth

When the progeny of women chronically alcoholic during gestation were compared to matched controls, significant differences were found[1]. The commonest finding was a borderline to moderate mental deficiency (44 %), but weight was below the third percentile in 33 % of infants, and length in 15 %. There were joint anomalies, strabismus, and cardiac murmurs in over 20 % of cases. Furthermore, growth deficiencies could still be demonstrated at the 7-year physical examination. These observations are in accord with previous studies in animals which indicated that ethanol does not support growth as well as sucrose[2,3]. It is also in accord with the finding in animals and in humans that adverse effects on growth that occur very early in life tend to be permanent. Dubos has coined the term 'biological Freudianism' to describe this phenomenon[4].

5.2.2 Animal growth

In rats, when 36 % of sucrose calories were isocalorically replaced by ethanol, the ethanol-fed animals grew more slowly than their pair-fed litter mates (Figure 5.1). It was calculated that, if all the animals lived indefinitely, the maximum weight that the ethanol animals could attain would be significantly less than that of the controls. It was also shown that skeletal mass was less in the alcohol-fed animals than in the controls but this change could be accounted for by the significant body weight differences between the two groups of animals[5]. At the time that these data were published, Lieber and I believed that this argument fully explained these skeletal changes. Subsequent studies on the effect of restricting a nutritionally adequate diet in rats revealed that simple dietary restriction led to *greater* skeletal mass, femur thickness, and bone-breaking strength than the litter mate controls at the same *weight*[6]. Thus, the failure of ethanol-fed rats to *increase* their skeletal characteristics, despite restricted growth, indicates that the restriction of growth resulting from isocaloric ethanol substitution for sucrose is of a different nature from a similar degree of growth retardation resulting from total diet restriction.

5.3 BONE DENSITY CHANGES

Standard bone plugs were taken from the left iliac crest of individuals who had died suddenly and unexpectedly in Manhattan (N.Y.) and had come to autopsy by the medical examiner. No individual with chronic diseases was examined.

Among the non-alcoholic individuals, bone density decreased after 50 years of age in women and after 70 years of age in men. Among the alcoholics, all of whom were under 45 years of age, bone density was about the same as that of non-alcoholic men and women over the age of 70[7] (see Figure 5.2).

When fractures occur, due to osteoporosis, they are usually found at the hip, the wrist, the upper humerus, and the vertebrae — the so-called

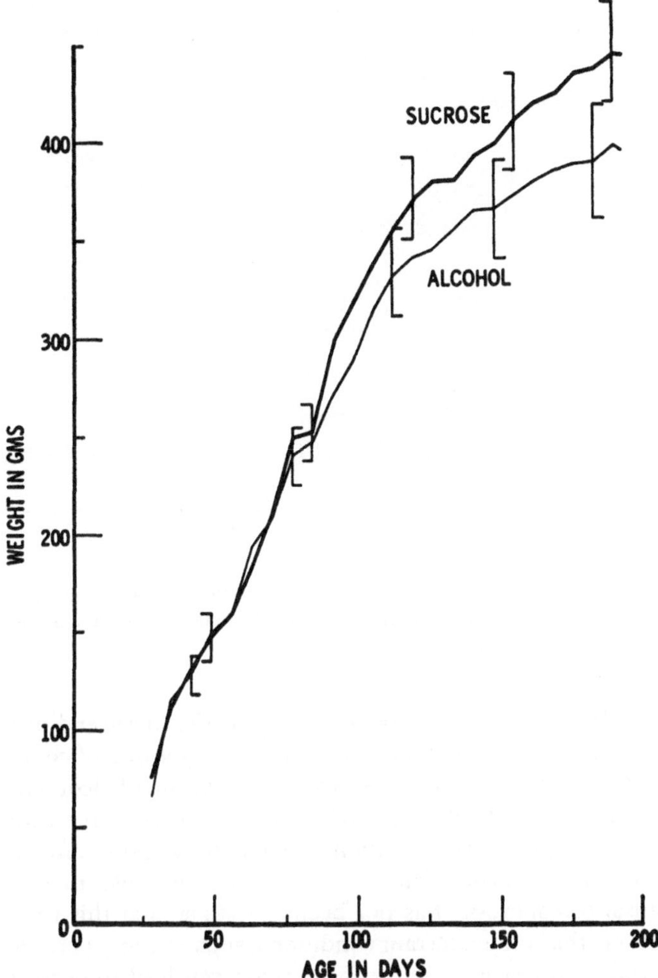

Figure 5.1 Growth curves from alcohol and sucrose pair-fed rat litter mates. Vertical bars represent ± two standard errors from the mean (from Saville and Lieber[5])

metabolic fractures. It is known that the factors which contribute to the production of femoral neck fractures include: increasing age, the female sex, and disease. Femoral neck fractures are uncommon in younger men when associated with only mild or moderate trauma. Nilsson compared 70 men under the age of 70 with fractures of the hip due to mild or moderate trauma to 125 age matched controls. In this series, if individuals with obvious causes for pathological fracture, such as paralysis, epilepsy, multiple sclerosis and polio were excluded, then about half of the remainder of men with fractured hips had either sustained partial gastrectomy or were chronic alcoholics[8]. This was significantly different from the controls.

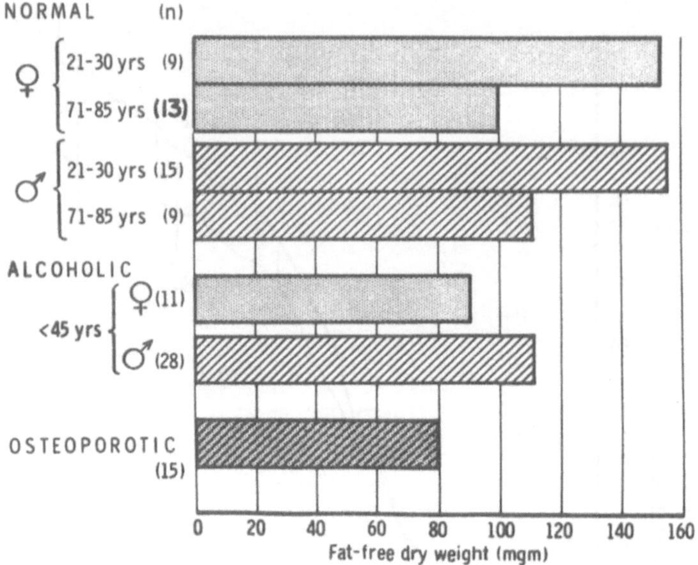

Figure 5.2 Average fat-free dry weight of standard-sized iliac crest bone plugs from normals, alcoholics, and osteoporotics. The normals and alcoholics had died suddenly and unexpectedly and had no chronic diseases

Nilsson and Westlin measured bone density at the lower end of the femur using a photon absorption method. They compared a group of control men to a group of chronic alcoholic men as well as a third group of alcoholic men who had sustained fractures. Table 5.1 shows the bone mass in the three groups. There were significant differences among them and these differences increased with increasing age[9]. Alcoholism, as a contributing cause to the so-called postmenopausal osteoporosis, has not been investigated at this time. It is apparent, however, that under certain conditions, such as those pertaining in the New York study, excessive alcohol consumption can lead to decreasing bone density and to metabolic types of fracture such as fractured hip, wrist, humerus and spine.

Table 5.1 Mineral mass at distal radius measured by photon absorption method in male controls and in male alcoholics with and without fractures of the wrist (data supplied by Nilsson and Westlin, Malmo, Sweden) (mean ± SD)

	Number	*Age*	*Distal radius* Mg/cm^2
Control	56	45 ± 11	459 ± 87
Alcoholic department	58	45 ± 11	408 ± 84
Orthopaedic department	35	52 ± 9	375 ± 90

5.3.1 Mechanism for alcohol changes in bone

Alcohol might affect skeletal metabolism in one of several ways: (1) by affecting calcium metabolism; (2) by affecting phosphorus metabolism; and (3) by affecting nitrogen metabolism.

5.3.1.1 Calcium metabolism

Alcohol satisfies caloric needs without satisfying calcium requirements. Alcoholics frequently have poor dietary habits and lack dietary calcium. Furthermore, fractional absorption of dietary calcium is believed to be impaired in alcoholics because of steatorrhea which may lead to malabsorption of vitamin D, or precipitation of calcium with fatty acids in the stools[10]. However, in rats, chronic ethanol ingestion has been shown to interfere with intestinal calcium transport, independent of hepatic and pancreatic dysfunction. A defect in calcium transport across the duodenal mucosa was demonstrated following 20 % ethanol ingestion and the defect could not be reversed by vitamin D or its more polar metabolites 25-hydroxycholecalciferol or 1,25-dihydroxycholecalciferol[11]. Kalbfleisch *et al.*[12] observed that 30 ml of ethanol given to controls and to alcoholics had a similar effect; within 20 minutes there was very nearly 100 % increase in urinary calcium excretion and a 167 % increase in magnesium excretion lasting for about 2 hours. Thus, the chronic alcoholic will have decreased dietary calcium, decreased fractional absorption of the diet, and increased urinary calcium, together resulting in prolonged periods of negative calcium balance. Since losses of calcium from the body tend to be greater than calcium absorbed into the body, hypocalcaemia will be the trend and will lead to stimulation of parathyroid hormone release; this in turn stimulates osteoclastic activity and bone resorption leading to a decrease in skeletal mass.

Alcohol consumption causes brisk magnesium diuresis and there is some evidence to show that the parathyroid glands are sensitive to the ionic concentrations of both magnesium and calcium[13]. Thus, alcohol-induced hypomagnesaemia could cause further chronic stimulation of the parathyroid glands, and increase bone resorption.

5.3.1.2 Phosphorus metabolism

Low serum inorganic phosphorus has been observed frequently in chronic alcoholics[14,15]. Inadequate dietary phosphorus seems the most likely cause of this finding, although magnesium depletion in the rat[16] induces excessive losses of phosphorus in the urine. Osteomalacia with pseudofractures has been described in patients suffering from phosphate depletion resulting from long-term ingestion of antacids for peptic ulcer[17]. A phosphorus depletion syndrome was induced in volunteers given low dietary phosphorus coupled with the administration of antacids. The syndrome induced experimentally was characterized by hypophosphataemia, hypophosphaturia, increased gastrointestinal absorption of calcium, hypercalciuria, increased resorption of skeletal calcium and phosphorus, and debility, with anorexia, weakness, bone pain, and malaise[18,19]. Low concentrations of inorganic phosphorus have been shown to increase the activity of osteoclastic bone resorption in tissue culture, while high concentrations have the opposite effect. Furthermore, high concentrations of phosphate in the tissue culture medium seem to stimulate osteoblastic activity as well as inhibiting osteoclastic activity[20]. Low serum inorganic phosphorus can be reduced even further when intravenous glucose is given to alcoholics by driving extracellular phosphorus into the cells. This is sometimes associated with widespread muscle damage and enormous elevations in the serum level of muscle enzymes which is then followed by hyperphosphataemia. This sequence of events suggests that acute hypophosphataemia results in muscle necrosis with liberation of phosphate from damaged muscle, thereby raising serum levels once more. Since bone mass and muscle mass are highly correlated, loss of muscle mass from phosphorus depletion must lead to a proportional decrease in bone mass[21].

5.3.1.3 Corticosteroid metabolism

There is some evidence in man and in animals that acute alcohol ingestion leads to corticosteroid hypersecretion; and increased urinary cortisol excretion has been noted in chronic alcoholics during the withdrawal phase[22]. What part, if any, hypercortisonism plays in the bone disease found in alcoholics is unknown.

5.4 NEUROPATHIC ARTHROPATHY IN ALCOHOLICS

In 1973, Thornhill and colleagues[23] reported ten alcoholics suffering from bone and joint changes in the feet associated with alcoholic neuropathy. All patients were males, even though these physicians also see chronic alcoholic females in their clinics in Harlem. Ages ranged from 29 to 59 and all individuals had been consuming alcohol for more than 10 years. There were severe soft tissue changes in all individuals, with ulcers, always painless, occurring usually beneath the first and fifth metatarsal heads. In addition, painless infected ulcers occurred on the undersurface of the first interphalangeal joint and the plantar surface of the toes in patients with clawing and fixed hammer toe deformities. Edema of the extremities with increased pigmentation and ulcers of the lower leg were frequent findings. All patients had warm feet with easily palpable pedal pulses. Eight patients had sustained amputation of one or more toes and in one case extensive infection occurred requiring an amputation below the knee. Roentgenographic changes included

(1) atrophy of phalanges, which was the most common bony change and included narrowing of the diaphysis in the anteroposterior view;

(2) phalangeal resorption occurred in some cases, with complete disappearance of some of the phalanges resulting in shrinkage of soft tissues, producing short toes;

(3) metatarsal resorption occurred in some cases showing tapering of the distal metatarsal, followed by gradual shortening of this bone. This change closely resembles the pencil and cup deformity seen in some psoriatic arthritics, as well as occasionally in diabetics;

(4) proximal migration of the sesamoids, which is a manifestation of resorption of either the proximal phalanx or the distal first metatarsal;

(5) in some cases there was subperiosteal new bone formation leading to thickening of the metatarsal cortex, most commonly seen in digits 3, 4, and 5. There was no other evidence of either bone destruction or active infection in these cases;

(6) interphalangeal joint destruction showing loss of joint space with sclerosis of the adjacent joint surfaces and subluxation thought to represent low-grade septic arthritis. There were also cases of interphalangeal fusion seen as bony arthrodesis reminiscent of fusion seen occasionally after untreated attacks of gonococcal arthritis.

5.5 NON-TRAUMATIC OSTEONECROSIS (ASEPTIC NECROSIS, AVASCULAR NECROSIS OF BONE)

Osteonecrosis may be defined as death of a volume of bone tissue within an anatomical bone. Osteonecrosis is referred to commonly in the English literature as *aseptic necrosis* or *avascular necrosis* of the bone. Since there are no counterparts of the descriptive adjective avascular, and while septic necrosis of bone is now hardly ever seen, the latter terms should be dropped. Osteonecrosis is best classified as either post-traumatic or non-traumatic in origin. The disease occurs most commonly in the head of the femur but may occur elsewhere, such as the head of the humerus, the medial femoral condyle, the talus, and other sites.

This article is concerned with the non-traumatic syndrome. It may occur from obstruction to the vascular supply of the femoral head or other sites, by air emboli in caisson workers; from macrophages in Gaucher's disease; by aggregated red cells in sickle cell anaemia; but in most cases, none of these conditions is present. Among the patients with non-traumatic osteonecrosis of unknown cause, a history of corticosteroid medication or chronic alcoholism will be elicited in the great majority[24]. Men outnumber women 4:1 and the disease occurs in both hips in somewhat more than 50 % of cases although symptoms are unilateral in the majority in the early stages.

5.5.1 Pathology

The blood supply to the femoral head consists of non-anastomosing terminal vessels. Obstruction to these vessels leads to necrosis of a small area of bone which, in turn, leads to attempts at a repair reaction. At first, dead bone is resorbed by osteoclastic activity and later there is invasion of blood vessels and osteocytes with new bone being laid down, often on old, unresorbed, dead bone.

5.5.2 Radiographic changes

There are no radiographic changes for at least 2 months after the onset of the disease. The earliest change seen is usually an area of resorption immediately beneath the cartilage within subchondral bone (Figure 5.3). This corresponds to resorption of dead bone. The next appearance is of increased bone density after some months, which correlates with the repair reaction (Figure 5.4). During this process the head of the femur loses its architectural integrity and may collapse under weight bearing. This results in an irregular shape to the head, contrasted to the smooth symmetrical roundness of a healthy head. The x-ray appearances may be difficult to visualize and may be better seen in a

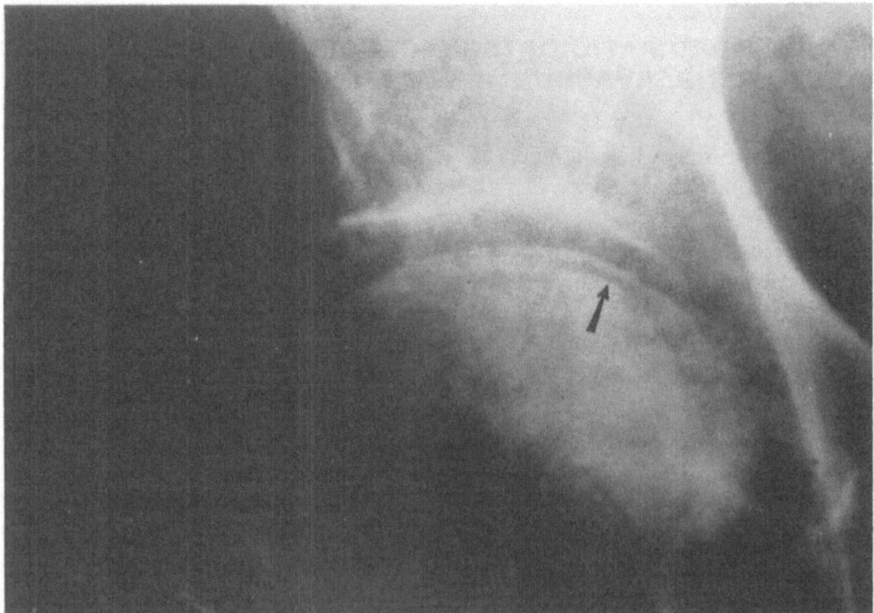

Figure 5.3 Shows the hip joint from a 65-year-old alcoholic with acute onset of pain in the hip of 12 weeks duration. Arrow marks a slit-like area of subchondral bone resorption, which is the earliest change seen in osteonecrosis. A radiograph taken 2 months earlier was normal

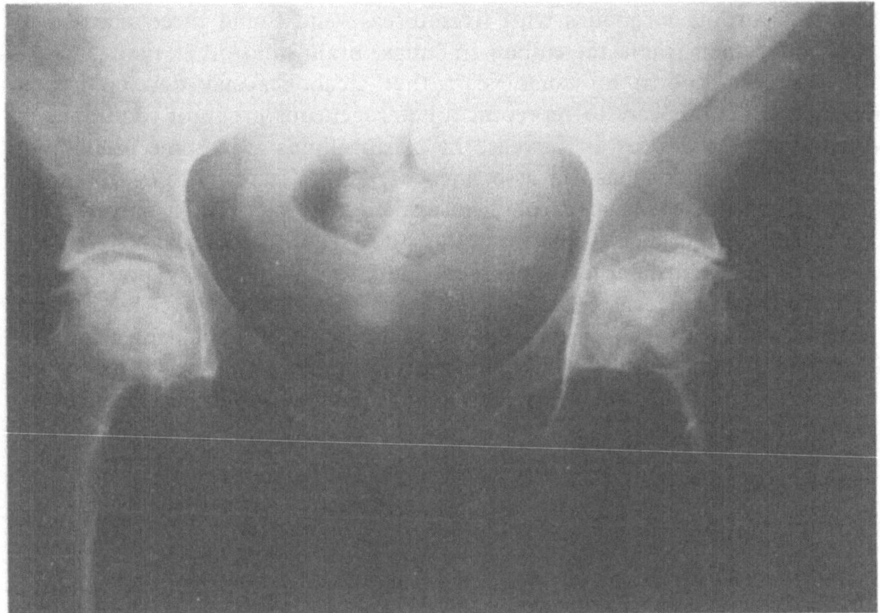

Figure 5.4 Shows bilateral well-established osteonecrosis of the hips with increased density, preservation of articular cartilage, and disruption of the articular surface of the femoral head from partial collapse of underlying bone

lateral view than an AP, or may be brought out best by planogram. Usually the joint space is maintained normally, as contrasted to osteoarthritic hips, but in a few patients a severe and rapid development of osteoarthritis will occur when the repair process, for some reason, invades the articular cartilage. At this stage, the radiographic appearance may be indistinguishable from any other type of osteoarthritis of the hip. Thus, among men, osteonecrosis of bone from alcoholism is one of the causes of osteoarthritis of the hip.

5.5.3 Etiology

Obstruction of small vessels by bubbles of nitrogen in deep sea divers is easy to comprehend, as is that due to Gaucher's disease or aggregates of red cells in sickle cell anaemia. In alcoholism and in corticosteroid administration, the mechanism by which osteonecrosis occurs remains obscure. However, in both of these conditions fatty infiltration of the liver as well as plasma lactescence are common findings in susceptible individuals. Jones and his colleagues[25] proposed that, in alcoholism, showers of fat emboli are released from the liver and obstruct vessels, and he claims to have found lipuria in 9 out of 30 of his patients and intravascular fat globules within two resected femoral heads. These investigators found liver disease in 87 % of their patients. Lynch *et al.*

examined chronic alcoholics with liver disease and found three-quarters of them had demonstrable fat emboli in lungs, brain, and other tissues[26].

It has been known for some years that alcoholics may develop hyperlipaemia, which appears to represent a heterogeneous group of conditions in which alcohol produces an increase in plasma lipids[27]. In some individuals hyperlipaemia of alcoholism is associated with gross lactescence of the serum following episodes of acute alcoholism and clearing again with abstinence[28]. The creamy appearance of plasma under these conditions indicates that the plasma is filled with large numbers of globules of fat which, presumably, might obstruct bone vasculature.

Fat embolization, as a common denominator linking alcoholism, corticosteroid administration and even recurrent pancreatitis (in all of which osteonecrosis may be found) remains an attractive hypothesis which, at present, is unproven.

5.5.4 Diagnosis

The diagnosis should be suspected when pain occurs in the groin, thigh, knee or buttock, accompanied by a limp, in individuals (especially men) over the age of 30 who are heavy drinkers. Physical examination will reveal an antalgic gait, associated with restriction of rotation and to a lesser extent of abduction as well. In about one-third of patients the symptoms come on with dramatic suddenness while in the remainder, symptoms occur gradually over several months, getting worse as time passes. The radiographic changes are quite unrelated to symptoms; conversely trivial radiographic changes may be associated with severe symptoms. Symptoms may be unilateral, though careful examination frequently reveals the disease to be bilateral. Treatment consists of taking the patient off weight bearing and stopping drinking. For severe disease, some authorities recommend the insertion of a bone graft up the femoral neck into the head to speed up the repair process. When serious deformity of the femoral head occurs, or when articular cartilage is involved with onset of secondary osteoarthritis, a total hip prosthesis becomes necessary.

5.6 SUMMARY

Excessive alcohol consumption has been shown to cause osteoporosis and an increased risk of fracture from mild to moderate trauma to the hip, the wrist, the upper humerus, and the spine. Alcohol ingestion has been shown to impair growth in rats and has been described as leading to impaired growth and mental development in children of alcoholic mothers. These changes may be permanent. A syndrome of neuropathic bone disease in the feet (Charcot's feet) has been described in chronic male alcoholics with severe peripheral

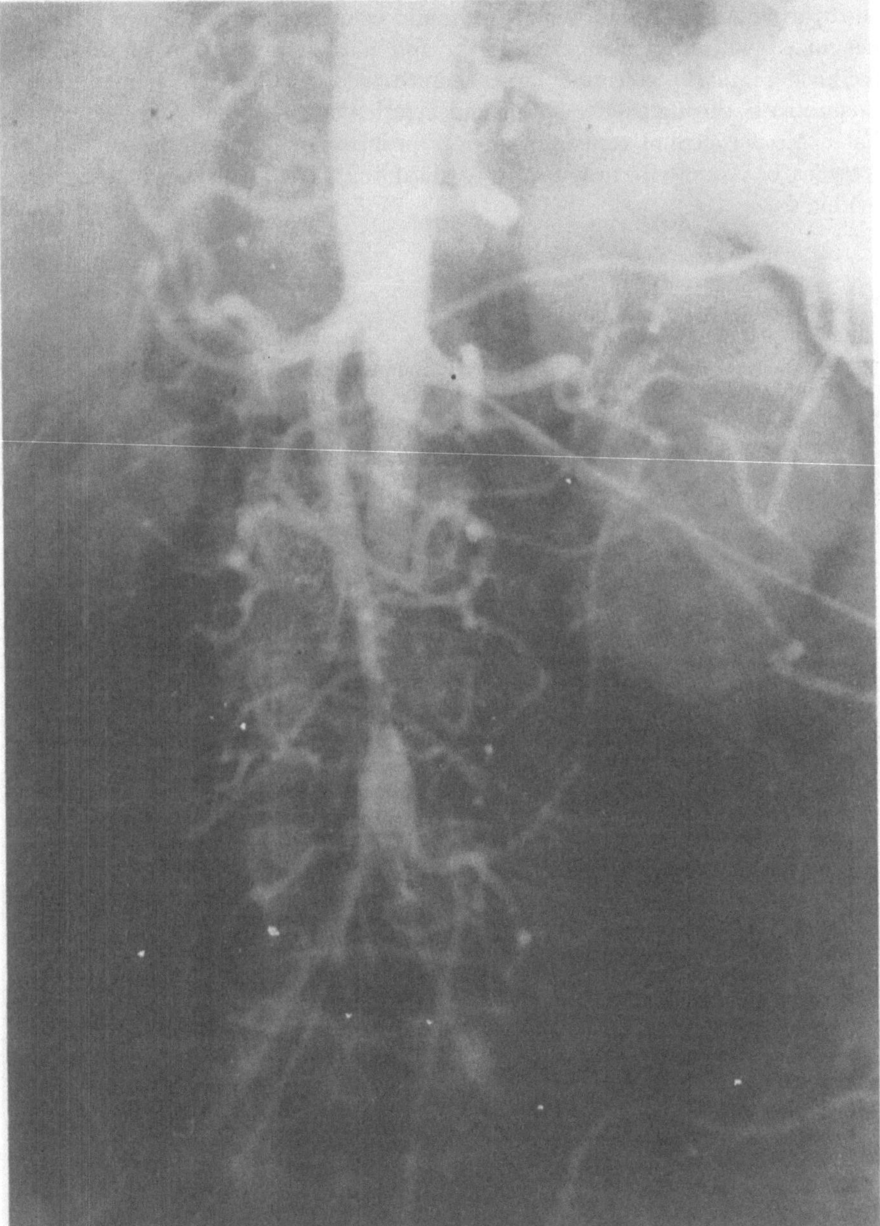

Figure 5.5 Shows aortogram revealing thrombosis of the terminal 50 mm of the abdominal aorta. This is the same alcoholic woman whose hip x-ray is shown in Figure 5.3. This woman also has osteoporosis and sustained a Colles fracture 5 years previously and a femoral neck fracture on the opposite hip 2 months subsequently and was readmitted to hospital with a severe polyneuropathy and a macrocytic anaemia, due to folic acid deficiency

neuropathy. A syndrome of non-traumatic osteonecrosis of the hip is being recognized with increasing frequency and a high proportion of these individuals regularly consume large quantities of alcohol which may cause osteonecrosis through blockage of end arteries by fat emboli. To the extent that excessive alcohol consumption is a problem in the western world, it is likely to be a contributing factor to disabling skeletal disease in older individuals.

References

1. Jones, K. L., Smith, D. W., Streissguth, A. P. and Myrianthopoulos, N. C. (1974). Outcome in offspring of chronic alcoholic women. *Lancet*, June 1, 1076
2. Morgan, A. F., Brinner, L., Plaa, D. B. and Stone, M. M. (1947). Utilization of calories from alcohol and wines and their effects on cholesterol metabolism. *Am. J. Physiol.*, **189,** 290
3. Mitchell, H. H. (1935). The food value of ethyl alcohol. *J. Nutr.* **10,** 311
4. Dubos, R., Savage, D. and Schaedler, R. W. (1966). Biological Freudianism: lasting effects of early environmental influences. *Pediatrics,* **38,** 789
5. Saville, P. D. and Lieber, C. S. (1965). Effect of alcohol on growth, bone density, and muscle magnesium in the rat. *J. Nutr.*, **87,** 477
6. Saville, P. D. and Lieber, C. S. (1969). Increases in skeletal calcium and femur cortex thickness produced by undernutrition. *J. Nutr.*, **99,** 141
7. Saville, P. D. (1965). Changes in bone mass with age and alcoholism. *J. Bone Joint Surg.*, **47A,** 492
8. Nilsson, B. E. (1970). Conditions contributing to fracture of the femoral neck. *Acta Chir. Scand.*, **136,** 383
9. Nilsson, B. E. and Westlin, N. E. (1973). Changes in bone mass in alcoholics. *Clin. Orthop. Rel. Res.*, **90,** 229
10. Mezey, E., Jow, E., Slavin, R. E. and Tobon, R. (1970). Pancreatic function and intestinal absorption in chronic alcoholism. *Gastroenterology,* **59,** 657
11. Krawitt, E. L. (1975). Effect of ethanol ingestion on duodenal calcium transport. *J. Lab. Clin. Med.*, **85,** 4
12. Kalbfleisch, J. M., Lindemann, R. D., Ginn, H. E. and Smith, W. O. (1963). Effects of ethanol administration on urinary excretion of magnesium and other electrolytes in alcoholic and normal subjects. *J. Clin. Invest.*, **42,** 1471
13. Targovnik, J. H. and Sherwood, L. M. (1969). Regulation by calcium and magnesium of parathyroid hormone production *in vitro. 51st Meeting of the American Endocrine Society, New York*
14. McCollister, R. J., Flink, E. B. and Doe, R. P. (1960). Magnesium balance studies in chronic alcoholism. *J. Lab. Clin. Med.*, **55,** 98
15. Stein, J. H., Smith, W. O. and Ginn, H. E. (1966). Hypophosphatemia in acute alcoholism. *Am. J. Med. Sci.*, **252,** 112
16. Smith, W. O., Baxter, D. J., Lindner, A. and Ginn, H. E. (1962). Effect of magnesium depletion on renal function in the rat. *J. Lab. Clin. Med.*, **59,** 211
17. Bloom, W. L. and Flinchum, D. (1960). Osteomalacia with pseudofractures caused by ingestion of aluminium hydroxide. *J. Am. Med. Ass.*, **74,** 327
18. Lotz, M., Zisman, E. and Bartter, F. C. (1968). Evidence for a phosphorus-depletion syndrome in man. *N. Engl. J. Med.*, **278,** 409
19. Lotz, M., Ney, R. and Bartter, F. C. (1964). Osteomalacia and debility resulting from phosphorus depletion. *Trans. Ass. Am. Physicians,* **77,** 281

20. Raisz, L. G. (1965). Bone resorption in tissue culture: factors influencing the response to parathyroid hormone. *J. Clin. Invest.*, **44,** 103
21. Saville, P. D. and Whyte, M. P. (1969). Muscle and bone hypertrophy: positive effect of running exercise in the rat. *Clin. Orthop. Rel. Res.*, **65,** 81
22. Santisteban, G. A. and Swinyard, C. A. (1956). The effect of ethyl alcohol on adrenal cortical activity in mice. *Endocrinology*, **59,** 391
23. Thornhill, H. L., Richter, R. W., Shelton, M. L. and Johnson, C. A. (1973). Neuropathic arthropathy (Charcot forefeet) in alcoholics. *Orthop. Clin. of N. Am.*, **4,** 7
24. Solomon, L. (1973). Drug-induced arthropathy and necrosis of the femoral head. *J. Bone Joint Surg.*, **55B,** 246
25. Jones, J. P., Jameson, R. M. and Engleman, E. P. (1968). Alcoholism, fat embolism, and avascular necrosis. *J. Bone Joint Surg.*, **50A,** 1065
26. Lynch, M. J. G., Raphael, F. S. and Dixeon, T. P. (1959). Fat embolism in chronic alcoholism. *Arch. Pathol.*, **67,** 68
27. Albrink, M. J. and Klatskin, G. (1957). Lactescence of serum following episodes of acute alcoholism and its probable relationship to acute pancreatitis. *Am. J. Med.*, **23,** 26
28. Losowsky, M. S., Jones, D. P., Davidson, C. S. and Lieber, C. S. (1963). Studies of alcoholic hyperlipemia and its mechanism. *Am. J. Med.*, **35,** 794

6
Metabolic Aspects of Alcoholism in the Brain

E. P. NOBLE and S. TEWARI

6.1 INTRODUCTION 149
6.2 ENERGY METABOLISM 151
6.3 NEUROTRANSMITTER SYSTEMS 152
6.3.1 *Serotonin* 152
6.3.2 *Catecholamines* 154
6.3.3 *Catecholamine-derived alkaloids* 157
6.3.4 *Acetylcholine* 159
6.3.5 *γ-Aminobutyric acid* 161
6.4 AMINO ACIDS, PROTEINS AND RIBONUCLEIC ACIDS 162
6.4.1 *Amino acids and proteins* 163
6.4.2 *Ribonucleic acids* 166
6.5 NEURAL MEMBRANES 167
6.5.1 *Theories of anaesthesia* 168
6.5.2 *Cation metabolism and adenosine triphosphate activity* 169
6.5.3 *Cyclic 3′,5′-adenosine monophosphate* 172
6.6 SUMMARY 173
6.6.1 *Energy metabolism* 173
6.6.2 *Neurotransmitter systems* 173
6.6.3 *Protein and RNA metabolism* 174
6.6.4 *Neural membranes* 175
Acknowledgments 175
References 175

6.1 INTRODUCTION

Biochemical studies on the central nervous system (CNS) are confounded by its extreme heterogeneity and complexity. Billions of cells of diverse types and

Dr Noble is currently Director National Institute on Alcohol Abuse and Alcoholism, Rockville, Maryland 20852, U.S.A.

sizes are distributed in cytoarchitecturally distinct regions and layers of the brain. The arrangement of these cells into a delicate network imparts to the brain an awesome communication system which leads to its unique properties of memory, cognition, motivation and emotions. What the underlying neurochemical mechanisms are that subserve the functional activity of the brain remain one of the great mysteries and challenges of the present century. Given the current state of the art regarding the brain, it is not surprising why knowledge of ethanol's action on this organ system is in such a rudimentary state. Nevertheless, given the accumulating information obtained from various disciplines including neurobiology, neuropharmacology and neurochemistry combined with the growing interest and willingness of investigators to participate in alcohol research, it would not be unduly optimistic to predict that deep inroads will be made into understanding brain–ethanol interactions within the next decade.

Most studies on the neurochemical effects of ethanol have been conducted on rodents, specifically rats and mice. The acute effects of this drug on a variety of biochemical systems have been studied in intact animals and in brain slices and homogenates. While such studies may be useful in identifying gross effects of ethanol, they have not too infrequently yielded negative or contradictory data. Treating the brain as an homogeneous organ ignores its richness and complexity and could obscure any important effect that ethanol may exert on small but discrete systems. The recently developed techniques for obtaining relatively pure subcellular fractions and the availability of neuronal and glial cell cultures as well as other simple neural systems should be employed more frequently in future research so as to discern more clearly and specifically ethanol's action on discrete components of the CNS.

The great bulk of the data in the literature relates to the acute actions of ethanol. Relatively few studies are available on the long-term effects of this drug. This situation has prevailed partly because acute studies require less attention and time than chronic studies and partly because the latter studies are often complicated by nutritional factors. The utilization of pair-feeding techniques and the availability of adequate nutritional diets as well as animal models of physical dependence have made more feasible and practicable much-needed studies on the chronic effects of ethanol on the brain.

In most fields of investigative endeavour, the preponderance of effort is generally expended on problems in which conceptual breakthroughs have occurred and where techniques and methodologies are already available. In this respect alcohol research is no exception. Thus, the cerebral effects of ethanol have been studied on energy metabolism, neurotransmitter systems and protein and nucleic acid metabolism. Furthermore, since it is generally acknowledged, though experimental proof is yet to be demonstrated, that neural membranes play a critical role in ethanol's central effects, some studies on ion metabolism, particularly as they relate to adenosine triphosphatase activity, are available. The present chapter will review, albeit selectively, the more recent findings in the above areas of research. No attempt at completeness is intended since the literature already contains numerous reviews on the specific topics covered.

6.2 ENERGY METABOLISM

The major pathway of ethanol metabolism in the body is via oxidation by alcohol dehydrogenase (ADH) and aldehyde dehydrogenase (AlDH) to produce acetate which in turn is oxidized via the tricarboxylic acid cycle to carbon dioxide and water. The liver is the major site of ethanol oxidation and this subject has been reviewed elsewhere in this volume.

Many of the earlier studies on the cerebral effects of ethanol have dealt with an assessment of respiratory and energy metabolism. Extensive reviews on these areas are available[1–5] and will not be detailed here again. More recently brain ADH activity (40 nmol/g/min) has been detected but this organ's capacity to oxidize ethanol is only one four-thousandth's that of the liver[6]. Thus, it is to be expected that ethanol's metabolic effects on the brain and liver will differ markedly[7]. Indeed, one of the consequences of ethanol's interaction with ADH in the liver is a large increase in the ratio of free $(NADH_2)/(NAD)$ in the cytoplasm with subsequent compensatory changes in metabolites linked to this reducto-oxidative nucleotide system[8,9]. With regard to the effects of ethanol on the brain, it has been reported that the oxidation of ethanol results in a small but significant increase in the $(NADH_2)/(NAD)$ ratio in mouse brain. Furthermore, pyrazole, an inhibitor of ADH, prevented the ethanol-induced increase in the reduced components of certain dehydrogenase-linked substrate pairs in brain[10]. On the other hand, using a very rapid brain-freezing technique, Veloso *et al.*[11] found that, whether given acutely or over a prolonged period, ethanol produces only minor effects in the levels of intermediary metabolites or on the redox states in brain. Their conclusions, therefore, do not support the contention of reports which attribute an important role in brain to the metabolism of ethanol by ADH[6,10,12].

In additional experiments, Raskin[13] has correlated changes in the activities of brain and liver ADH and AlDH to the development of tolerance to ethanol. He found no changes in liver ADH and AlDH nor in brain AlDH activity in animals introduced to ethanol for a 9-week period as compared to controls. However, modest increases in brain ADH were found in the ethanol-tolerant rats. He suggested a possible causal relationship between the increase in brain ADH activity and the development of tolerance. On the other hand, Rawat *et al.*[10] found no significant differences in the rate of ethanol utilization and ADH activity in brains of control mice and mice chronically imbibing ethanol. However, in this latter study, no assessment of behavioural tolerance to ethanol was made.

In conclusion, the acute and chronic effects of ethanol on brain ethanol and energy metabolism appear to be small, if present at all. More likely, ethanol induced CNS depression and possibly the development of tolerance and physical dependence are products of functional alteration in neural membranes[14,15]. However, the possibility has not been ruled out that discrete metabolic changes in brain regions, cell types or subcellular fractions induced by either ethanol or its metabolic product, acetaldehyde, could influence brain activity and hence behaviour. Additional, more refined, studies are, therefore, warranted to settle this issue.

6.3 NEUROTRANSMITTER SYSTEMS

The past 20 years have witnessed great strides in our understanding of the neurotransmitters, both in the peripheral and the CNS. Such advances have been made possible largely through the development of analytical techniques, sufficiently sensitive and accurate to measure the very low amounts of these substances in nervous tissue; the development of methods to separate subcellular components and thus determine the localization of the neurotransmitters; and finally the increasing availability of drugs that modify both neurotransmitter function and behaviour. Thus, at this time, firm knowledge exists regarding the biosynthesis and disposition of the neurotransmitters, and intense efforts are being expended on how these substances may control neural function. Because of the important part the neurotransmitters seem to play in the CNS, several speculations have arisen as to their role in modifying behaviour. It was, therefore, not surprising that, in view of ethanol's effect on behaviour, studies on the neurotransmitters would be undertaken. Indeed, the alcohol literature is replete with such studies and this field currently represents one of the most intensive areas investigated.

6.3.1 Serotonin

Although the effects of ethanol on brain serotonin (5-HT) metabolism have received considerable attention, few consistent findings are available. Levels of brain 5-HT following acute administration of ethanol have been measured by several investigators. Some have reported decreases[16,18], others have found increases[18–21], while a large number have found unchanged 5-HT levels[22–33].

The rate of 5-HT biosynthesis following acute ethanol administration has been estimated in several laboratories. In this measure also conflicting data prevail. Thus, some reports show that the rate of accumulation of 5-HT after pretreatment with pargyline, a monoamine oxidase (MAO) inhibitor, to be depressed after single doses of ethanol[32,34]. Another study finds increased levels of 5-HT following ethanol administration[21], while other investigators find no effects of acute ethanol on brain 5-HT turnover[30,31,35].

Given the disparate observations of ethanol's acute effects on brain 5-HT levels and turnover rate, it would not be surprising to predict discordant findings on other aspects of brain 5-HT metabolism. On the other hand, in the periphery, studies of 5-HT metabolism have shown unequivocally that ethanol induces a shift in 5-HT metabolism from the oxidative, as measured by formation of 5-OH indole acetic acid (5-HIAA), to the reductive pathway, as measured by 5-OH tryptophol (5-HTOL) production[36,37]. With respect to the central effects of ethanol on these metabolic pathways, conflict again abounds although it is generally acknowledged that if ethanol induces a shift in brain 5-HT pathways its extent is not at all comparable to that found in the periphery. Arguments persist as to which of the two 5-HT metabolites, 5-HIAA or 5-HTOL, is increased with ethanol in the CNS. The reports that indicate increased 5-HTOL levels may have ignored the peripheral contribution of 5-HTOL to the CNS. That differences between central and peripheral 5-HT metabolism exist were shown by Huff *et al.*[38] who found that in both control and ethanol-treated animals, the level of 5-HTOL was more than twice as high when [^{14}C]-5HT was administered intravenously than when given intracranially. Furthermore, incubation of rat brain slices in the presence of ethanol failed to produce an increase in the amount of 5-HTOL production[39].

In recent *in vivo* experiments utilizing push–pull perfusions of localized areas in the caudate nucleus, lateral hypothalamus or midbrain reticular formation, the introduction of [^{14}C]-5HT into rats given acute ethanol and controls resulted in no sigificantly greater production of [^{14}C]-5HTOL in the ethanol-treated animals in any of the three areas examined[40]. Despite the lack of convincing evidence that ethanol induces an increase in CNS synthesis of 5-HTOL, this metabolite could still, by virtue of its production in the peripheral system, mediate the soporific effects of ethanol[31,41]. However, additional evidence is required to establish more conclusively this notion.

Data are also available regarding the acute effects of ethanol on brain 5-HIAA levels. Tyce *et al.*[34] report that, although ethanol did not alter the brain concentration of 5-HIAA, it slightly but significantly blocked the pargyline-induced decrease in 5-HIAA. Similarly Feldstein[31] found no changes in 5-HIAA levels in rat brain following acute ethanol administration. Ahtee and Ericksson[42] report that alcohol-preferring rats, given a free choice of ethanol or water for a month, showed 10 % greater levels of 5-HIAA than that of non-alcohol-preferring animals. However, no changes in 5-HIAA were noted in non-alcohol-preferring rats when they were forced to drink the same amount of ethanol as the alcohol-preferring rats drank voluntarily. Tytell and Myers[40] found that intracranial injection of [^{14}C]-5HT resulted in a significant increase in [^{14}C]-5HIAA levels in three localized brain areas. Tabakoff and Boggan[33] describe short-lived increases in brain 5-HIAA levels after a single ethanol injection and significant elevation in 5-HIAA levels in physically dependent mice during withdrawal period. However in contrast to the above studies, Palaić *et al.*[21] found a decrease in brain 5-HIAA levels with ethanol and an acceleration of the pargyline-induced decrease in 5-HIAA.

There are also some studies available on the long-term effects of ethanol on the turnover of brain 5-HT but again discrepancies exist. Kuriyama *et al.*[30] found a marked acceleration in the turnover of 5-HT after chronic administration of ethanol in mice. However, using rats, Hunt and Majchrowicz[32] found no changes in 5-HT turnover in animals undergoing an alcohol withdrawal syndrome and conclude that the activity of the serotoninergic pathways is not related to alcohol-dependence in these animals.

In an attempt to further clarify ethanol's effects on the serotoninergic system, recent studies have dealt with enzymes involved in the biosynthesis and catabolism of 5-HT. Kuriyama *et al.*[30] could not find any effects on the activity of brain tryptophan hydroxylase, the rate-limiting step in the biosynthesis of 5-HT, following an anaesthetic dose of ethanol to mice. However, an increase in the activity of this enzyme was found in animals chronically treated with ethanol. They interpret these observations as consonant with the lack of effects of acute ethanol on 5-HT turnover and in line with increases in 5-HT turnover in animals chronically treated with ethanol. The findings on the acute effects of ethanol were corroborated by the studies of Carlsson and Lindqvist[43] who found that the injection of an aromatic amino acid decarboxylase inhibitor following ethanol administration to rats did not alter the accumulation of brain 5-HT. On the other hand, Rogawski *et al.*[44], using rat striate synaptosomes *in vitro*, found that ethanol in a concentration of 460 mg/% and higher inhibited the conversion of tryptophan to 5-HT. They attribute this effect not to a decrease in tryptophan uptake but rather to a non-competitive inhibition of tryptophan hydroxylase activity.

The catabolic enzymes involved in 5-HT metabolism have received meagre attention. Recently, Tabakoff and Boggan[33] found that in mice exposed chronically to ethanol vapour, no significant differences in brain MAO, cytosol and mitochondrial aldehyde dehydrogenase or aldehyde reductase activities were found when compared to untreated controls.

In summary, the studies of ethanol's action on the serotoninergic system, up to this time, show no clear-cut consistent and reproducible effects. However, this is not to imply that this system does not mediate in the actions of ethanol on the brain. The present confusion and lack of concordance may in part be related to species differences, modes of ethanol administration, whole *v.* discrete brain elements, *in vivo v. in vitro* conditions and other experimental variables. Until a clearer appreciation of these factors is achieved, the literature will continue to amass seemingly contradictory data.

6.3.2 Catecholamines

Norepinephrine (NE), dopamine (DA) and epinephrine are the three major catecholamines found in mammalian systems. Of these three, NE and DA constitute the main catecholamines in the brain. As in the case of 5-HT, there is a significant amount of work done on the effects of ethanol on the catecholamines, particularly NE, but the available information, in general, is more consistent than the findings on 5-HT. Ethanol–catecholamine interactions have been reviewed by many authors[2,45–51] and this section will deal essentially with work done subsequent to these reviews.

It is generally acknowledged that an acute dose of ethanol exerts no significant effect on the steady state levels of brain NE and DA[18,23,52]. However, the turnover rate of these biogenic amines appear to be influenced by ethanol administration. Corrodi *et al.*[53] using an inhibitor of catecholamine biosynthesis, α-methyl-*p*-tyrosine, found that ethanol accelerates the depletion of NE content of the brain but not that of DA. These authors suggest that ethanol acts as a specific activator of noradrenergic neurons. Carlsson and Lindqvist[43] measuring the accumulation of 3,4-dihydroxyphenylalanine (dopa) after the administration of an inhibitor of aromatic amino acid decarboxylase found that ethanol increased further the accumulation of brain dopa. This effect was found both in a DA- and NE-dominated area of the brain. In another study, Carlsson *et al.*[54] studied the synthesis of [^{3}H]catecholamines from [^{3}H]tyrosine in brain. They found an increase in [^{3}H]DA and [^{3}H]NE and the ratio of [^{3}H]DA/[^{3}H]NE was significantly increased by ethanol. On the other hand, Thadani and Truitt[55] observed that a single oral dose of ethanol resulted in a small decrease in the turnover of intracisternally injected [^{3}H]NE. In a more recent detailed study of NE and DA turnover in rat brains, Hunt and Majchrowicz[56] investigated the effect of time after ethanol administration on the turnover rates of these catecholamines. They found that in animals given a single dose of ethanol, NE turnover was increased, while DA turnover was unaffected during the first few hours after treatment. However, after that time the turnover of both NE and DA was reduced. This study may help to explain some of the apparent discrepancies observed by previous investigators and it is in accord with the known behavioural and physiological biphasic effects of ethanol on the CNS, namely initial stimulation and later depression.

In order to gain an understanding into the *in vivo* effects of ethanol on catecholamine turnover rates, recent studies have dealt with specific mechanisms involved in the subsequent fate of these neurotransmitters. Roach *et al.*[57] studied the effects of ethanol on synaptosomes obtained from rat brain homogenates. At an ethanol concentration (3000 mg/%) which would be several folds greater than the dose lethal in animals, a 30–40 % inhibition in the uptake of NE, 5-HT and γ-aminobutyric acid was found. As would be expected, ethanol was a non-competitive inhibitor of [^{3}H]NE uptake. At a lower, but still physiologically very high concentration (500 mg/%), ethanol exerted much lesser effects on the uptake of these putative neurotransmitters. These authors used other aliphatic alcohols and found that the observed inhibition of synaptosomal uptake was a function of the hydrophobic character of the alcohol. Using synaptosomes obtained from mouse brain, similar results were obtained by Israel *et al.*[58]. They also found a 25 % inhibition of NE uptake with slices of guinea-pig brain cortex but at a concentration considered lethal to these animals (1000 mg/%). On the other hand, when guinea-pig cerebral cortex slices were preloaded with [^{3}H]NE, spontaneous or electrically stimulated release of [^{3}H]NE was uninfluenced by the presence of ethanol (1000 mg/%). In a more recent study using rat brain cortical slices, Israel *et al.*[59] determined the concentration of ethanol required to inhibit the electrically stimulated release of neurotransmitters by 50 % (IC 50). With this tissue, the IC 50 for NE was approximately 1900 mg/%, but lesser concentrations of ethanol were required for an equivalent effect on acetylcholine or 5-HT release. However, in *in vivo* studies, Thadani and Truitt[55] found that the injection of low doses of ethanol (0.3 g/kg i.p. × 2) into rats whose brains were prelabelled with [^{3}H]NE had no effect on the release of [^{3}H]NE.

Seeman and Lee[60] have investigated the DA-releasing actions of neuroleptics and ethanol. Using rat caudate synaptosome fractions, they found that ethanol as well as neuroleptics, enhanced the spontaneous release of DA at threshold concentrations which were one-half to one-twentieth those required to inhibit the uptake of DA. Specifically with ethanol, the threshold concentration required to promote the spontaneous release of DA was 230 mg/%, a high but nevertheless a non-lethal concentration in animals. These authors reason that if the DA-releasing effect also occurs *in vivo*, then the increased spontaneous release of DA induced by ethanol and neuroleptics would diminish DA levels, thus disinhibiting tyrosine hydroxylase[61–63]. The resultant effect of the DA-releasing action of these drugs would lead to increased turnover of DA from the hypothesized intraneuronal feedback mechanism. While this concept is intriguing and may well account for the enhanced turnover rate induced by some neuroleptics[64–67] it is not generally supported by studies on ethanol where most of the data (see above) show unchanged or decreased DA turnover rates following acute ethanol administration.

There are relatively few studies available on the long-term effects of ethanol on the brain catecholamine system. Using mice, Rawat[68] found that the chronic administration of ethanol in a liquid diet for 4 weeks resulted in a decrease in brain NE content, but after withdrawal of ethanol for 1 day, the levels of NE returned to normal. Hunt and Majchrowicz[56] on the other hand used rats and induced physical dependence over a 5-day period by ethanol intubation. They observed no differences in the steady-state levels of brain NE and DA among control, ethanol-dependent rats under intoxication and also in animals during the withdrawal syndrome. However, when the turnover rates of these biogenic amines were determined, ethanol-dependent rats, whether intoxicated or undergoing a withdrawal syndrome, showed an increase NE turnover, while DA turnover was reduced. These interesting findings do not support the hypothesis that the activity of the catecholamine system differentiates the withdrawal from the ethanol (non-withdrawal) state in the *in vivo* condition. Nevertheless, before any such clear conclusion is reached additional studies are required to validate or refute the above findings.

In summary, the catecholamine system appears to be affected by both the acute and chronic administration of ethanol *in vivo*. *In vitro* studies also demonstrate an effect of ethanol on the uptake and the release of catecholamines by brain slices and fractions, but mostly at high and supralethal concentrations of the drug. Whether in fact these changes play a significant role in the variety of behaviours manifested by ethanol will be dependent on the outcome of a great deal more of future investigations.

6.3.3 Catecholamine-derived alkaloids

Since 1968 there has been increasing research efforts focused on the role of condensation produces of aldehydes and biogenic amines in alcoholism. Two principal theories related to these condensation products have emerged.

First, ethanol-derived acetaldehyde may produce 'simple' (1-alkyl) tetrahydroisoquinoline (TIQ) alkaloids from its biomolecular condensation with catecholamines[69–72]. The major products of these reactions are salsolinol derived from DA, and the corresponding 4,6,7-trihydroxy-TIQ alkaloids derived from epinephrine and NE.

The second theory postulates that ethanol-derived acetaldehyde, acting as a substrate for aldehyde dehydrogenase, may inhibit the oxidation and thereby elevate the steady-state levels of phenylacetaldehydes, compounds which normally arise from DA and 3-methoxy-DA deaminations. It is suggested[73] that the cyclization of the phenylacetaldehydes with DA then would lead to the formation of tetrahydropapaverolines (1-benzyl-substituted TIQs). Both these theories have in common the proposition that the above reaction products and their derivatives would exert important pharmacological effects on the CNS thus inducing altered behavioural states. This topic has been reviewed recently by Erwin and Deitrich[74] and Davis *et al.*[75].

In 1934 Schöpf and Bayerle[76] showed that acetaldehyde could condense at neutral pH and room temperature with DA or its *N*-methyl congener (epinine) to yield the corresponding TIQs. In fact this pathway was suggested as the route for synthesis of TIQ alkaloids in plants. More recently, accumulating evidence is supporting the notion that these alkaloids can also be formed in animal tissues. Perfusion of cow adrenal glands *in situ* with an unphysiologically high concentration of acetaldehyde (10 mg/%) as well as with a more physiological level of this metabolite (0.1 mg%) leads to the formation of small amounts of TIQ alkaloids[71,77]. *In vitro* studies have shown that incubation of brain or liver homogenates with dopamine and acetaldehyde or ethanol results in the formation of salsolinol[72]. Very recently Collins and Bigdeli[78,79] demonstrated that salsolinol could be detected under *in vivo* conditions in brains of pyrogallol–ethanol treated rats. However, this alkaloid was not found in rats given acute ethanol in the absence of pyrogallol, nor in pyrogallol controls given saline in place of ethanol.

Cohen and co-workers[80,81] have shown that TIQ compounds accumulated by rat adrenergic tissues, inhibit the uptake and also cause the release of catecholamines. It is suggested that the TIQs fit the description of 'false transmitters'[82]; however, the rate of the uptake process is lower for these compounds than for the catecholamines, and they have a lower affinity for the uptake process than the biogenic amines. These observations indicate that, to be effective as competitive inhibitors of the uptake process, they would have to be present at an equal or higher concentration than that of the catecholamines, a situation that is difficult to achieve under physiological conditions[74].

The second theory, advocated primarily by Davis and her co-workers, proposes that ethanol administration induces the formation of even more complex alkaloids (the 1-benzyl substituted TIQs) than the first theory. These compounds are the biogenic precursors in plants of a diverse array of highly complex alkaloids that belong to the protoberberine, morphine and the papaverine classes. *In vitro* studies have shown that the formation of tetrahydropapaveroline (THP), one such compound with pharmacological activity[83,84], is enhanced when ethanol or acetaldehyde is added to brain homogenates[73,85]. Furthermore, THP decreased the accumulation of [^{14}C]NE and increased its release in rat brain synaptosomal preparations[86] suggesting complex effects on adrenergic function.

In vivo studies on animals, thus far, have not demonstrated increased formation of THP with ethanol administration. However, this compound can be formed *in vivo* in brains of rats treated with L-dopa[85]. On the other hand, when animals received a 10 % solution of ethanol instead of L-dopa, no detectable levels of THP were found. Recent studies by Davis *et al.*[75] have shown that THP is further converted by rats *in vivo* and by rat liver and brain preparations to the more complex alkaloid, tetrahydroprotoberberine.

Studies on humans also have demonstrated their ability to form TIQ alkaloids, but this occurs during pharmacological manipulation unrelated to ethanol. Thus, Sandler *et al.*[87] have detected both THP and salsolinol in urine of patients receiving L-dopa therapy for Parkinson's disease and Davis *et al.*[75] have reported in similarly treated patients the presence of tetrahydroprotoberberine alkaloids.

In conclusion, the evidence at hand indicates that mammals, including humans, are capable of forming alkaloids with pharmacological properties, including addictive liability. However, the TIQs formed *in vivo* from the initial condensation of catecholamines and aldehydes require the presence of drugs; pyrogallol, for salsolinol formation and L-dopa, for the production of THP. Thus far, no reports are available which indicate that ethanol alone enhances TIQ formation in the whole animal, although under *in vitro* conditions, ethanol promotes TIQ alkaloid synthesis. Furthermore, it should be stated that despite some unique effects of the TIQs on biological systems, as for example their possible role as 'false transmitters', there is no evidence as yet that they contribute in any significant way to the acute or chronic effects of ethanol. Moreover, the above theories have been criticized on the basis that the withdrawal symptoms in opiate addicts are dissimilar to those of alcohol addicts[88,89], that naloxone administration to mice made physically dependent upon ethanol failed to produce withdrawal symptoms[90] and that *t*-butanol displays both the acute and chronic actions of ethanol[91] even though it is presumed to be a metabolically stable molecule. Despite these criticisms the two theories, in the opinion of these reviewers, remain not only interesting but still viable. Additional stronger evidence is required to either refute or make them tenable.

6.3.4 Acetylcholine

The effects of ethanol on the acetylcholine (Ach) system have been reviewed earlier[51,92] and in this system also controversy prevails. Thus, ethanol concentrations of 230 mg/% or less appear to inhibit Ach output from unstimulated cerebral cortex slices *in vitro*[93,94] but increase the spontaneous and impulse-stimulated output of Ach from motor nerve endings[95–97]. This apparent discrepancy may in large part be related to the nature of the systems (peripheral *v.* central) studied since more recent reports confirm ethanol's properties of decreasing Ach output from the CNS. Erickson and Graham[98] found that the *in vivo* administration of ethanol to rabbits, depressed, in a dose-dependent manner, the amount of Ach collected from the parietal cortex and mesencephalic reticular formation with the effect being greater on the parietal cortex. Israel *et al.*[59] studying rat brain cortical slices preloaded with [^{3}H]choline found enhanced efflux of Ach after electrical stimulation but obtained significant inhibition with 250 mg/% ethanol. When other putative neurotransmitters, including 5-HT, NE and glutamate, were tested their output was found to be less sensitive to ethanol than Ach. Furthermore, the inhibitory effect of ethanol on Ach output was not found to be unique for this drug since two higher alcohols and barbiturates also influenced the efflux of Ach from electrically stimulated tissue.

Many factors could account for the decrease in brain Ach output induced by ethanol. Ethanol may inhibit the rate of Ach synthesis and/or enhance its degradation. It is also possible that ethanol may act directly or indirectly on presynaptic cholinergic nerve terminals inhibiting the release of Ach.

Rawat[68] has recently reported that the amount of Ach and the total incorporation of [^{3}H]choline into Ach in brain was depressed upon acute administration of ethanol to mice. Because acetaldehyde also decreases the cerebral levels of Ach, Rawat reasons that this effect of ethanol is mediated through acetaldehyde, perhaps by reaction with sulphydryl groups of coenzyme A (CoA) to form the biological inactive thiohemiacetal. A similar suggestion was made in 1965 by Heim *et al.*[99]. Presumably the lowered levels of CoA thus attained would adversely affect Ach synthesis. Furthermore, Rawat explains the decreased incorporation of [^{3}H]choline into Ach on the basis of increased degradation of Ach by the acute ethanol administration. However, no convincing data is provided to substantiate this point of view. Indeed, other investigators[93,98] have found that ethanol, if anything, causes small increases in total brain Ach levels and has no significant effect on the activity of acetylcholinesterase[93,100]. Similarly, no decrease by ethanol of choline acetyltransferase activity was found[93] and a recent study[101] even reports a modest stimulation of this enzyme in homogenates of rat brain but only at high, supralethal, ethanol concentrations.

It has been suggested that the effects of ethanol on decreasing Ach output are exerted primarily on the release process[102], most probably occurring at the presynaptic level[59,98]. However, Nikander and Wallgren[103] have reported that ethanol also inhibits the intracellular changes in Na^+ and K^+ that are evolved by electrical stimulation. On this basis, they propose that ethanol inhibits the action potential in brain tissue. Recently, Israel *et al.*[59] have confirmed the findings of Nikander and Wallgren. Thus it is entirely feasible that the observed changes in Ach release may be a consequence of altered ion metabolism, particularly Na^+ conductance, induced by ethanol. However, a specific effect at the presynaptic level cannot yet be excluded[59].

From the above studies, it is tempting to conclude that Ach could play an important role in ethanol-mediated behaviour, particularly CNS depression. In fact, cholinergic involvement in ethanol intoxication has been suggested by Erickson and Burnam[104] who showed that physostigmine antagonizes ethanol-induced sleep-time in mice. However, ethanol-induced EEG synchrony, a frequently used indicator of CNS depression, could not be correlated with the depression of cerebral output of Ach prompted by ethanol[98]. Furthermore, more recent studies by Graham and Erickson[105], utilizing drugs which would reverse or enhance reported effects of ethanol in reducing free cerebral Ach, failed to alter ethanol-induced behavioural depression. These authors suggest that during ethanol intoxication, the decrease of free Ach is more probably a reflection of decreased neuronal activity rather than being the critical factor in the resulting CNS depression.

There are also some studies available on the chronic effects of ethanol on the Ach system. Long-term ethanol ingestion has been reported to result in a decline[106,107] or unchanged activity of brain acetylcholinesterase[68]. With regard to choline acetyltransferase, forced ethanol consumption for 26 weeks caused a decrease in enzyme activity in female rats, but not in males[107], whereas only 2 weeks of ethanol ingestion in male mice resulted in a decline in choline acetyltransferase activity[68].

The functional significance of changes in Ach enzyme activity in chronic ethanol-induced behaviour is not clear. Kalant and Grose[94] found that the administration of ethanol for 1–5 weeks did not alter the brain levels of Ach but abolished the ability of ethanol *in vitro* to block Ach release. This study implies that the chronic effects of ethanol are not related *per se* to the activity of the

Ach enzymes but rather that the development of tolerance to ethanol was accompanied by a development of cellular resistance to the direct Ach-releasing action of ethanol. Rawat[68], on the other hand, found unchanged levels of choline but decreased levels of Ach in brains of mice allowed to consume ethanol in a liquid diet for 2 weeks. Furthermore, Ach returned to normal levels 4 days after ethanol withdrawal. Finally, Goldstein[108] found that drugs that affect the cholinergic system had no significant effect in modifying the ethanol withdrawal syndrome in mice. It is difficult to resolve these conflicting findings which, in part, may be related to the experimental design, including the species of animals used and the nature of ethanol administration. Obviously, additional experiments are necessary to establish whether or not Ach plays any significant role in the chronic effects of ethanol.

6.3.5 γ-Aminobutyric acid

There has been and continues to be much interest in the role played by γ-aminobutyric acid (GABA) in the acute and chronic effects of ethanol. The possible function of GABA as an inhibitory transmitter in the CNS[109,110], and its implication in neuronal excitability including convulsive disorders[111–113] have, in part, attracted this interest. Furthermore, the pathway of GABA biosynthesis and its unique connection with the tricarboxylic acid cycle via the GABA 'shunt' makes for an intriguing relationship in the brain between the synthesis of a neurotransmitter and energy metabolism.

There is a fairly extensive, yet inconsistent, literature regarding ethanol's effect on the GABA system. The earlier work on this interaction has been previously reviewed[2,45,51]. Unfortunately more recent data has not done much to reduce this confusion.

As with the other neurotransmitters, one approach has been to measure the levels of GABA after ethanol administration. However, in the earlier studies, increase[114,115], decrease[116–118] or no change[119] in brain concentrations were found during acute or chronic ethanol administration. More recent studies have left these apparent contradictory findings unresolved. Thus, Sutton and Simmonds[120] report no changes in GABA concentrations following acute ethanol injection in rats, whereas Rawat[68] found increased concentrations in mice. With chronic ethanol ingestion, both Sutton and Simmonds[120] and Rawat[68] found increased levels of brain GABA, with the latter reporting that GABA returns to normal levels 2 days after withdrawal of ethanol. However, using another mode of chronic ethanol administration, namely inhalation, Patel and Lal[121] found no changes in GABA levels when the mice were still under the influence of chronic ethanol but significant decreases occurred 8 hours after withdrawal when symptoms were maximum.

In order to investigate the dynamic aspects of GABA system in brain, the enzymes involved in its biosynthesis, L-glutamate 1-carboxylase (GAD), and in its subsequent metabolism, 4-aminobutyrate:2-oxoglutarate aminotransferase (GABA-T), were studied as a function of ethanol administration. Sutton and Simmonds[120] found a small increase in GAD activity in rats following the acute injection of ethanol but the activity of GABA-T remained unchanged. However, when ethanol was presented for 3 weeks in the drinking solution, GAD activity was unaffected whereas GABA-T activity increased. Rawat[68], using mice given ethanol chronically in a liquid diet, obtained very different results. He found a decrease in GAD activity, but unchanged GABA-T activity following 3 weeks of ethanol ingestion.

Turnover studies of GABA in the brain are rare. However, Sutton and Simmonds[120] found that neither acute nor chronic ethanol treatment affected the fractional rate constants of [^{3}H]GABA that were intracisternally injected. Based on this observation and their above described changes in GAD and GABA-T activities and GABA levels, they suggest that the acute and chronic effects of ethanol are likely influencing the metabolic pool of GABA rather than the transmitter pool. However, it should be borne in mind that in this study a 14 % ethanol solution in water was given as the drinking fluid for 3 weeks. Since, under these conditions, withdrawal symptoms have not been reported to occur, further studies are necessary on brain GABA turnover rates in animals made physically dependent upon ethanol.

There is some evidence from behavioural studies implicating the GABA system in the development of the ethanol withdrawal reaction. Goldstein[108], using mice made physically dependent upon ethanol by a combination of inhalation of this drug and pyrazol injection, found that aminooxyacetic acid, an inhibitor of GABA breakdown, decreased whereas picrotoxin, a GABA antagonist, increased convulsions. Unfortunately, both amino-oxyacetic acid and picrotoxin were toxic since mortality was significantly increased by their use. More recently Noble *et al.*[122] have tested the effects of *n*-dipropyl acetate (*n*-DPA), a drug that increases brain GABA levels and inhibits GABA transaminase activity[113], on rats made physically dependent upon ethanol. With this drug, no mortality or observable morbidity was found; however, significant decreases in audiogenically induced withdrawal symptoms were noted. These findings should stimulate further investigations on the precise role the GABA system plays in physical dependence upon ethanol.

6.4 AMINO ACIDS, PROTEINS AND RIBONUCLEIC ACIDS

There is growing interest in the role amino acids, proteins and ribonucleic acids (RNA) play in brain function and how ethanol acts to modify the metabolism of these molecules. Besides their general role in metabolic process, including protein synthesis, some amino acids may have neurotransmitter function. Similarly proteins and RNA, beyond their generalized and well-established functional and structural role in cells, are thought also to have distinctive functions in the CNS[123–125]. For example, alterations in protein and RNA have been demonstrated in memory and learning process[126–128].

Clinical observations and investigations have described memory defects and a variety of behavioural and other CNS dysfunctions in man as a consequence of acute and chronic ethanol ingestion[129–132]. Furthermore, since recent studies on rodents[133,134] have shown that long-term ethanol exposure leads to decrements in associative learning processes, increasing interest has been directed to the effects of ethanol on CNS macromolecular metabolism.

6.4.1 Amino acids and proteins

The studies on the effects of ethanol on brain amino acid metabolism have been reviewed by Israel[1] and Wallgren and Barry[2,45]. Unfortunately, since these reviews have appeared, relatively little new and useful information has been obtained regarding amino acid–ethanol interactions.

In peripheral systems it is known that the active transport of amino acids is inhibited by ethanol[135,136]. While claims have been made that ethanol also affects the transport of amino acids into the CNS, convincing data are lacking. However, in a recent study using α-aminoisobutyric acid (a non-metabolizable amino acid), Freund[137] found that acute administration of ethanol inhibited the transport of this amino acid into the brain of mice. On the other hand this effect was absent in animals given ethanol for prolonged periods provided that no ethanol remained in their system.

The effects of ethanol on amino acid biosynthesis and catabolism are perplexing and at times contradictory. Roach[138] reported that acute ethanol administration led to a decrease in the *in vivo* incorporation of ^{14}C from [^{14}C]glucose into glutamate, glutamine, aspartate and GABA in hamster brain. On the other hand, Häkkinen and Kulonen[139] found that ethanol increased the levels of glutamate, asparate and GABA, while the level of glutamine was decreased in rat brains. In a more recent investigation, these authors[140] explained their earlier finding by suggesting that ethanol decreased the catabolism of glutamate and GABA and the biosynthesis of glutamine. Obviously, additional studies are needed to clarify the acute and chronic effects of ethanol on brain amino acid metabolism.

There is more consistent information concerning the acute effects of ethanol on amino acid incorporation into brain protein. Kuriyama *et al.*[141] reported that 1.5–3 hours after the injection of ethanol into mice, the *in vitro* incorporation of [^{14}C]leucine into brain ribosomal protein was depressed. However, they found this system to be insensitive to the *in vitro* addition of ethanol. Choy *et al.*[142] injected [^{3}H]lysine into rats rendered unconscious with ethanol. They found that the incorporation of [^{3}H]lysine into protein was decreased in the cerebral white, hypothalamus and cerebellum. However, this study did not clarify whether the observed effect was a consequence of decreased lysine transport into the brain or depressed amino acid incorporation into protein. Jarlstedt and Hamberger[143] found that the injection of ethanol into rats resulted in a decreased *in vitro* incorporation of [^{3}H]leucine into protein by cerebral cortex slices. When the brain was fractionated into neuronal and glial-enriched components, they observed the neuronal specific radioactivity was unaffected by ethanol, whereas the radioactivity in the glial fraction was significantly depressed.

There are a growing number of studies on the effects of chronic ethanol administration on protein metabolism in the brain of rodents. Jarlstedt[144] injected [^{3}H]leucine into rats that had ingested a 15 % ethanol solution for 8 weeks. He found a minor overall depression of protein synthesis in the cerebellum and cortex cerebri. If ethanol was withdrawn for 24 hours before the injection of isotope, the incorporation of labelled amino acid into protein was increased when compared to the brain regions obtained from control or non-withdrawn animals. Kuriyama *et al.*[141] found that contrary to the acute effect of ethanol, mice maintained on a liquid diet containing ethanol showed a stimulation of protein synthesis in a ribosomal preparation obtained from brain. However, Friedhoff and Miller[145] found that prolonged ingestion of ethanol in a liquid diet resulted in a depression in the activity of a specific protein, tryptophan hydroxylase, in brain.

The laboratory of the present authors has conducted extensive and detailed studies of the chronic effects of ethanol on the brain protein-synthesizing system of physically dependent and non-dependent mice and rats[146–150]. The details of the findings are presented below. The data obtained, under both *in vitro* and *in vivo* conditions, indicate that a significant inhibition in brain protein synthesis occurs in the animals maintained for prolonged periods on ethanol.

A strain of mice that prefers ethanol over water (C57BL/6J), were maintained on a 10 % ethanol solution, as their sole drinking fluid, for various periods. Under this condition the animals showed no gross nutritional deficiency, gained weight comparable to the control water-drinking mice, but experienced no abstinence syndrome upon withdrawal of ethanol. Twenty-four hours prior to sacrifice the ethanol solution was replaced by water. Our first studies were directed at the initial steps of the brain protein synthesizing system. The data indicated that the protein content of the pH5 enzymes fraction decreased as a function of duration on ethanol[148]. When the pH5 enzymes fraction was incubated with ribosomes in the presence of [^{14}C]leucine, an inhibition in ribosomal protein synthesis was found in the fractions obtained from ethanol-imbibing mice when compared to control animals drinking water. To determine whether this inhibition involved the pH5 enzymes fraction, the ribosomes, or both, a crossover experiment was performed. The results showed an increase in [^{14}C]leucine incorporation when ribosomes derived from the control mice were substituted for ribosomes of ethanol-treated animals. However, an even greater enhancement of incorporation occurred when the control pH5 enzymes fraction was substituted for the ethanol pH5 enzymes fraction. These findings suggested that, while a major defect in the cerebral protein-synthesizing system of ethanol-imbibing mice is located in the pH5 enzymes fraction, alterations in ribosomal function were also induced by ethanol.

Tewari and Noble[148] and Noble and Tewari[147] next studied the components of the pH5 enzymes fraction. They found that the *in vitro* synthesis of [^{14}C]leucyl-tRNA and [^{14}C]phenylalanyl-tRNA by the pH5 enzymes fraction was inhibited in ethanol-drinking animals. To determine whether aminoacyl-tRNA synthetases were affected by ethanol, incubations were carried out by crossmatching tRNA from control rat brain with synthetases obtained from control or ethanol-drinking mice. The results showed a decreased ability for aminoacylation when the source of enzymes was derived from ethanol-treated animals. On the other hand, minimal effects were obtained when the source of tRNA was used as a variable. The data indicated that the major effect of ethanol ingestion on the aminoacylation reaction is exerted on the aminoacyl-tRNA synthetases[151].

Since earlier studies indicated that the brain ribosomal fraction was also affected by chronic ethanol ingestion, an assessment was made of this subcellular component. Free and membrane-bound polysomes were obtained from the mixed ribosomal population and their capacity to synthesize protein was investigated[150]. Free polysomes from ethanol-drinking mice and rats had a diminished capacity to incorporate [^{14}C]leucine into protein when compared to free polysomes obtained from control animals. Similarly, a diminished incorporation was observed in the membrane-bound polysomes from ethanol-ingesting animals but not to as great an extent as found in the free polysomes.

What the underlying biochemical mechanisms are that affect the free and bound polysomes in alcohol-ingesting animals remain unknown. Despite a common source of the pH5 enzymes fraction obtained from control animals, decreased incorporation of amino acid still occurred in free and bound polysomal proteins of the ethanol-ingesting animals. Furthermore, in the presence of a synthetic mRNA (poly U) and a common source of control pH5 enzymes fraction, stimulation of polypeptide synthesis by poly U was much less in the ribosomes of ethanol-treated animals than those of controls. These and other findings suggested, not only the possibility of a paucity of mRNA and/or a decrease in its function, but are also indicative of a defect in the capacity of ethanol-treated ribosomes to synthesize polypeptides in the presence of exogenous mRNA. Thus at this time, it does not seem unlikely that chronic ethanol exposure alters polysomal composition and/or conformation to such an extent as to render them, particularly the free species, unstable and/or inefficient in the process of initiation, elongation or termination of protein synthesis. Additional studies, however, are necessary to locate more precisely the site of the polysomal defect induced by ethanol.

The above experiments were performed on animals that had chronically ingested a 10 % ethanol solution. As indicated earlier, under this condition the abstinence syndrome did not develop when ethanol was withdrawn. To assess the functional state of the cerebral protein-synthesizing system in physically dependent animals, two recent models of physical dependence upon ethanol were used. The first described by Lieber and DeCarli[152] consists of administering ethanol in a liquid diet to rats. The second described by Wallgren *et al.*[153] involves the technique of delivering ethanol to rats by intragastric intubation. Utilizing both these procedures, we have observed that the *in vitro* incorporation of either [^{14}C]leucine or [^{14}C]phenylalanine into brain ribosomal protein was inhibited in animals rendered physically dependent upon ethanol[154]. Furthermore, when ethanol was withheld for 24 hours, a period during which the abstinence syndrome is at a maximum, an even greater inhibition was attained. On the other hand, 7 days after ethanol administration had ceased, no differences were observed in the *in vitro* capacity to synthesize proteins between control and the ethanol-withdrawn ribosomal system. The site of the biochemical lesion(s) underlying the changes in the protein synthesis in brains of physically dependent animals is currently under intensive investigation in the present authors' laboratory.

6.4.2 Ribonucleic acids

Aside from studies conducted in the present authors' laboratory, no significant data are available in the literature on the effects of ethanol on brain RNA metabolism. Our studies have been reported previously[147,149,155,156], and have included both *in vitro* and *in vivo* studies on mice and rats chronically drinking a 10 % solution of ethanol. No data is yet available on brain RNA metabolism of physically dependent animals. A summary of our findings is presented below.

In vivo studies have shown that when a radioactive precursor of RNA, [5^{3}H]orotic acid, is injected intraventricularly into the brain of mice, a marked decrease, at all subsequent time periods, was observed in the incorporation of precursor label into transfer tRNA, ribosomal rRNA and polysomal RNA of the ethanol-ingesting animals. The inhibition was more pronounced in the polysomal fraction than the ribosomal fraction suggesting a more pronounced effect on messenger mRNA. In the nucleus, a biphasic effect of chronic ethanol ingestion was demonstrated in the nuclear nRNA fraction where increased incorporation of precursor label occurred at the early time points, but this was followed by a marked depression at later time points.

Various experiments were conducted to define more clearly the effects of chronic ethanol ingestion on brain RNA metabolism. Since the availability of nucleotides in the ethanol-treated animals could influence RNA synthesis,

[5^3H]orotic acid or another radioactive RNA precursor, [5^3H]uridine, was injected intraventricularly into the brains of mice. No significant differences in the labelling pattern and pool sizes of UMP, GMP, AMP or CMP were found in the brains of control and ethanol-treated animals indicating that altered availability of nucleotides was not a factor in the observed changes in RNA metabolism.

The above described data on the biphasic RNA labelling pattern of nuclear RNA which was not reflected in the cytoplasmic RNA fractions is suggestive of a possible defect in the transport of RNA from the nucleus to the cytoplasm resulting in the accumulation of RNA in the nucleus. As the homopolynucleotide, polyadenylic acid (poly A), is thought to be an essential part of the mRNA processing mechanism, the reduced availability of mRNA in the ethanol-treated brains may be a function of decreased synthesis and/or defective modification of this RNA. To determine the influence of poly A on the observed changes in RNA metabolism, studies were conducted on the effects of chronic ethanol ingestion on the *in vitro* synthesis of poly A by rat brain. The data showed a significant inhibition of poly A formation in the brains of ethanol-ingesting animals.

The findings on poly A coupled with earlier observations of reduced protein synthesis by both mixed population of ribosomes as well as free and bound ribosomes in the brains of ethanol-drinking animals[147,149] suggest that the reduced incorporation of precursor label into mRNA may in part be related to the poly A synthesizing system at the preribosomal level. Since the presence of the poly A tail in the mRNA molecules is also a prerequisite for successful production of this latter RNA[157–159], the severe inhibition of poly A synthesis induced by ethanol could cause an imbalance in the brain cell's capacity to synthesize proteins[155]. Of course, chronic ethanol administration was also shown to affect tRNA and rRNA metabolism. Additional studies are currently in progress on the critical role of other aspects of the RNA system to the observed alterations induced by ethanol on brain macromolecules.

6.5 NEURAL MEMBRANES

Biomembranes constitute an interphase through which all cells interact with the extracellular environment. Besides this vital function, neural membranes contain the additional property of excitability which constitutes one of the distinctive features of intercellular communication in the brain. The interaction of various neural cell types, for example glia and neurons, the mechanism of which is not yet fully understood, is thought to occur through the juxtaposition of their respective membranes. Because of these considerations as well as recent experimental evidence, cited below, many investigators[2,4,5,45,160] have proposed that ethanol's effect on the brain is mediated primarily through cellular membranes.

6.5.1 Theories of anaesthesia

The classic work of Meyer and Overton[161,162] established that the potency of an anaesthetic is directly proportional to its lipid/water partition coefficient. These investigators suggested that anaesthetics acted when dissolved in a lipid phase of the cell, which is now generally believed to be the cell membrane. Further refinements to this concept were offered by Ferguson[163] who found that anaesthetic potency is more accurately predicted if the concentration of each alcohol was multiplied by its respective thermodynamic activity coefficient. Mullins[164] predicted that equinarcotic effects should occur at equal-volume occupation of anaesthetics within the membrane phase. Recent studies on neural systems support these views. Thus, using a variety of alcohols, Roach *et al.*[57] observed that increasing carbon number caused a progressively greater inhibition of [^{3}H]DL-norepinephrine transport by rat brain synaptosomes while Israel *et al.*[59] found a very good correlation between the relative volume of occupation of various alcohols in the lipid phase and their inhibition of efflux of [^{3}H]DL-norepinephrine and [^{3}H]acetylcholine.

Other theories of anaesthesia have also been proposed. Of interest is the notion of Pauling[14] suggesting a general correlation between the anaesthetic potency of a compound, including ethanol, and the Van der Waals interaction. He argues for an aqueous site for anaesthesia by proposing that anaesthetic molecules stabilize aqueous clathrates among the protein side chains. However, no strong experimental evidence is available to support this theory. Miller *et al.*[165], studying the behaviour of the fluorine-substituted hydrocarbons, decided that the evidence favoured the hydrocarbons rather than the aqueous phase as the site of anaesthesia.

It is now well established, by using a variety of approaches including proton relaxation[166], permeability studies[167] and electron resonance[168,169], that an important effect of anaesthetic molecules on membranes is to increase the fluidity, disorder or entropy of the membrane. However, there is some controversy as to which one of the membrane components, lipids or proteins, is the most critically affected by alcohol.

Gage *et al.*[170] have found that some aliphatic alcohols, but not ethanol, cause synaptic currents in the sartorius muscle of toads to become briefer. They suggest that this may be due to an effect of the alcohols on the fluidity of the lipid environment of the acetylcholine receptor. However, they do not exclude the participation of proteins in the conductance change. Noble *et al.*[171] have assessed the effects of ethanol on neuraminidase releasable sialic acid (NRSA) of intact cultured neural cells. Utilizing a clonal line (NN) of hamster astroblasts, the results indicate that the effect of acute addition of ethanol (250 mg/%) upon NRSA of cultured neural cells is minimal, whereas chronic contact of cells with this drug leads to enhanced exposure of membrane sialolipids and/or sialoproteins rendering them more susceptible to attack by neuraminidase.

Bangham and co-workers[172,173] showed that general anaesthetics such as the *n*-alcohols from butanol to octanol increased the K^+ permeability of liposomes (a protein-free system) at anaesthetic concentrations. From these studies, they conclude that the cation permeability barrier to be located at the aqueous–lipid interface, and that anaesthetics sterically impede the rearrangement of the groups near the surface of the lipid which produces the sudden increase in Na^+ permeability. Additional studies by Hill[174], again using liposomes, have shown that the introduction of anaesthetic molecules alters their Gibbs-free energy, as measured by changes in boiling or freezing point temperatures. This and other findings led Hill[174] to propose a hypothesis of general anaesthesia based on the changes in the thermodynamic state of the lipids induced by the anaesthetic agents. More recently, Hill and Bangham[175] have elaborated on the original biophysical hypothesis of Hill[174] to explain the phenomenon of drug dependence.

Seeman[176] on the other hand argues for proteins as the critical determinant for the action of depressants. He reasons that in contrast to the increased permeability of cations in liposomes observed by Bangham and co-workers[172], anaesthetics, including ethanol, decreased cation permeability in natural membranes by blocking the channels through which Na^+ rapidly enters the cell during polarization (see Section 6.5.2). In addition, utilizing a high-precision density meter, Seeman[177] found that at concentrations of ethanol known to block nerve fibres, the membrane expands 2–3 % and, significantly, the expansion is about 10 times what would be predicted from the amount of ethanol known to enter the membrane. In contrast, when the same experiments were conducted on liposomes, in which protein is not present, no such amplification occurs. Based on these and other findings, Seeman[178] has elaborated the concepts of Meyer and Overton[161,162] and has proposed a hypothesis of anaesthesia based on membrane expansion. While these studies implicate the protein component of membranes in the actions of ethanol, it is also possible that ethanol-induced perturbations of the lipid matrix may in turn affect protein structure.

6.5.2 Cation metabolism and adenosine triphosphatase activity

Since the electrical properties of the neuron are intimately related to ion metabolism, much attention, both direct and indirect, has been devoted to this topic in an attempt to delineate the central actions of ethanol. Of special interest has been the membrane-bound $[Na^+ + K^+]$-activated adenosine triphosphatase (ATPase), an enzyme believed to represent the carrier system in the active translocation of Na^+ and K^+ across cell membrane[179,180]. The proposed mechanism of reaction for $[Na^+ + K^+]$-activated ATPase involves the formation of a phosphorylated intermediate (E–P). Sodium ions are necessary for the formation of the E–P compound; K^+ ions promote its hydrolysis thus liberating inorganic phosphate.

It has been reported that the acute administration of ethanol inhibits brain microsomal[181–183] and synaptosomal[146] [Na^+ + K^+]-activated ATPase of animals and whole homogenates and synaptosomes obtained from human brain[184]. Kalant[4] has suggested that one effect of impairment of cell membrane [Na^+ + K^+]-activated ATPase would be to reduce the resting potential (partial depolarization) by lowering the intracellular K^+ concentration. Since ethanol, at different concentrations, may reduce the resting potential of neural tissue and skeletal muscle fibres, Kalant proposes that depolarization in these tissues is not an instantaneous effect of exposure to ethanol, but a slowly developing change which would presumably be in keeping with a progressive reduction in intracellular K^+ concentration through inhibition of [Na^+ + K^+]-activated ATPase activity. Furthermore, Kalant *et al.*[102] indicate that although gross analysis of tissue electrolyte content shows little effect of ethanol, inhibition of active transport might still be important in ethanol-induced depression of nerve function because only a minute fraction of total Na^+ might be involved in the very rapid local ion movements of nerve activity.

Wallgren and co-workers[15,185,186] find the above hypothesis difficult to reconcile with the finding that a large proportion of cerebral K^+ and Na^+ is involved in the response to electrical stimulation. In more recent studies Wallgren *et al.*[187] have helped to define a probable ethanol-sensitive site in the complex structure of the excitable membrane. In studying the effects of ethanol (~500 mg/%) on Na^+ and K^+ movement in cerebral tissue, Wallgren *et al.*[187] found inhibition of Na^+ entry with very little effect on K^+ loss during electrical sitmulation. On the other hand, during recovery, it is the K^+ movement that is predominantly influenced. More specifically, a depression of the inward movement of K^+ was found.

The above observations are of interest in view of recent electrophysiological experiments which have established that during the excitation cycle, Na^+ and K^+ move through separate channels in excitable membranes. The increase in Na^+ conductance, which involves both an activation and an inactivation mechanism[188] is blocked by the neuropoison, tetrodotoxin. This substance acts on the external surface of the membrane, inhibiting the activation of the Na^+ channel[189]. The K^+ channel seems to be less direct than the Na^+ channel, involves an activation step but not a rapid distinct inactivation, and is selectively blocked, for instance by tetraethylammonium ions[189,190]. Rojas and Armstrong[191] obtained additional support for the location of the Na^+ activation mechanism on the outside of the membrane and for the existence of separate Na^+ and K^+ channels by treating the external and internal surface of the squid axon with a proteolytic enzyme.

In view of the findings of Nikander and Wallgren[103] that ethanol inhibits the intracellular changes in Na^+ and K^+ evoked by electrical stimulation, data which have been confirmed recently by Israel *et al.*[59], the suggestion that ethanol inhibits the action potential in brain tissue becomes quite tenable. Furthermore, the fairly selective effect of ethanol on the net influx of Na^+

supports the notion that influencing the activation mechanism of the Na^+ channel may be a more critical factor in ethanol-induced CNS depression than the inhibition of [Na^+ + K^+]-activated ATPase.

The effects of chronic ethanol exposure has been determined on a number of phosphate-cleaving enzymes in neural tissues. Israel *et al.*[192] found that ethanol increases the activity of [Na^+ + K^+]-activated ATPase in homogenates of whole rat brains while Israel and Kuriyama[193] observed enhanced activity of [Mg^{2+}]-activated ATPase in the mitochondrial fraction isolated from the mouse brain. Similarly, Knox *et al.*[194] found that the chronic administration of ethanol to cats by means of a stomach tube enhanced the activities of [Na^+ + K^+]-activated ATPase as well as that of [Mg^{2+}]-activated ATPase in several areas of the cat brain. Roach *et al.*[195] administered ethanol by inhalation of ethanol vapour to rats for 1 week. Brain subcellular fractionation revealed an increase in [Na^+ + K^+]-activated ATPase activity in the microsomes and to a smaller extent in the crude mitochondrial fraction. Gradient centrifugation of the crude mitochondrial preparation showed, however, that the increase in the [Na^+ + K^+]-activated ATPase activity was in the synaptosomes. Wallgren *et al.*[196] using rats found that with increasing degree of ethanol withdrawal excitability a proportional increase in [Na^+ + K^+]-activated ATPase and decrease in [Mg^{2+}]-activated ATPase activities occur in brain. It is not known in which cell type the enhanced phosphate-cleaving enzyme activity occurs, although in a recent study[197] on glioblastoma cells (C_6) grown in culture, chronic ethanol exposure resulted in more than a 30 % increase in the activities of 5′-nucleotidase and [Ca^{2+}]-activated ATPase.

Israel *et al.*[192] suggest that an increase in the [Na^+ + K^+]-activated ATPase activity responding to the initial inhibition by ethanol may be related to the development of tolerance after chronic administration of this drug. This phenomenon was later proposed as a biochemical model for the central tolerance to depressant agents[4]. Unfortunately other findings have not corroborated this view. Akera *et al.*[198] tested the effects of chronic ethanol administration in a liquid diet on the subsequent development of behavioural tolerance and brain ATPase activity in rats. Despite the development of tolerance to the depressant effects of ethanol as measured by conditioned avoidance behaviour and Rotarod performance, [Na^+, Mg^{2+}, ATP]-dependent binding of [^{3}H]ouabain of brain region (cerebrum, midbrain, medulla oblongata and cerebellum) homogenates were unchanged in control and ethanol-withdrawn animals. Goldstein and Israel[199] measured ATPase activity in brains of mice rendered physically dependent upon ethanol by introducing them to a constant atmosphere of ethanol vapour. [Na^+ + K^+]-activated ATPase activity of brain homogenates was not increased at the end of the intoxication period nor at 10 hours later when the withdrawal reaction was at its peak. These authors conclude from their data that physical dependence in the mouse does not involve ATPase and indicate that the [Na^+ + K^+]-activated

ATPase enzyme does not fit the 'depression theory' of tolerance and dependence[200,201].

It appears then that conflict abounds as to the role of ATPase in the phenomenon of ethanol tolerance and dependence. The discrepancies may in part be related to the fractions, species and conditions of assay that have been used. The present reviewers consider the alterations in ATPase more as a function of general perturbation in membrane structure and hence function that has been induced by chronic ethanol rather than being a critical contributory factor in the development of the above phenomena.

6.5.3 Cyclic 3′,5′-adenosine monophosphate

With the discovery of cyclic 3′,5′-adenosine monophosphate (cAMP) and its presumptive role as a 'second messenger' for the action of biogenic amines and hormones[202–204], studies have been directed as to its involvement in the function of neural cells. Indeed there is growing evidence that such an involvement prevails[205–209]. Because ethanol induces changes in the endocrine system[210] and in view of its actions on biogenic amines (see section 6.3), recent studies have assessed the effects of ethanol on brain cAMP metabolism.

Israel *et al.*[211,212] report that i.p. injection of ethanol (4 g/kg) into mice did not affect adenylate cyclase and phosphodiesterase enzymes respectively involved in the synthesis and degradation of cAMP activities in the cerebral cortex. Furthermore cAMP content remained unchanged. On the other hand, when these animals were chronically fed ethanol in a liquid diet, changes occurred in adenylate cyclase activity and cAMP content but not phosphodiesterase activity when compared to controls receiving isocaloric sucrose as a substitute for ethanol in the liquid diet. Specifically, 1, 2 and 3 weeks after the introduction of ethanol, adenylate cyclase activity increased 50, 39 and 44 % respectively while cAMP content increased 64, 49, and 14 %. The authors aptly suggest that since similar activation of brain adenylate cyclase activity was observed by them following morphine administration[213] the present findings are not specific for chronic ethanol administration. On the other hand, they do offer that continuous activation of the hypothalamic–pituitary adrenal axis by ethanol induces an increase in brain cAMP level which in turn, they believe, contributes to the establishment of physical dependence. Unfortunately, the authors do not present data on the chronic effects of ethanol administered for periods of less than 1 week. Since these authors found maximum changes in the cAMP system at 1 week of ethanol administration, these changes probably are more a reflection of the CNS depressant effects of this drug and as such would probably play no significant role in the development of dependence.

Volicer and Gold[214] studied the effect of ethanol on cAMP levels in isolated brain regions including: cerebrum, cerebellum and pons and medulla oblongata and whole rat brain. Following acute ethanol administration (6 g/kg, p.o.), brain cAMP levels decreased to 40 % that of controls and this effect lasted for 8 hours. Furthermore, the decrease was found to be dose-dependent and limited to the cerebellum. It is not clear through what biochemical mechanism ethanol exerts its influence on cAMP nor is it known which cell types are most susceptible to the ethanol effects. A possible target is the Purkinje cells, given that ethanol[215] and cAMP[216] inhibit their activity and cerebellar dysfunction is a major sign of ethanol intoxication.

6.6 SUMMARY

The neurochemical effects of ethanol have been examined on: energy metabolism, neurotransmitter systems, protein and nucleic acid metabolism and membrane structure and function.

6.6.1 Energy metabolism

Ethanol is metabolized primarily via alcohol dehydrogenase (ADH) and aldehyde dehydrogenase in the liver and recently the brain was found to contain a low ADH activity. Oxidation of ethanol results in a greater increase in the ratio of cytoplasmic free ($NADH_2$)/(NAD) for hepatic tissue than the brain. A causal relationship has been suggested between the increase in brain ADH activity following ethanol consumption and the development of tolerance. However, more recent data do not support such a contention.

6.6.2 Neurotransmitter systems

The effects of ethanol on central neurotransmitter systems are thus far confusing and few consistent findings are available.

Ethanol's action on the serotoninergic system has been the subject of numerous studies. Discordant results have been reported on levels and turnover of brain serotonin and its subsequent metabolism to 5-OH indole acetic acid and 5-OH tryptophol. Enzyme studies have shown that acute administration of ethanol did not affect the activity of brain tryptophan hydroxylase, whereas chronic treatment increased its activity. Furthermore, chronic exposure to ethanol did not alter brain MAO, cytosol and mitochondrial aldehyde dehydrogenase or aldehyde reductase activities.

The catecholamine system appears to be affected by both the acute and chronic administration of ethanol *in vivo. In vitro* studies also demonstrate an effect of ethanol on the uptake and the release of catecholamines by brain slices and fractions but mostly at high and supralethal concentrations of the drug. In addition, recent findings suggest that ethanol acts as a specific activator of noradrenergic neurons and also as a non-competitive inhibitor of [^{3}H]norepinephrine uptake. The role of condensation products of aldehydes and catecholamines in alcoholism has been examined and, despite their possible role as 'false transmitters', there is no strong evidence, thus far, of their involvement in the acute and chronic effects of ethanol.

With the acetylcholine (Ach) system ethanol was shown to decrease the output of Ach from the CNS. It has been suggested that the effects of ethanol on Ach are primarily exerted on the release process by altering ion metabolism, particularly Na^+ conductance. The functional significance of the Ach system, however, remains controversial since drugs that modify this system fail to alter ethanol-induced behavioural depression. Knowledge relating to the chronic effects of ethanol on Ach system is meagre.

A confusing array of findings have been obtained on the effects of ethanol on neurochemical aspects of the γ-aminobutyric acid (GABA) system. Despite this prevailing uncertainty, evidence is accumulating to suggest that drugs which modify the GABA-minergic system alter the course of physical dependence upon ethanol.

6.6.3 Protein and RNA metabolism

There are a few studies on the effects of acute ethanol administration on brain protein synthesis. The data show consistently that such treatment significantly depresses the incorporation of amino acids into protein. More detailed investigations are available on the long-term effects of ethanol ingestion. *In vitro* and *in vivo* studies show a decreased capacity for cerebral synthesis of proteins. This effect of ethanol was not only due to a reduced capacity of the aminoacylation reaction but also was a product of altered polyribosomal function.

Chronic ingestion of ethanol also led to alterations in RNA metabolism. *In vivo* studies showed a diminished incorporation of labelled precursor into tRNA, rRNA and polysomal RNA. No significant differences in the labelling pattern and pool sizes of UMP, GMP, AMP and CMP were found in the brains of control and ethanol-drinking animals indicating that altered availability of nucleotides was not a factor in the observed changes in RNA metabolism. *In vitro* studies showed a significant inhibition of polyadenylic acid synthesis in the brain of ethanol-ingesting animals suggesting a possible defect in the processing of transport of RNA from the nucleus to the cytoplasm. It is feasible then that the disturbed RNA metabolism may in part be related to the polyadenylation process at the preribosomal level thereby causing an imbalance in the brain's capacity to synthesize proteins.

6.6.4 Neural membranes

It is generally acknowledged that neural membranes represent the primary site of ethanol's action on the CNS. However, what the ethanol-induced changes in membranes are or how they contribute to CNS depression or the development of tolerance and physical dependence remain enigmatic.

Ethanol is thought to expand membranes and also to increase the fluidity or disorder of membrane components. Such changes have been linked to the altered ionic permeability, the inhibition of the action potential and the functional blockage of nervous tissue induced by ethanol. Chronic treatment of neural cells with this drug enhances the exposure of certain functional groups in membranes rendering them more susceptible to hydrolytic cleavage.

Much interest has been focused upon the observation that acute ethanol exposure inhibits the activity of $[Na^+ + K^+]$-activated ATPase, a membrane-associated enzyme. However, the fairly selective effect of ethanol on the net influx of Na^+ supports the notion that influencing the activation mechanism of the Na^+ channel may be a more critical factor in ethanol-induced CNS depression than the inhibition of $[Na^+ + K^+]$-activated ATPase. Furthermore, the changes in ATPase activity induced by chronic ethanol exposure is now thought to be more a product of general perturbation in membrane structure affecting this enzyme rather than being a critical contributing factor in the development of tolerance and dependence.

A few studies are available on another membrane-associated system, adenylate cyclase. Chronic ethanol ingestion increased the activity of adenylate cyclase and cAMP content. However, of special interest is the observation that acute ethanol administration resulted in a decrease in cAMP levels which was dose-dependent and limited to the cerebellum. This finding needs to be replicated and extended since cerebellar dysfunction is a major sign of ethanol intoxication.

Acknowledgements

This work was supported in part by a research grant (AA00252) from the National Institute on Alcohol Abuse and Alcoholism (NIAAA), ADAMHA. One of us (E.P.N.) was a Guggenheim Fellow (1974–1975) while the other (S.T.) is a recipient of a Research Scientist Development Award from the NIAAA (AA70899).

References

1. Israel, Y. (1970). Cellular effects of alcohol. A review. *Q. J. Stud. Alc.*, **31,** 293
2. Wallgren, H. and Barry, H., III (1970). *Actions of Alcohol, Vol. 1, Biochemical, Physiological, and Psychological Aspects*. Amsterdam: Elsevier

3. Kalant, H. (1971). Absorption, diffusion, distribution, and elimination of ethanol: effects on biological membranes. In B. Kissin and H. Begleiter, eds. *The Biology of Alcoholism, Vol. 1, Biochemistry,* p. 1. New York: Plenum Press
4. Wallgren, H. (1971). Effect of ethanol on intracellular respiration and cerebral function. In B. Kissin and H. Begleiter, eds. *The Biology of Alcoholism, Vol. 1, Biochemistry,* p. 103. New York: Plenum Press
5. Grenell, R. G. (1971). Effects of alcohol on the neuron. In B. Kissin and H. Begleiter, eds. *The Biology of Alcoholism, Vol. 2, Physiology and Behavior,* p. 1. New York: Plenum Press
6. Raskin, N. H. and Sokoloff, L. J. (1972). Enzymes catalysing ethanol metabolism in neural and somatic tissues of the rat. *J. Neurochem.,* **19,** 273
7. Krebs, H. A. (1969). The effects of ethanol on the metabolic activities of the liver. *Adv. Enzym. Regulation,* **6,** 467
8. Rawat, A. K. (1970). Effect of ethanol on glycerol metabolism in rat liver during different hormonal conditions. *Biochem. Pharmacol.,* **19,** 2791
9. Veech, R. L., Guynn, R. H. and Veloso, D. (1972). The time-course of the effects of ethanol on the redox and phosphorylation states of rat liver. *Biochem. J.,* **127,** 387
10. Rawat, A. K., Kuriyama, K. and Mose, J. (1973). Metabolic consequences of ethanol oxidation in brains from mice chronically fed ethanol. *J. Neurochem.,* **20,** 23
11. Veloso, D., Passonneau, J. V. and Veech, R. (1972). The effects of intoxicating doses of ethanol upon intermediary metabolism in rat brain. *J. Neurochem.,* **19,** 2679
12. Mushahwar, I. K. and Koeppe, R. E. (1972). Incorporation of label from [1-^{14}C]ethanol into the glutamate–glutamine pools of rat brain *in vivo. Biochem. J.,* **126,** 467
13. Raskin, N. H. (1973). Alcohol dehydrogenase in brain: a toxicological role? *Ann. N.Y. Acad. Sci.,* **215,** 49
14. Pauling, L. (1961). A molecular theory of general anesthesia. *Science,* **134,** 15
15. Wallgren, H. and Barry, H., III (1970). *Actions of Alcohol, Vol. 1, Biochemical, Physiological and Psychological Aspects,* p. 209. Amsterdam: Elsevier
16. Gursey, D. and Olson, R. E. (1960). Depression of serotonin and norepinephrine levels in brain stem of rabbit by ethanol. *Proc. Soc. Exp. Biol. Med.,* **104,** 280
17. Gursey, D., Vester, J. W. and Olson, R. E. (1959). Effect of ethanol administration upon serotonin and norepinephrine levels in rabbit brain. *J. Clin. Invest.,* **38,** 1008
18. Bonnycastle, D. D., Bonnycastle, M. F. and Anderson, E. G. (1962). The effect of a number of central depressant drugs upon brain 5-hydroxytryptamine levels in the rat. *J. Pharmacol. Exp. Ther.,* **135,** 17
19. Passonen, M. K. and Giarman, N. J. (1958). Brain levels of 5-hydroxytryptamine after various agents. *Arch. Intern. Pharmacodyn. Ther.,* **114,** 189
20. Reichle, F. A., Goodman, P. M., Reichle, R. M., Labinsky, L. S. and Rosemond, G. P. (1971). The effect of acute alcohol administration on brain dopamine, serotonin and norepinephrine. *Fed. Proc.,* **30,** 382
21. Palaić, D. J., Desaty, J., Albert, J. M. and Painsset, J. C. (1971). Effect of ethanol on metabolism and subcellular distribution of serotonin in rat brain. *Brain Res.,* **25,** 381
22. Efron, D. H. and Gessa, G. L. (1961). Failure of ethanol and barbiturates to alter the content of brain 5-HT and NE. *Biochem. Pharmacol.,* **8,** 172
23. Efron, D. H. and Gessa, G. L. (1963). Failure of ethanol and barbiturates to alter brain monoamine content. *Arch. Intern. Pharmacodyn. Ther.,* **142,** 111
24. Haggendal, J. M. and Lindqvist, M. (1961). Ineffectiveness of ethanol on noradrenaline, dopamine or 5-hydroxytryptamine levels in brain. *Acta Pharmacol. Toxicol.,* **18,** 278
25. Pscheidt, G. R., Issekutz, B., Jr. and Himwich, H. E. (1961). Failure of ethanol to lower brain stem concentration of biogenic amines. *Q. J. Stud. Alc.,* **22,** 550
26. Rudas, N. and Vacca, L. (1964). Influenza dell'alcool sul contenuto di monoamine del sistema nervoso centrale. *Acta Neurol.,* **19,** 848
27. Truitt, E. B., Jr. and Duritz, G. (1966). The role of acetaldehyde in the actions of ethanol. In R. P. Maickel, ed. *Biochemical Factors in Alcoholism,* p. 61. Oxford: Pergamon Press

28. Tyce, G. M., Flock, E. V. and Owen, C. A., Jr. (1968). Effect of ethanol on serotonin (5-HT) metabolism in brain and in isolated perfused liver. *Fed. Proc.*, **27**, 400
29. Tyce, G. M., Flock, E. V. and Owen, C. A., Jr. (1968). 5-Hydroxytryptamine metabolism in brains of ethanol-intoxicated rats. *Mayo Clin. Proc.*, **43**, 668
30. Kuriyama, K., Rauscher, G. E. and Sze, P. Y. (1971). Effect of acute and chronic administration of ethanol on the 5-hydroxytryptamine turnover and tryptophan hydroxylase activity of the mouse brain. *Brain Res.*, **26**, 450
31. Feldstein, A. (1973). Ethanol-induced sleep in relation to serotonin turnover and conversion of 5-hydroxyindoleacetaldehyde, 5-hydroxytryptophol, and 5-hydroxyindoleacetic acid. *Ann. N.Y. Acad. Sci.*, **215**, 71
32. Hunt, W. A. and Majchrowicz, E. (1974). Turnover rates and steady-state levels of brain serotonin in alcohol-dependent rats. *Brain Res.*, **72**, 181
33. Tabakoff, B. and Boggan, W. O. (1974). Effects of ethanol on serotonin metabolism in brain. *J. Neurochem.*, **22**, 759
34. Tyce, G. M., Flock, E. V., Taylor, W. F. and Owen, C. A., Jr. (1970). Effect of ethanol on 5-hydroxytryptamine turnover in rat brain. *Proc. Soc. Exp. Biol.*, **134**, 40
35. Frankel, D., Khanna, J. M., Kalant, H. and LeBlanc, A. E. (1974). Effect of acute and chronic ethanol administration on serotonin turnover in rat brain. *Psychopharmacologia*, **37**, 91
36. Feldstein, A., Hoagland, H., Freeman, H. and Williamson, O. (1967). The effects of ethanol ingestion on serotonin-C^{14} metabolism in man. *Life Sci.*, **6**, 53
37. Davis, V. E., Brown, H., Huff, J. A. and Cashaw, I. L. (1967). The alteration of serotonin metabolism of 5-hydroxytryptophol by ethanol ingestion in man. *J. Lab. Clin. Med.*, **69**, 132
38. Huff, J. A., Davis, V. E., Brown, H. and Clay, M. M. (1971). Effects of chloral hydrate, paraldehyde, and ethanol on the metabolism of [^{14}C]serotonin in the rat. *Biochem. Pharmacol.*, **20**, 476
39. Eccleston, D., Reading, W. H. and Ritchie, I. M. (1969). 5-Hydroxytryptamine metabolism in brain and liver slices and the effects of ethanol. *J. Neurochem.*, **16**, 274
40. Tytell, M. and Myers, R. D. (1973). Metabolism of [^{14}C]serotonin in the caudate nucleus, hypothalamus and reticular formation of the rat after ethanol administration. *Biochem. Pharmacol.*, **22**, 361
41. Blum, K., Calhoun, W., Merritt, J. H. and Wallace, J. E. (1973). Synergy of ethanol and alcohol-like metabolites: tryptophol and 3,4-dihydroxyphenylethanol. *Pharmacology*, **9**, 294
42. Ahtee, L. and Ericksson, K. (1972). 5-Hydroxytryptamine and 5-hydroxyindolylacetic acid content in brain of rat strains selected for their alcohol intake. *Physiol. Behav.*, **8**, 123
43. Carlsson, A. and Lindqvist, M. J. (1973). Effect of ethanol on the hydroxylation of tyrosine and tryptophan in rat brain *in vivo*. *J. Pharm. Pharmacol.*, **25**, 437
44. Rogawski, M. A., Knapp, S. and Mandell, A. J. (1974). Effect of ethanol on tryptophan hydroxylase activity from striate synaptosomes. *Biochem. Pharmacol.*, **23**, 1955
45. Wallgren, H. and Barry, H., III (1970). *Actions of Alcohol, Vol. 2, Chronic and Clinical Aspects*. Amsterdam: Elsevier
46. von Wartburg, J. P. (1970). Biochemical and enzymatic changes induced by chronic ethanol intake. In J. Trémolières, ed. *International Encyclopedia of Pharmacology and Therapeutics, Section 20, Vol. II, Alcohol and Derivatives*, p. 301. Oxford: Pergamon Press
47. Schenker, V. J. (1970). Effects of ethanol on the endocrines. In J. Trémolières, ed. *International Encyclopedia of Pharmacology and Therapeutics, Section 20, Vol. I, Alcohol and Derivatives*, p. 261. Oxford: Pergamon Press
48. Mendelson, J. H. (1970). Biological concomitants of alcoholism. *N. Engl. J. Med.*, **283**, 24 and 71
49. Hawkins, R. D. and Kalant, H. (1972). The metabolism of ethanol and its metabolic effects. *Pharmacol. Rev.*, **24**, 67

50. Walsh, M. J. (1971). Role of acetaldehyde in the interactions of ethanol with neuroamines. In M. K. Roach, W. M. McIsaac, and P. J. Creaven, eds. *Biological Aspects of Alcohol,* p. 233. Austin and London: University of Texas Press
51. Feldstein, A. (1971). Effect of ethanol on neurohumoral amine metabolism. In B. Kissin and H. Begleiter, eds. *The Biology of Alcoholism, Vol. 1, Biochemistry,* p. 127. New York: Plenum Press
52. Duritz, G. and Truitt, E. B., Jr. (1966). Importance of acetaldehyde in the action of ethanol on brain norepinephrine and 5-hydroxytryptamine. *Biochem. Pharmacol.,* **15,** 711
53. Corrodi, H., Fuxe, K. and Hökfelt, T. (1966). The effects of ethanol on the activity of central catecholamine neurones in rat brain. *J. Pharm. Pharmacol.,* **18,** 821
54. Carlsson, A., Magnusson, T., Svensson, T. H. and Waldeck, B. (1973). Effect of ethanol on the metabolism of brain catecholamines. *Psychopharmacologia,* **30,** 27
55. Thadani, P. V. and Truitt, E. B. (1973). Norepinephrine turnover effects of ethanol and acetaldehyde in rat brain. *Fed. Proc.,* **32,** 697
56. Hunt, W. A. and Majchrowicz, E. (1974). Alterations in the turnover of brain norepinephrine and dopamine in alcohol-dependent rats. *J. Neurochem.,* **23,** 549
57. Roach, M. K., Davis, D. L., Pennington, W. and Nordyke, E. (1973). Effect of ethanol on the uptake by rat brain synaptosomes of [^{3}H]DL-norepinephrine, [^{3}H]5-hydroxytryptamine, [^{3}H]GABA and [^{3}H]glutamate. *Life Sci.,* **12,** 433
58. Israel, Y., Carmichael, F. J. and Macdonald, J. A. (1973). Effect of ethanol on norepinephrine uptake and electrically stimulated release in brain tissue. *Ann. N.Y. Acad. Sci.,* **215,** 38
59. Israel, Y., Carmichael, F. J. and Macdonald, J. A. (1975). Effects of ethanol on electrolyte metabolism and neurotransmitter release in the CNS. In M. Gross, ed. *Advances in Experimental Medicine and Biology, Vol. 59,* p. 55. New York: Plenum Press
60. Seeman, P. and Lee, T. (1974). The dopamine-releasing actions of neuroleptics and ethanol. *J. Pharmacol. Exp. Ther.,* **190,** 131
61. Spector, S., Gordon, R., Sjoerdsma, A. and Udenfriend, S. (1967). End-product inhibition of tyrosine hydroxylase as a possible mechanism for regulation of norepinephrine synthesis. *Mol. Pharmacol.,* **3,** 549
62. Javoy, F., Agid, Y., Bouvet, D. and Glowinski, J. (1972). Feedback control of dopamine synthesis in dopaminergic terminals of the rat striatum. *J. Pharmacol. Exp. Ther.,* **182,** 454
63. Weiner, N., Cloutier, G., Bjur, R. and Pfeffer, R. I. (1972). Modification of norepinephrine synthesis in intact tissue by drugs and during short-term adrenergic nerve stimulation. *Pharmacol. Rev.,* **24,** 203
64. Da Prada, M. and Pletscher, A. (1966). Acceleration of the cerebral dopamine turnover by chlorpromazine. *Experientia,* **22,** 465
65. Anden, N.-E., Bédard, P., Fuxe, K. and Ungerstedt, U. (1972). Early and selective increase in brain dopamine levels after axotomy. *Experientia,* **28,** 300
66. Nybäck, H. (1972). Effect of brain lesions and chlorpromazine on accumulation and disappearance of catecholamines formed *in vivo* from [^{14}C]tyrosine. *Acta Physiol. Scand.,* **84,** 54
67. Kehr, W., Carlsson, A., Lindqvist, M., Magnusson, T. and Atack, C. J. (1972). Evidence of a receptor–mediator feedback control of striatal tyrosine hydroxylase activity. *J. Pharm. Pharmacol.,* **24,** 744
68. Rawat, A. K. (1974). Brain levels and turnover rates of presumptive neurotransmitters as influenced by administration and withdrawal of ethanol in mice. *J. Neurochem.,* **2,** 915
69. Collins, M. and Cohen, G. (1968). Tissue catecholamines condense with acetaldehyde to form isoquinoline alkaloids. *Amer. Chem. Soc. 156th Nat. Meeting, Abstr.* **274**
70. Robbins, J. H. (1968). Alkaloid formation by condensation of biogenic amines with acetaldehyde. *Clin. Res.,* **16,** 350

71. Cohen, G. and Collins, M. (1970). Alkaloids from catecholamines in adrenal tissue: possible role in alcoholism. *Science*, **167**, 1749
72. Yamanka, Y., Walsh, M. J. and Davis, V. E. (1970). Salsolinol, an alkaloid derivative of dopamine formed *in vitro* during alcohol metabolism. *Nature* (*London*), **227**, 1143
73. Davis, V. E. and Walsh, M. (1970). Alcohol, amines and alkaloids: a possible biochemical basis for alcohol addiction. *Science*, **167**, 1005
74. Erwin, V. G. and Deitrich, R. A. (1975). Involvement of biogenic amine metabolism in ethanol addiction. Unpublished findings
75. Davis, V. E., Cashaw, J. L. and McMurtrey, K. D. (1975). Disposition of catecholamine-derived alkaloids in mammalian systems. In M. Gross, ed. *Advances in Experimental Medicine and Biology. Vol. 59*, p. 65. New York: Plenum Press
76. Schopf, C. and Bayerle, H. (1934). Zur Frage der Biogenese der Isochinolinalkaloide: Die Synthese des 1-methyl-6,7-dioxy-1,2,3,4-tetrahydro-isochinolins unter physiologischen Bedingungen. *Liebig Ann. Chem.*, **513**, 190
77. Cohen, G. (1971). Tetrahydroisoquinoline alkaloids in the adrenal medulla after perfusion with 'blood concentrations' of [^{14}C]acetaldehyde. *Biochem. Pharmacol.*, **20**, 1757
78. Collins, M. A. and Bigdeli, M. G. (1975). Biosynthesis of tetrahydroisoquinoline alkaloids in brain and other tissues of ethanol-intoxicated rats. In M. Gross, ed. *Advances in Experimental Medicine and Biology*, *Vol. 59*, p. 79. New York: Plenum Press
79. Collins, M. A. and Bigdeli, M. G. (1975). Tetrahydroisoquinolines *in vivo*. 1. Rat brain formation of salsolinol, a condensation product of dopamine and acetaldehyde under certain conditions during ethanol intoxication. *Life Sci.*, **16**, 584
80. Heikkila, R., Cohen, G. and Dembiec, D. (1971). Tetrahydroisoquinoline alkaloids: uptake by rat brain homogenates and inhibition of catecholamine uptake. *J. Pharmacol. Exp. Ther.*, **179**, 250
81. Mytilineou, C., Cohen, G. and Barrett, R. (1974). Tetrahydroisoquinoline alkaloids: uptake and release by adrenergic nerve *in vivo*. *Eur. J. Pharmacol.*, **25**, 390
82. Cohen, G. (1973). Tetrahydroisoquinoline alkaloids: uptake, storage, and secretion by the adrenal medulla and by adrenergic nerves. *Ann. N.Y. Acad. Sci.*, **215**, 116
83. Laidlaw, P. P. (1910). The action of tetrahydropapaveroline hydrochloride. *J. Physiol.* (*London*), **40**, 480
84. Santi, R., Ferrari, M., Tóth, C. E., Contessa, A. R., Fassina, G., Bruni, A. and Luciani, S. (1967). Pharmacological properties of tetrahydropapaveroline. *J. Pharm. Pharmacol.*, **19**, 45
85. Turner, A. J., Baker, K. M., Algeri, S., Frigerio, A. and Garattini, S. (1974). Tetrahydropapaveroline: formation *in vivo* and *in vitro* in rat brain. *Life Sci.*, **14**, 2247
86. Alpers, H. S., McLaughlin, B. R., Nix, W. M. and Davis, V. E. (1974). Tetrahydroisoquinoline and tetrahydroprotoberberine alkaloids: inhibition of catecholamine accumulation by rat brain synaptosomal preparation. *Fed. Proc.*, **33**, 511
87. Sandler, M., Carter, S. B., Hunter, K. R. and Stern, G. M. (1973). Tetrahydroisoquinoline alkaloids: *in vivo* metabolites of L-dopa in man. *Nature* (*London*), **241**, 439
88. Halushka, P. V. and Hoffman, P. C. (1970). Alcohol addiction and tetrahydropapaveroline. *Science*, **169**, 1104
89. Seevers, M. H. (1970). Morphine and ethanol physical dependence: a critique of a hypothesis. *Science*, **170**, 1113
90. Goldstein, A. and Judson, B. A. (1971). Alcohol dependence and opiate dependence: lack of relationship in mice. *Science*, **172**, 290
91. Wallgren, H. (1973). Neurochemical aspects of tolerance to and dependence on ethanol. In M. Gross, ed. *Advances in Experimental Medicine and Biology*, *Vol. 35*, p. 15. New York: Plenum Press
92. Kalant, H. (1970). Effect of ethanol on the nervous system. In J. Trémolières, ed. *International Encyclopedia of Pharmacology, Section 20, Vol. I, Alcohols and Their Derivatives*, p. 189. Oxford: Pergamon Press

93. Kalant, H., Israel, Y. and Mahon, M. A. (1967). The effect of ethanol on acetylcholine synthesis, release, and degradation in brain. *Can. J. Physiol. Pharmacol.*, **45,** 172
94. Kalant, H. and Grose, W. (1968). Effects of ethanol and pentobarbital on release of acetylcholine from cerebral cortex slices. *J. Pharmacol. Exp. Ther.*, **158,** 386
95. Gage, P. W. (1965). The effect of methyl, ethyl, *n*-propyl alcohol on neuromuscular transmission in the rat. *J. Pharmacol. Exp. Ther.*, **150,** 236
96. Okada, K. (1967). Effects of alcohols and acetone on the neuromuscular junction of frog. *Jap. J. Physiol.*, **17,** 245
97. Inoue, F. and Frank, G. B. (1967). Effects of ethyl alcohol on excitability and on neuromuscular transmission in frog skeletal muscle. *Br. J. Pharmacol. Chemother.*, **30,** 186
98. Erickson, C. K. and Graham, D. T. (1973). Alteration of cortical and reticular acetylcholine release by ethanol *in vivo*. *J. Pharmacol. Exp. Ther.*, **185,** 583
99. Heim, F., Ammon, H. P. T., Estler, C.-J. and Mikschiczek, D. (1965). Funktion und Stoffwechsel des Gehirns unter Finwirkung niedriger alkoholkonzentrationen. *Med. Pharmacol. Exp.*, **13,** 361
100. Modak, A. T. and Stavinoha, W. B. (1971). Effects of ethanol on the cholinesterase activity in the brain of the rat. *Pharmacologist,* **13,** 219
101. Reisberg, R. B. (1974). Stimulation of choline acetyltransferase activity by ethanol in *in vitro* preparations of rat cerebrum. *Life Sci.*, **14,** 1965
102. Kalant, H., Mons, W. and Mahon, M. A. (1966). Acute effects of ethanol on tissue electrolytes in the rat. *Can. J. Physiol. Pharmacol.*, **44,** 1
103. Nikander, P. and Wallgren, H. (1970). Ethanol, electrical stimulation, and net movements of sodium and potassium in rat brain tissue *in vitro*. *Acta Physiol. Scand.*, **80,** 27A
104. Erickson, C. K. and Burnam, W. L. (1971). Cholinergic alteration of ethanol-induced sleep and death in mice. *Agents Actions*, **2,** 8
105. Graham, D. T. and Erickson, C. K. (1974). Alteration of ethanol-induced CNS depression: ineffectiveness of drugs that modify cholinergic transmission. *Psychopharmacologia,* **34,** 173
106. Kinard, F. W. and Hay, M. G. (1960). Effect of ethanol administration on brain and liver enzyme activities. *Am. J. Physiol.*, **198,** 657
107. Smyth, R. D., Martin, G. J., Moss, J. N. and Beck, H. (1967). The modifications of various enzyme parameters in brain acetylcholine metabolism by chronic ingestion of ethanol. *Exp. Med. Surg.*, **25,** 1
108. Goldstein, D. B. (1973). Alcohol withdrawal reactions in mice: effects of drugs that modify neurotransmission. *J. Pharmacol. Exp. Ther.*, **186,** 1
109. Curtis, D. R. and Watkins, J. C. (1965). The pharmacology of amino acids related to gamma-aminobutyric acid. *Pharmacol. Rev.*, **17,** 347
110. Krnjević, K. (1971). Glutamate and γ-aminobutyric acid in brain. *Nature* (*London*), **228,** 119
111. Killam, K. F. and Bain, J. A. (1957). Convulsant hydrazides. I. *In vitro* and *in vivo* inhibition of vitamin B_6 enzymes by convulsant hydrazides. *J. Pharmacol. Exp. Ther.*, **19,** 255
112. Wood, J. D. and Peesker, S. J. (1973). The role of GABA metabolism in the convulsant and anticonvulsant actions of aminooxyacetic acid. *J. Neurochem.*, **20,** 379
113. Simler, S., Ciesielski, I., Maitre, M., Randrianarisoa, H. and Mandel, P. (1973). Effects of sodium *n*-dipropylacetate on audiogenic seizures and brain γ-aminobutyric acid level. *Biochem. Pharmacol.*, **22**, 1701
114. Häkkinen, H.-M. and Kulonen, E. (1963). Comparison of various methods for the determination of γ-aminobutyric acid and other amino acids in rat brain with reference to ethanol intoxication. *J. Neurochem.*, **10,** 489
115. Sytinski, I. A. and Priyathina, T. N. (1964). Effects of certain drugs on gamma-aminobutyric acid content of the central nervous system. *Fed. Proc.* (*Trans. Suppl*)., **23,** T879
116. Ferrari, R. A. and Arnold, A. (1961). Effects of central nervous system agents on rat brain gamma-aminobutyric acid level. *Biochim. Biophys. Acta,* **52,** 361

117. Gordon, E. R. (1967). The effect of ethanol on the concentration of γ-aminobutyric acid in the rat brain. *Can. J. Physiol. Pharmacol.*, **45,** 915
118. Higgins, E. S. (1962). The effect of ethanol on GABA content of rat brain. *Biochem. Pharmacol.*, **11,** 394
119. Hagen, D. W. (1967). GABA levels in rat brain after prolonged ethanol intake. *Q. J. Stud. Alc.*, **28,** 613
120. Sutton, I. and Simmonds, M. A. (1973). Effects of acute and chronic ethanol on the γ-aminobutyric acid system in rat brain. *Biochem. Pharmacol.*, **22,** 1685
121. Patel, G. J. and Lal, H. (1973). Reduction in brain γ-aminobutyric acid and in barbital narcosis during ethanol withdrawal. *J. Pharmacol. Exp. Ther.*, **186,** 625
122. Noble, E. P., Gillies, R., Vigran, R. and Mandel, P. (1976). The modification of the ethanol withdrawal syndrome in rats by di-*n*-propylacetate. *Psychopharmacologia*, **46,** 127
123. Moore, B. W. (1968). Specific acid proteins of the nervous system. In F. D. Carlson, ed. *Physiological and Biochemical Aspects of Nervous Integration*, p. 343. Englewood Cliffs, N.J.: Prentice Hall
124. Barondes, S. H. and Jarvik, M. E. (1964). The influence of actinomycin-D on brain RNA synthesis and on memory. *J. Neurochem.*, **11,** 187
125. Bondy, S. C. (1966). The ribonucleic acid metabolism of the brain. *J. Neurochem.*, **13,** 955
126. Hyden, H. and Lange, P. W. (1965). A differentiation in RNA response in neurons early and late during learning. *Proc. Nat. Acad. Sci. USA*, **353,** 946
127. Faiszt, J. and Adam, G. (1968). Role of different RNA reactions from the brain in transfer effect. *Nature (London)*, **220,** 367
128. Glassman, E. (1969). The biochemistry of learning: an evaluation of the role of RNA and protein. *Ann. Rev. Biochem.*, **38,** 605
129. Parker, E. S., Alkana, R. L., Birnbaum, I. M., Hartley, J. T. and Noble, E. P. (1974). Alcohol and the disruption of cognitive processes. *Arch. Gen. Psychiatry*, **31,** 824
130. Jones, B. and Parsons, O. A. (1971). Impaired abstracting ability in chronic alcoholics. *Arch. Gen. Psychiatry*, **24,** 71
131. Parsons, O. A. (1974). Brain damage in alcoholics: altered states of unconsciousness. Paper presented at the *20th International Institute of the Prevention and Treatment of Alcoholism, Manchester, England,* **June 24–28, 1974**
132. Goodwin, D. W. (1971). Blackouts and alcohol-induced memory dysfunction. In N. K. Mello and J. H. Mendelson, eds. *Recent Advances in Studies of Alcoholism*, p. 508. Washington, D.C.: U.S. Government Printing Office
133. Freund, G. (1970). Impairment of shock avoidance learning after long-term alcohol ingestion in mice. *Science*, **168,** 1599
134. Freund, G. (1973). The prevention of ethanol withdrawal seizures in mice by lidocaine. *Neurology*, **23,** 91
135. Chang, T. , Lewis, J. and Glazko, A. J. (1967). Effect of ethanol and other alcohols on the transport of amino acids and glucose by everted sacs of rat small intestine. *Biochim. Biophys. Acta*, **135,** 1000
136. Israel, Y., Salazar, I. and Rosenmann, E. (1968). Inhibitory effects of alcohol on intestinal amino acid transport *in vivo* and *in vitro*. *J. Nutr.*, **96,** 499
137. Freund, G. (1972). The effect of ethanol and ageing on the transport of α-aminoisobutyric acid into the brain. *Brain Res.*, **46,** 363
138. Roach, M. K. (1970). The effect of ethanol on the synthesis of amino acids from glucose in hamster brain. *Life Sci.*, **9: Part II,** 437
139. Häkkinen, H.-M. and Kulonen, E. (1967). Amino acid metabolism in various fractions of rat-brain homogenates with special reference to the effect of ethanol. *Biochem. J.*, **105,** 261
140. Häkkinen, H.-M. and Kulonen, E. (1972). Ethanol and the metabolic interactions of carbohydrates and amino acids in brain preparations. *Biochem. Pharmacol.* **21,** 1171

141. Kuriyama, K., Sze, P. Y. and Rauscher, G. E. (1971). Effects of acute and chronic ethanol administration on ribosomal protein synthesis in mouse brain and liver. *Life Sci.*, **10: Part II,** 181
142. Choy, O. G., Ford, D. H. and Rhines, R. K. (1972). The effect of ethanol anesthesia on the accumulation of [^{3}H]lysine into different brain regions, plasma, muscle and liver in the rat. *Acta Neurol. Scand.*, **48,** 341
143. Jarlstedt, J. and Hamberger, A. (1972). Experimental alcoholism in rats. Effect of acute ethanol intoxication on the *in vitro* incorporation of [^{3}H]leucine into neuronal and glial proteins. *J. Neurochem.*, **19,** 2299
144. Jarlstedt, J. (1972). Experimental alcoholism in rats: protein synthesis in subcellular fractions from cerebellum, cerebral cortex and liver after long-term treatment. *J. Neurochem.*, **19,** 603
145. Friedhoff, A. J. and Miller, J. A. (1973). Effect of ethanol on biosynthesis of dopamine. *Ann. N.Y. Acad. Sci.*, **215,** 183
146. Noble, E. P. and Tewari, S. (1972). The effects of chronic ethanol ingestion on the protein-synthesizing system of C57BL/6J mice. In O. Forsander and K. Eriksson, eds. *Biological Aspects of Alcohol Consumption,* Vol. 20, p. 273. Helsinki: The Finnish Foundation for Alcohol Studies
147. Noble, E. P. and Tewari, S. (1973). Protein and ribonucleic acid metabolism in brains of mice following chronic alcohol consumption. *Ann. N.Y. Acad. Sci.*, **215,** 333
148. Tewari, S. and Noble, E. P. (1971). Ethanol and brain protein synthesis. *Brain Res.*, **26,** 469
149. Tewari, S. and Noble, E. P. (1975). Chronic ethanol ingestion by rodents: effects on brain RNA. In M. A. Rothschild, M. Oratz, and S. S. Schreiber, eds. *Alcohol and Abnormal Protein Biosynthesis*, p. 421. New York: Pergamon Press (In press)
150. Noble, E. P. and Tewari, S. (1975). Ethanol and brain ribosomes. *Fed. Proc.*, **34,** 1942
151. Fleming, E. W., Tewari, S. and Noble, E. P. (1975). Effects of ethanol ingestion on brain aminoacyl-tRNA. *J. Neurochem.*, **24,** 553
152. Lieber, C. S. and De Carli, L. M. (1973). Ethanol dependence and tolerance: a nutritionally controlled experimental model in the rat. *Res. Commun. Chem. Pathol. Pharmacol.*, **6,** 983
153. Wallgren, H., Kosyen, A. -L. and Ahtee, L. (1972). Techniques for producing an alcohol-withdrawal syndrome in rats. Paper presented at the joint meeting of the *European Brain and Behaviour Society and Israel Center for Psychobiology, Jerusalem,* **April, 18–19, 1972**
154. Tewari, S., Goldstein, M. A. and Noble, E. P. (1975). Unpublished findings
155. Tewari, S. and Noble, E. P. (1975). Alteration in cerebral polynucleotide metabolism following chronic ethanol ingestion. In M. Gross, ed. *Advances in Experimental Medicine and Biology, Vol. 59*, p. 37. New York: Plenum Press
156. Tewari, S., Fleming, E. W. and Noble, E. P. (1975). Alterations in brain RNA metabolism following chronic ethanol ingestion. *J. Neurochem.*, **24,** 561
157. Gabrielli, F. and Baglioni, C. (1974). Translation of histone messenger RNA by homologus cell-free systems from synchronized HeLa cells. *Eur. J. Biochem.*, **42,** 121
158. Adesnik, M., Salditt, M., Thomas, W. and Darnell, J. E. (1972). Evidence that all messenger RNA molecules (except histone messenger RNA) contain poly (A) sequences and that the poly (A) has a nuclear function. *J. Mol. Biol.*, **71,** 21
159. Mendecki, J., Lee, S. Y. and Brawerman, G. (1972). Characteristics of polyadenylic acid segment associated with messenger ribonucleic acid in mouse sarcoma 180 ascites cells. *Biochemistry,* **11,** 792
160. Quastel, J. H. (1965). Effects of drugs on metabolism of the brain *in vitro. Br. Med. Bull.*, **21,** 49
161. Meyer, K. H. (1937). Contributions to the theory of narcosis. *Trans. Faraday Soc.*, **33,** 1062

162. Overton, E. (1901). *Studien uber die Narkose: zugleich ein Beitrag zur allgemeinen Pharmakologie,* Jena: Verlag von Gustaf Fisher
163. Ferguson, J. (1939). The use of chemical potentials as indices of toxicity. *Proc. R. Soc. Lond. (Biol.),* **127,** 387
164. Mullins, L. J. (1954). Some physical mechanisms in narcosis. *Chem. Rev.,* **54,** 289
165. Miller, K. W., Patton, W. D. M. and Smith, E. B. (1965). Site of action of general anesthetics. *Nature (London),* **206,** 574
166. Metcalfe, J. C., Seeman, P. and Burgen, A. S. V. (1968). The proton relaxation of benzyl alcohol in erythrocyte membranes. *Mol. Pharmacol.,* **4,** 87
167. Johnson, S. M. and Bangham, A. D. (1969). The action of anesthetics on phospholipid membranes. *Biochim. Biophys. Acta,* **193,** 92
168. Paterson, S. J., Butler, K. W., Huang, P., Labelle, J., Smith, I. C. P. and Schneider, A. (1972). The effects of alcohols on lipid bilayers: a spin label study. *Biochim. Biophys. Acta,* **266,** 597
169. Trudell, J. R., Hubbell, W. L. and Cohen, E. N. (1973). The effect of two inhalation anesthetics on the order of spin-labeled phospholipid vesicles. *Biochim. Biophys. Acta,* **291,** 321
170. Gage, P. W., McBurney, R. N. and Van Helden, D. (1974). Endplate currents are shortened by octanol: possible role of membrane lipid. *Life Sci.,* **14,** 2277
171. Noble, E. P., Syapin, P. J., Vigran, R., Gombos, G., Vincendon, G. and Rosenberg, A. (1975). The effects of ethanol on neuraminidase releasable sialic acid of cultured neural cells. Paper presented at the *5th International Meeting of the International Society for Neurochemistry, Barcelona, Spain,* **September 2–6**
172. Bangham, A. D., Standish, M. M. and Miller, N. G. A. (1965). Cation permeability of phospholipid model membranes: effect of narcosis. *Nature (London),* **208,** 1295
173. Johnson, S. M. and Bangham, A. D. (1969). The action of anesthetics on phospholipid membranes. *Biochim. Biophys. Acta,* **193,** 92
174. Hill, M. W. (1974). The Gibbs-free energy hypothesis of general anesthesia. In M. J. Halsey, J. A. Sutton and R. A. Miller, eds. *Molecular Mechanisms of General Anesthesia,* p. 132. Edinburgh: Churchill, Livingston
175. Hill, M. W. and Bangham, A. D. (1975). General depressant drug dependency: a biophysical hypothesis. In M. Gross, ed. *Advances in Experimental Medicine and Biology, Vol. 59,* p. 1. New York: Plenum Press
176. Seeman, P. (1974). The actions of nervous system drugs on cell membranes. *Hospital Practice,* **Sept.,** 93
177. Seeman, P. (1974). The membrane expansion theory of anesthesia: direct evidence using ethanol and a high-precision density meter. *Experientia,* **30,** 759
178. Seeman, P. (1972). The membrane actions of anesthetics and tranquilizers. *Pharmacol. Rev.,* **24,** 583
179. Albers, R. W. (1967). Biochemical aspect of active transport. *Ann. Rev. Biochem.,* **36,** 727
180. Whittman, R. and Wheeler, K. P. (1970). Transport across cell membranes. *Ann. Rev. Physiol.,* **32,** 21
181. Jarnefelt, J. (1961). Inhibition of the brain microsomal adenosinetriphosphatase by depolarizing agents. *Biochim. Biophys. Acta,* **48,** 111
182. Israel, Y., Kalant, H. and Laufer, I. (1965). Effects of ethanol on [Na^+, K^+, Mg^{++}]-stimulated microsomal ATPase activity. *Biochem. Pharmacol.,* **14,** 1803
183. Israel, Y. and Salazar, I. (1967). Inhibition of brain microsomal adenosine triphosphatases by general depressants. *Arch. Biochem. Biophys.,* **122,** 310
184. Sun, A. Y. and Samorajski, T. (1975). The effects of age and alcohol on [$Na^+ + K^+$]-ATPase activity of whole homogenate and synaptosomes prepared from mouse and human brain. *J. Neurochem.,* **24,** 161
185. Wallgren, H. and Barry, H., III. (1970). *Actions of Alcohol, Vol. 1, Biochemical, Physiological, and Psychological Aspects,* p. 273. Amsterdam: Elsevier

186. Keesey, J. C., Wallgren, H. and McIlwain, H. (1965). The sodium potassium and chloride of cerebral tissues: maintenance, change on stimulation and subsequent recovery. *Biochem. J.*, **95**, 289
187. Wallgren, H., Nikander, P., von Boguslawsky, P. and Linkola, J. (1974). Effects of ethanol, *tert.* butanol, and clomethiazole on net movements of sodium and potassium in electrically stimulated cerebral tissue. *Acta Physiol. Scand.*, **91**, 83
188. Moore, J. W. and Narahashi, T. (1967). Tetrodotoxin's highly selective blockage of an ionic channel. *Fed. Proc.*, **26**, 1655
189. Hille, B. (1970). Ionic channels in nerve membranes. *Prog. Biophys. Mol. Biol.*, **21**, 1
190. Armstrong, C. M. (1971). Interaction of tetraethylammonium ion derivatives with the potassium channels of giant axons. *J. Gen. Physiol.*, **58**, 513
191. Rojas, E. and Armstrong, C. (1971). Sodium conductance activation without inactivation in pronase-perfused axons. *Nature* (*New Biol.*), **229**, 177
192. Israel, Y., Kalant, H., LeBlanc, A. E., Bernstein, J. C. and Salazar, I. (1970). Changes in cation transport and [Na^+ + K^+]-activated adenosine triphosphatase produced by chronic administration of ethanol. *J. Pharmacol. Exp. Ther.*, **174**, 330
193. Israel, M. A. and Kuriyama, K. (1971). Effects of *in vivo* ethanol administration on adenosinetriphosphatase activity of subceullar fractions of mouse brain and liver. *Life Sci.*, **10: Part II**, 591
194. Know, W. H., Perrin, R. G. and Sen, A. K. (1972). Effect of chronic administration of ethanol on [Na^+ + K^+]-activated ATPase activity in six areas of the cat brain. *J. Neurochem.* **19**, 2881
195. Roach, M. K., Khan, M. M., Coffman, R., Pennington, W. and Davis, D. L. (1973). Brain [Na^+ + K^+]-activated adenosine triphosphatase activity and neurotransmitter uptake in alcohol-dependent rats. *Brain Res.*, **63**, 323
196. Wallgren, H., Nikander, P. and Virtanen, P. (1975). Ethanol-induced changes in cation stimulated adenosine triphosphatase activity and lipid-proteolipid labeling of brain microsomes. In M. Gross, ed., *Advances in Experimental Medicine and Biology*, *Vol. 59*, 23. New York: Plenum Press
197. Syapin, P. J., Stefanovic, V., Ciesielski-Treska, J., Mandel, P. and Noble, E. P. (1975). The effects of ethanol on growth and on ecto-enzymatic activity of cultured cells. Paper presented at the *5th International Meeting of the International Society for Neurochemistry, Barcelona, Spain,* **September 2–6**
198. Akera, T., Rech, R. H., Marquins, W. J., Tobin, T. and Brody, T. M. (1973). Lack of relationship between brain [Na^+ + K^+]-activated adenosine triphosphatase and the development of tolerance to ethanol in rats. *J. Pharmacol. Exp. Ther.*, **185**, 594
199. Goldstein, D. B. and Israel, Y. (1972). Effects of ethanol on mouse brain [Na^+ + K^+]-activated adenosine triphosphatase. *Life Sci.*, **11: Part II**, 957
200. Goldstein, D. B. and Goldstein, A. (1961). Possible role of enzyme inhibition and repression in drug tolerance and addiction. *Biochem. Pharmacol.*, **8**, 48
201. Shuster, L. (1961). Repression and de-repression of enzyme synthesis as a possible explanation of some aspects of drug action. *Nature* (*London*), **189**, 314
202. Sutherland, E. W. and Rall, T. W. (1960). The relation of adenosine-3′,5′-phosphate and phosphorylase to the actions of catecholamines and other hormones. *Pharmacol. Rev.*, **12**, 265
203. Butcher, R. W., Robison, G. A., Hardman, J. G. and Sutherland, E. W. (1968). The role of cyclic AMP in hormone actions. *Adv. Enzyme Regul.*, **6**, 357
204. Breckenridge, B. McL. (1970). Cyclic AMP and drug action. *Ann. Rev. Pharmacol.*, **10**, 19
205. Bloom, F. E., Hoffer, B. J. and Siggins, G. R. (1972). Norepinephrine-mediated cerebellar synapses: a model system for neuropsychopharmacology. *Biol. Psychiatry*, **4**, 157
206. Greengard, P., McAfee, D. A. and Kebabian, J. E. (1972). On the mechanism of action of cyclic AMP and its role in synaptic transmission. *Adv. Cyclic Nucleotide Res.*, **1**, 337

207. McAfee, D. A. and Greengard, P. (1972). Adenosine 3′,5′-monophosphate: electrophysiological evidence for a role in synaptic transmission. *Science*, **178**, 310
208. Kebabian, J. W., Petzold, G. L. and Greengard, P. (1972). Dopamine-sensitive adenylate cyclase in caudate nucleus of rat brain and its similarity to the 'dopamine receptor'. *Proc. Nat. Acad. Sci. USA*, **69**, 2145
209. Siggins, G. R., Hoffer, R. J. and Bloom, F. E. (1969). Cyclic adenosine monophosphate possible mediator for norepinephrine effects on cerebellar Purkinje cells. *Science*, **165**, 1018
210. Noble, E. P. (1973). Alcohol and adrenocortical function of animals and man. In P. G. Bourne and R. Fox, eds. *Alcoholism: Progress in Research and Treatment*, p. 105. New York: Academic Press
211. Israel, M. A., Kimura, H. and Kuriyama, K. (1972). Changes in activity and hormonal sensitivity of brain adenyl cyclase following chronic ethanol administration. *Experientia*, **28**, 1322
212. Kuriyama, K. and Israel, M. A. (1973). Effect of ethanol administration on cyclic 3′,5′-adenosine monophosphate metabolism in brain. *Biochem. Pharmacol.*, **22**, 2919
213. Naito, K. and Kuriyama, K. (1973). Effect of morphine administration on adenyl cyclase and 3′,5′-cyclic nucleotide phosphodiesterase activities in brain. *Jap. J. Pharmacol.*, **23**, 274
214. Volicer, L. and Gold, B. I. (1973). Effect of ethanol on cyclic AMP levels in the rat brain. *Life Sci.*, **13**, 269
215. Eidelberg, E., Bond, M. L. and Kelter, A. (1971). Effects of alcohol on cerebellar and vestibular neurones. *Arch. Intern. Pharmacodyn. Ther.*, **192**, 213
216. Siggins, G. R., Oliver, A. P., Hoffer, B. J. and Bloom, F. E. (1971). Cyclic adenosine monophosphate and norepinephrine: effect on transmembrane properties of cerebellar Purkinje cells. *Science*, **171**, 192

7
The Effect of Alcohol on Striated and Smooth Muscle

S. A. GELLER and E. RUBIN

7.1 INTRODUCTION 188
7.2 ALCOHOLIC CARDIOMYOPATHY 188
7.2.1 *Clinical aspects* 188
7.2.1.1 Preclinical alcoholic cardiomyopathy 189
7.2.1.2 Acute cardiac disease in chronic alcoholics 189
7.2.1.3 Chronic alcoholic cardiomyopathy 190
7.2.2 *Pathology* 192
7.2.2.1 Gross pathology 192
7.2.2.2 Microscopic pathology 192
7.2.2.3 Electronmicroscopy 192
7.2.2.4 Cardiac triglycerides 194
7.2.2.5 Functional studies 195
7.3 ALCOHOLIC MYOPATHY 196
7.3.1 *Clinical aspects* 197
7.3.1.1 Subclinical alcoholic myopathy 197
7.3.1.2 Acute alcoholic myopathy 198
7.3.1.3 Chronic alcoholic myopathy 198
7.3.2 *Pathology* 199
7.3.2.1 Subclinical myopathy 199
7.3.2.2 Acute alcoholic myopathy 199
7.3.2.3 Chronic alcoholic myopathy 200
7.3.3 *Electronmicroscopy* 200
7.3.3.1 Acute alcoholic myopathy 200
7.3.3.2 Chronic alcoholic myopathy 201
7.3.3.3 Experimental studies 202
7.4 SMOOTH MUSCLE 204
7.5 SUMMARY 205
References 205

Who hath wounds without cause? .....
They that tarry long at the wine
Proverbs 23:29

7.1 INTRODUCTION

The association of alcohol abuse and liver injury was well known before the time of Hippocrates. By contrast, clinical recognition of disease involving the heart or skeletal muscle due to excess alcohol consumption is less than 150 years old. In this paper we review the historical, clinical, morphological and experimental aspects of alcoholic cardiomyopathy and myopathy, together with the effects of alcohol on smooth muscle.

7.2 ALCOHOLIC CARDIOMYOPATHY

The current concept of a primary myocardial disease associated with chronic abuse of alcoholic beverages was developed in the last two decades[1–4], a century after Wood[5] first suggested alcohol ingestion as a contributing factor. A number of investigators in the late nineteenth century also considered chronic alcohol consumption as a possible cause of heart disease, and Strumpell's description in 1890[6] of the heart at autopsy is in keeping with those cases we now recognize as alcoholic cardiomyopathy. Steel, in 1893, described 25 cases of heart failure that he ascribed to chronic alcoholism and stated: 'Not only do I now recognize alcoholism as one of the causes of muscle failure of the heart, but I find it to be comparatively a common one'[7]. Despite these reports the importance of alcoholic heart disease was not widely appreciated. The delay in the recognition of alcohol as a cardiotoxin may have been caused by the occurrence of thiamine deficiency among chronic alcoholics, with the resultant development of beriberi heart disease[4,8–12]. Chronic alcoholics with cardiomyopathy were considered to have nutritional heart disease, and the possible effects of alcohol were often overlooked, even though many of the cases did not respond to the administration of thiamine. Occasionally an alcoholic patient may manifest a cardiomyopathy that is both thiamine-dependent (alcoholic beriberi) and thiamine-independent (alcoholic cardiomyopathy)[13]. The absence of nutritional deficiency or hepatic disease in chronic alcoholics with cardiac dysfunction was clearly documented by Eliaser and Giansiracusa[1]. It now appears clear that alcohol exerts a direct effect on the myocardium[14–17] and that alcoholic cardiomyopathy is produced by chronic damage to the myocardium[12].

7.2.1 Clinical aspects

The typical patient with the condition is male, in the third to the sixth decade of life, and has generally been drinking an excess of alcoholic beverages for more than 10 years[2,4,10,11,15,18–26]. The onset of disease is often gradual, manifesting as both left and right-sided congestive heart failure, with a rapid pulse and narrowed pulse pressure. The diastolic blood pressure is somewhat elevated. Neck veins are distended, the heart is enlarged, and a protodiastolic gallop rhythm is heard. Pulmonary and peripheral edema may be present, while evidence of hepatic disease is usually absent. In some instances the onset may be sudden, or the previously gradual onset of signs and symptoms may suddenly be exacerbated[4,20,27,28]. This acute alcohol-induced cardiomyopathy is distinct from that encountered in the epidemics of fulminant heart disease which occurred in beer drinkers during the fall and winter of 1965–66[29–31]. That syndrome was directly related to a toxic effect of cobalt sulphate, which had been added to the beer during its manufacture[32]. Beer drinkers' cardiomyopathy has been reviewed elsewhere[33,34].

7.2.1.1 *Preclinical alcoholic cardiomyopathy*

It has been apparent in recent years that morphological and physiological alterations of the myocardium in chronic alcoholics may precede the development of the clinical signs and symptoms of myocardial damage. Haemodynamic studies of right ventricular function were not remarkable in 17 alcoholics without cardiomyopathy[35]. In a later study two of eleven chronic alcoholics, all without clinical heart disease or abnormal results of haemodynamic studies, had electrocardiographic changes after the ingestion of alcohol[36]. In contrast to studies in which objective evidence of altered cardiac haemodynamics was not demonstrated, Spodick found abnormal results of cardiac function tests in chronic alcoholics without overt heart disease[37]. The results in the alcoholics were similar to, but less severe than, those in a group of patients with alcoholic cardiomyopathy. The preinjection period and ejection time of the left ventricle were both prolonged in the group of chronic alcoholics without symptoms or signs of heart disease. A similar study of chronic alcoholics without objective evidence of heart disease, but with unexplained symptoms (fatigue, dyspnea on exertion, non-specific chest pain), demonstrated elevated mean left ventricular end-diastolic pressure, low mean cardiac output, and depressed myocardial contractility[38].

7.2.1.2 *Acute cardiac disease in chronic alcoholics*

The great majority of patients in whom indiscreet use of alcoholic beverages leads to cardiac disease present[5] with gradually occurring signs and symptoms. In some, however, an acute illness develops, which may mimic coronary artery disease[27,28]. Angina at rest (Prinzmetal variant angina) was directly associated with alcohol ingestion in a 47-year-old man in whom coronary angiography revealed coronary artery disease[27]. Saphenous vein bypass grafts resulted in complete relief of alcohol-related symptoms. Regan *et al.* described seven chronic alcoholics who presented with the typical syndrome of acute myocardial infarction[28]. The patients were all between 34 and 50 years of age, and histories of alcoholism ranged from 15 to 20 years. Three patients died within the year, and four underwent coronary arteriography. No obstructive lesions of the coronary arteries could be documented in any patient. Interstitial fibrosis around intramural coronary arteries was found, and was interpreted as secondary to chronic ethanol consumption. The authors suggested that this fibrosis may limit vasodilation during periods when high coronary flow is required, and thus lead to myocardial infarction.

7.2.1.3 Chronic alcoholic cardiomyopathy

Alcoholic cardiomyopathy has been the subject of many clinical reports[1–4,9–15,17,21–28,35–47] and numerous reviews[16,18,19,48–51]. The incidence of alcoholic cardiomyopathy is difficult to ascertain. Eliaser and Giansiracusa found electrocardiographic changes and/or evidence of left ventricular enlargement in more than half of the 94 chronic alcoholics they evaluated[1]. Evidence of myocardial disease was similarly found in 63 % of chronic alcoholics admitted to a psychiatric ward[24]. In hearts of chronic alcoholics studied at autopsy, cardiomegaly was documented in more than 90 % of cases, and irregular myocardial fibrosis in more than 85 %[42,46]. Death from clinically obvious myocardial disease occurred in 8.5 to 15 % of the chronic alcoholics studied. However, alcoholic cardiomyopathy is not an inevitably fatal condition and improvement frequently follows abstinence from alcohol, particularly in those patients in whom cardiac symptoms are of recent onset[47].

Most patients present with a syndrome of heart failure, most often right-sided[4,9–11,13,20,22–25,35,38,39,41,42,45,47,52,53]. The illness is often heralded by insidious or abrupt shortness of breath or cough[52]. These symptoms may spontaneously improve[2,39]. Edema of lower extremities follows, and may be the dominant complaint[4,10,11,13,20,39,47]. Fatigue on effort is more common than in other forms of heart failure[2,9,10,39] a finding which suggests the possibility of concomitant myopathy. Palpitations, either in association with sinus rhythm or atrial fibrillation are common[2,9,10,20,39,47]. Chest pain has been emphasized in many reports[2,4,9,10,20,22,35,41,47,53], but was conspicuously absent in one large series[52]. Some patients have occasional haemoptysis[4,10,47]. Although evidence of hepatic disease is said usually to be absent[12,54], many cases of alcoholic cardiomyopathy with fatty liver or cirrhosis are reported[10,42,46,52].

Cardiomegaly is almost universal[2,9,10,22,24,41,42,47,52]. Distended neck veins, pulmonary rales, hepatomegaly and peripheral edema reflect the heart failure[2,4,10,52]. The gallop rhythm tends to disappear with clinical improvement, and may be accompanied by a reduction in heart size, or slowing of the cardiac rate[52]. Blood pressure may be low, normal, or elevated and the pulse is characteristically weak and sometimes difficult to palpate[2,52]. Systolic murmurs may be heard[10,47,52]. Venous pressure is elevated although circulation time may be normal or shortened[10,52]. Cardiomegaly of varying degrees is usually confirmed on chest roentgenograms[2,4,9,10,20,22–24,39,41,47,52], although cardiomyopathy may rarely occur without cardiomegaly[38]. Enlargement usually reflects ventricular and atrial hypertrophy and, in addition, prominence of the aortic and pulmonary arteries may be seen[41,52]. Pulmonary congestion, hydrothorax and pericardial effusion are often demonstrable[2,41,52], and may persist even after adequate therapy results in improvement of myocardial status[41].

Electrocardiographic findings in chronic alcoholics are varied[1,3,4,9,10,20,39,41,52,55] and include disturbances of cardiac rhythm and conduction[3,20,24–26,39,47]. Infrequently, the electrocardiographic pattern may be normal in a patient with cardiomyopathy[4,38]. In chronic alcoholics in whom the electrocardiograph has been normal the acute ingestion of alcohol may induce flattening and inversion of T waves[36]. Seelig has pointed to similarities between the electrocardiographs of alcoholics and those seen in human and experimental forms of magnesium depletion[56], and, in some cases, the electrocardiographic abnormalities were reported to have improved after magnesium was administered[57]. By contrast, no electrocardiographic correlation could be made with the level of serum magnesium in dogs rendered severely hypomagnesaemic[58].

Cardiac dynamics have been evaluated in many chronic alcoholics using cardiac catheterization techniques[2,10,13,15,17,37,38,42,45,52,59,63]. In cardiomyopathy without associated beriberi heart disease, cardiac output is usually decreased[2,10,13,38,42,52,59–63]. Right atrial pressure, wedged pulmonary artery pressure[2] and right and left ventricular diastolic and systolic pressures may be increased[2,10,38,63], and the isometric phase of left ventricular contraction may be prolonged[45]. This latter finding has been reported in rats chronically intoxicated with alcohol[64].

An increase in the concentration of mitochondrial-derived enzymes, isocitric and malic dehydrogenase, was found in coronary sinus blood of alcoholic subjects consuming large amounts of alcohol, whether or not clinical manifestations of heart disease were present[35]. Potassium and phosphates were elevated in coronary sinus blood, serum transaminase was increased and triglyceride uptake was reduced after alcohol ingestion, both in man[15] and in the dog[65]. Histochemical observations on samples of myocardium obtained at autopsy have similarly documented mitochondrial damage. There was a pronounced decrease in the histochemical reaction for succinic dehydrogenase, isocitric dehydrogenase, and lactic dehydrogenase[40]. Dogs given alcohol for 14 weeks[66] or for several years[50] displayed few changes in functional parameters of the heart. Oxidative enzymes and the respiratory control ratio of mitochondria were decreased. Myocardial ATP content was also reduced. The authors concluded that chronic ethanol acts by damaging cardiac mitochondria.

7.2.2 Pathology

7.2.2.1 Gross pathology

The heart is enlarged in most cases of alcoholic cardiomyopathy[9,10,20,28,39–42,46,52,67]. Reported cardiac weights range up to 1100 g[52]. In most cases left ventricular hypertrophy is conspicuous, but the usual case demonstrates biventricular hypertrophy and dilatation[10,52]. The heart is often pale and flabby[9,20,40]. However, fibrosis frequently imparts a firm consistency[10,39,40,52]. Endocardial mural thrombosis, particularly involving the atria, is common, and systemic emboli may be found[10,20,39,40,52]. Coronary and systemic atherosclerosis is generally mild. Uncommonly, a myocardial infarct, without significant coronary disease, has been described[28].

7.2.2.2 Microscopic pathology

Myocardial fibre hypertrophy and fibrosis are most often seen[20,39–42,46,52,67]. Necrosis is variable[39]. Fatty change may be prominent[9] and fibres may show lipid or glycogen vacuolization[40,42]. Myocytes tend to lose their striations, and nuclei are pyknotic, with varying degrees of inflammatory cell infiltration[46,42]. Fibrosis is characteristically subendocardial, interstitial, and perivascular[46]. Small coronary artery branches may be occluded[20], perhaps as a secondary response to local areas of myocardial degeneration and fibrosis[12] (see Figures 7.1, 7.2 and 7.3).

7.2.2.3 Electronmicroscopy

Ultrastructural changes of the myocardium in alcoholic cardiomyopathy have been studied at autopsy[67,68] or by cardiac biopsy[44,67,69–71] in man and in animals fed diets rich in alcohol[72–74]. Mitochondrial and sacroplasmic swelling in man are frequent[68–70], although evidence of mitochondrial damage was conspicuously lacking in one study[44]. Mitochondria may show degenerative changes with loss of cristae and accumulation of inclusion bodies[68–70]. Undamaged mitochondria were reported to be increased in man[67,69–71] and rats[72]. The sarcoplasmic reticulum is often swollen and vesicular[67–70] and damage to myofibrils may be seen[68]. Glycogen may be dramatically increased[44,67–69,72], perhaps because the systems necessary for glycogen formation remain intact while other systems are damaged[44]. Accumulation of lipids, lipochromes and lysosomes may also be seen[68–70]. Ultrastructural evidence of cardiomyopathy

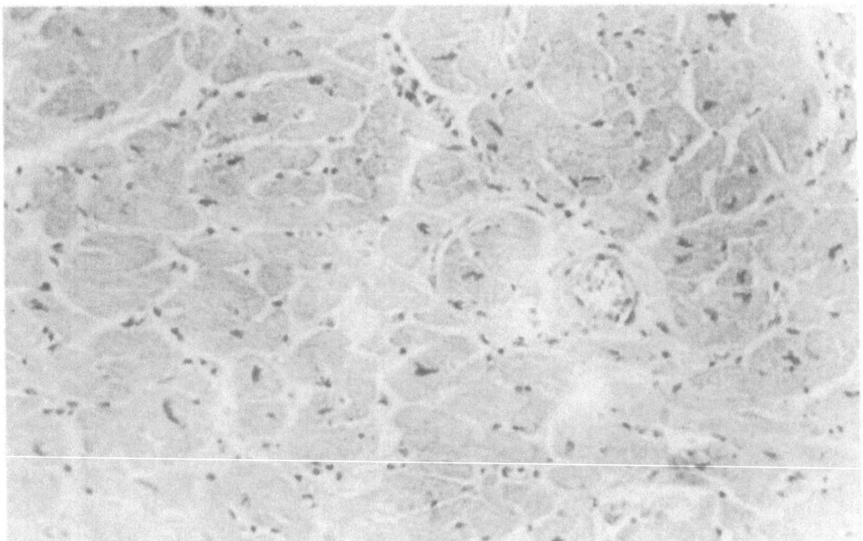

Figure 7.1 Myocardium from a patient with alcoholism without heart failure demonstrates significant accumulation of Alcian Blue material in the interstitium. Alcian positive material was also seen in the myocardium of alcoholics with heart failure

Figures 7.1, 7.2 and 7.3 are courtesy of Dr Timothy Regan of the College of Medicine and Dentistry of New Jersey and are from *Circulation,* **51,** 453 (1975)

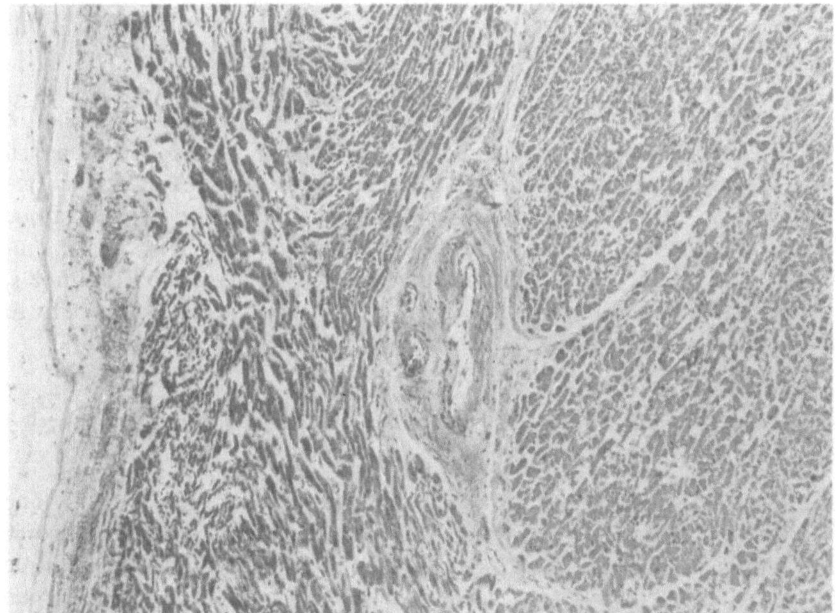

Figure 7.2 This section of left ventricular myocardium from an area of the muscle in an alcoholic patient who had had acute infarction shows concentric periarterial fibrosis

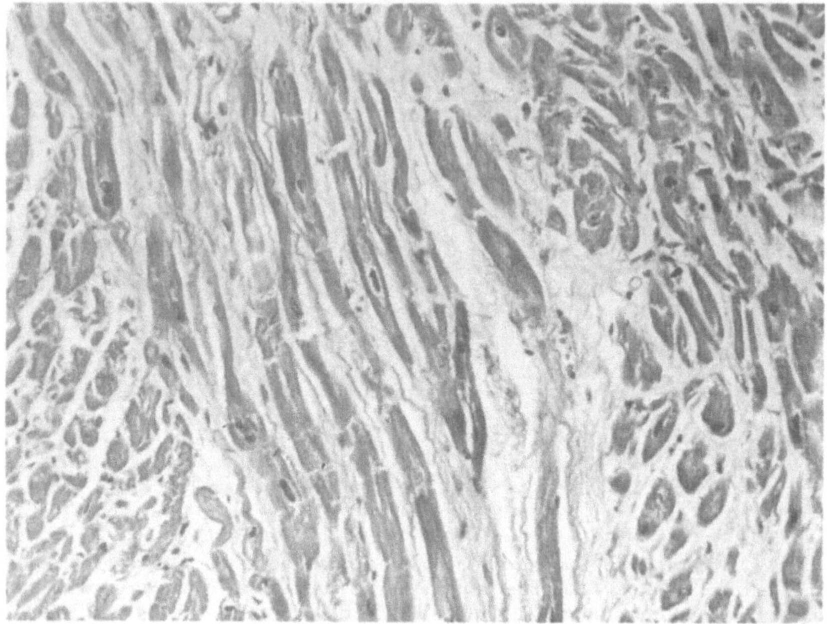

Figure 7.3 More extensive fibrosis is seen with infiltrates of collagen between myofibres and loss of contractile units

was found in a chronic alcoholic who had been clinically without evidence of heart disease, and who had a normal electrocardiogram[75]. The morphological changes in this case were similar to those in fatal cases of alcoholic cardiomyopathy[68–70]. Although the ultrastructural changes observed in alcoholic cardiomyopathy have been reported experimentally[72,73,76,77], most investigators have found few morphological alterations in experimental animals, and those that have been demonstrated were not comparable in severity to those in alcoholics with alcoholic cardiomyopathy[78].

7.2.2.4 Cardiac triglycerides

Ingestion of ethanol by rats for 24 days doubled cardiac triglycerides[79]. The increase in cardiac triglycerides (350 %) was confirmed in dogs given chronic alcohol administration for 10 weeks[80]. Infusion of ethanol into rabbits led to a doubling in heart triglyceride content, whereas norepinephrine had no effect[81]. In this study lipoprotein lipase activity of the heart was unchanged[81]. The accumulation of triglycerides was said not to involve the activity of cardiac lipoprotein lipase, since this activity is increased after acute ethanol intoxication[82]. Fatty acid oxidation was decreased in the heart, whereas fatty acid esterification was increased. The authors concluded that the increase in cardiac triglycerides results from decreased fatty acid oxidation rather than increased triglyceride uptake or fatty acid synthesis. The accumulation of fatty acids in the heart after chronic ethanol ingestion in rats was characterized by an increase in linoleic acid and a decrease in arachidonic acid[83]. These changes are not caused by the metabolism of ethanol, since the heart does not appear to metabolize ethanol[84,85].

Webb *et al.* suggested that the effects of alcohol on the heart represented secondary effects of alcohol intoxication, because alcohol had little effect in an isolated heart–lung preparation[86]. Other investigators suggested on the basis of direct perfusion of the sinus node of anaesthetized dogs that the acute and chronic cardiac effects of alcoholism may be caused, in part, by the release of myocardial norepinephrine by acetaldehyde[87].

7.2.2.5 Functional studies

In acutely intoxicated dogs low concentrations of alcohol had no effect on coronary blood flow, whereas levels over 190 mg per 100 cc increased effective coronary blood flow, but diminished velocity of left ventricular contraction[88]. Infusion of alcohol in dogs significantly increased the work load of the heart, while reducing the coronary flow and functional capacity of the myocardium. This increased the susceptibility to shock in these inebriated animals[89]. In dogs infused with alcohol, cardiac output declined, while coronary vascular resistance fell. However, despite the decrease in cardiac output, myocardial oxygen consumption increased, suggesting that alcohol exerted a direct effect on the myocardium[90]. The function of the left ventricle was diminished as shown by a decline in stroke output and a rise in end-diastolic pressure in dogs infused with alcohol. A direct negative ionotropic effect on the left ventricle of dogs infused with ethanol was found, which was more marked in the presence of autonomic blockade. The effect, however, was small in the absence of this blockade[91]. Depression of ventricular dynamics by infusions of alcohol in dogs was reversed by ouabain[92]. Perfusion of guinea-pig hearts *in vitro* with ethanol did not alter cardiac function or protein synthesis in the myocardium. By contrast, acetaldehyde produced a positive chronotropic and ionotropic effect on the perfused heart and decreased protein synthesis in the myocardium[93].

A negative ionotropic effect of alcohol was claimed by Nakano and Moore[94] and confirmed by Fisher and Kavaler[95], who showed the effect, in the frog, to be due to shortening of the action potential and lowering of its plateau, and, in the cat, due to direct effect of alcohol on the contractile mechanism. *In vitro,* low concentrations of ethanol depressed the contractility of rat atrium, the effect being reversible when ethanol was removed. The action potential was shortened, simultaneous with the reduction in contractility, owing to a more rapid rate of repolarization[96]. In rats given alcohol chronically for 4 months a decrease in potential ventricular contractile force was reported[64].

Few studies have been carried out on the effects of ethanol on the organelles of heart muscle cells. Ethanol, *in vitro,* was shown to inhibit calcium uptake and calcium binding by canine cardiac microsomes[97]. Since the release and uptake of calcium by microsomes modulates myocardial contractility, this effect may play a role in the negative ionotropic effect on ethanol. The effects of ethanol were reversible upon removal of ethanol from the incubation medium. Both ethanol and acetaldehyde, *in vitro*, inhibited the $[Na^+ + K^+]$-activated ATPase of isolated cardiac plasma membranes, suggesting that ethanol may interfere with the transport of ions across the cell membrane[98].

7.3 ALCOHOLIC MYOPATHY

In 1837 James Jackson in commenting on a 'peculiar disease resulting from the use of ardent spirits' described a progressive weakness of the limbs[99]. Despite the resemblance to other forms of paralysis, he suggested that the disorder was due to 'some affection of the muscles'. Magnus Huss, in 1849, described muscular weakness in chronic alcoholics[100]. The illustration in a study of peripheral nerves and muscles in a chronic alcoholic, by Siemerling in 1889, clearly shows a chronic myositis[101]. Gudden, in 1896, described three alcoholics in whom histological changes suggested a myopathy[102]. A half-century passed before Hed, Larssen and Wahlgren reported a 53-year-old alcoholic who developed sudden pain, tenderness and swelling of the legs[103]. This condition resolved spontaneously, but recurred several times during the next 3 years. The patient died 4 days after the onset of severe calf pain and myoglobinuria. At autopsy the muscle fibres of the calf were swollen and fragmented, had lost their striations, and were infiltrated by polymorphonuclear leukocytes.

Hed's (1955) report of acute myoglobinuria renewed interest in the study of myopathy in alcoholics[104], and by 1962 he had collected data on twelve such cases, five of which were fatal[105]. Muscle aching and local tenderness were the most frequent complaints, although some had intense pain. Several of the cases presented with signs and symptoms suggesting the diagnosis of deep-vein thrombosis. Five of the twelve presented in renal failure; myoglobinuria was demonstrated spectrographically in four of these. Varying degrees of muscle damage were seen in muscle biopsies and severe rhabdomyolysis could be demonstrated in all of the muscles studied at autopsy. Ekbom, in 1964, described a condition of insidiously progressive weakness in alcoholics, without evidence of acute disease[106]. Of the sixteen patients, eight were without symptoms of muscle disease. However, evidence of myopathy was demonstrable in all by electromyography and, in some, by muscle biopsy. Several forms of alcoholic myopathy have been recognized in recent years. These have been documented by studies of clinical syndromes, evaluation of muscle function, demonstration in the serum of biochemical abnormalities representative of muscle derangement, studies of muscle metabolism *in vitro,* and morphological studies of the muscles of alcoholics[107–135]. The administration of alcohol with an adequate diet to normal non-alcoholic volunteers resulted in ultrastructural changes of skeletal muscle and increased activity of serum creative phosphokinase (CPK)[136].

7.3.1 Clinical aspects

Alcoholic myopathy may be classified as subclinical, acute, and chronic[137,138].

7.3.1.1 Subclinical alcoholic myopathy

Elevated activity of serum creatine phosphokinase (CPK) is common in chronic alcoholics who do not display other evidence of myopathy[109,114,122,139]. Of the 59 alcholics studied by Perkoff, none of whom had muscular complaints, more than half gave a history of muscle cramps or weakness, and six described episodes of dark urine[120]. In 36 the serum CPK determination was elevated. In addition, the majority displayed a diminished rise in blood lactic acid after ischaemic exercise. Nygren, however, has cast doubt on the specificity of this finding[127]. Dimberg reported raised values for serum CPK, GOT, and GPT after feeding a low carbohydrate diet to alcoholics[118]. In those cases of alcoholic myopathy in which both serum CPK and GOT activities were increased, the latter returned to normal before the former[115]. This pattern of response contrasts with that usually observed in cases of myocardial ischaemia[115]. Combined electromyographic and histological studies were performed on 24 alcoholics without overt evidence of muscle disease[119]. Electromyographic evidence of proximal myopathy was present in almost half, and in most of these biopsy disclosed a myopathy. Muscle action potentials were compared in chronic alcoholics and non-alcoholic individuals[140]. The electromyographically recorded action potentials were significantly shorter in the alcoholics, none of whom had manifestations of muscle disease. Lactic dehydrogenase isoenzyme-5 (LDH-5) may be low in the skeletal muscle of alcoholics[127]. A correlation could not be made between increased serum activity of this isoenzyme and CPK, although skeletal muscle contains predominantly LDH-5[141]. Such a correlation could be found between CPK and LDH-1[127]. Hed *et al.* found elevated serum activity of LDH-1 and LDH-2 in healthy volunteers given alcohol and maintained on a carbohydrate-poor diet, whereas normal levels were found in those volunteers given alcohol and a normal diet, and the authors suggested a nutritional basis for alcoholic myopathy[133]. It has been clearly demonstrated, however, that serum CPK activity may be increased and ultrastructural alterations of skeletal muscle induced in healthy volunteers given alcohol with an entirely adequate diet[136]. Oh reviewed the literature and his own experience, and suggested that subclinical alcoholic myopathy, as manifested by elevation of serum CPK, is present in about 38 % of chronic alcoholics[138]. It is likely that subclinical alcoholic myopathy is a reversible disorder, and that morphological changes in this condition are not permanent[136].

7.3.1.2 Acute alcoholic myopathy

Acute alcoholic myopathy may present only as weakness, without paralysis[120,127,130,142]. On the other hand it may be characterized by the sudden onset of muscular pain or by the rapid progression of a previous chronic myopathy[111,120,126,142,143]. It may be accompanied by myoglobinuria, and may even progress to death[103–105,107,108,111,124,131].

Muscles may be exquisitely tender[105,120], and weakness is often confined to one limb or group of muscles[113,123,130,142], although it may be diffuse[103,126]. A proximal weakness is most common. Rhabdomyolysis may prove life-threatening, and may be complicated by renal failure[131]. Myoglobin is often demonstrable in the urine and/or the serum[107,108,111,117,120,144,145]. The presence of marked swelling of one or more extremities may suggest thrombophlebitis[105,135]. A subnormal blood lactic acid response to ischaemic exercise is a frequent finding[109,129], and electromyographic studies are virtually always abnormal[132].

The signs and symptoms may disappear and complete restoration of function may occur with the cessation of alcohol intake[109,137,138]. Hyperkalaemia is well documented in alcoholics with acute rhabdomyolysis[104,105,107,124,144–146], and is often accompanied by renal failure. Electrocardiographic changes are common and hyperkalaemia has often been incriminated as the direct cause of death. Schneider has suggested that hyperkalaemia may be a non-specific phenomenon following acute necrosis of muscle[144], but this has not been documented in all forms of rhabdomyolysis[147]. The elevated K^+ may reflect renal insufficiency rather than a release of K^+ from damaged muscle cells. Knochel *et al.* have recently reviewed the mechanisms cited as potential bases for muscle injury in chronic alcoholism and have suggested phosphate deficiency as a cause[148].

7.3.1.3 Chronic alcoholic myopathy

Some alcoholics exhibit a gradual, insidious development of muscle weakness, which may be associated with atrophy[104,106,120,126,149], and which may become incapacitating. Muscle involvement is generally symmetrical, and the proximal muscles, particularly those of the lower extremities, are most conspicuously involved. An undetermined number of alcoholics complain of no symptoms, but have evidence of myopathy, demonstrable either by muscle tenderness, by objective evaluation of muscle strength[106], or by various biochemical parameters[150]. Occasionally, episodes of acute myopathy, particularly when precipitated by a drinking spree, will complicate the course of chronic myopathy[120]. Discontinuation of excessive intake of alcohol leads to improvement[109,117,120].

7.3.2 Pathology

7.3.2.1 Subclinical myopathy

Ekbom found only a minor increase in fat between degenerated muscle fibres[106]. These changes were confirmed by others[119] and, in addition, an increased number of sarcolemmal nuclei, vacuolization of fibres, macrophage infiltration, and atrophy of fibres have been described in patients without overt evidence of muscle disease[119,125]. The findings, in the absence of acute inflammation, suggest a recent bout of mild acute myositis.

7.3.2.2 Acute alcoholic myopathy

The histological features of muscle obtained from alcoholics presenting with the acute onset of pain, swelling, and tenderness are particularly dramatic, although not pathognomonic. Muscle swelling, fragmentation of muscle fibres, hyalin and granular degeneration, and loss of striations are features of acute rhabdomyolysis[103,104,106,108,111,121,122,124,139,143,149]. Inflammation with polymorphonuclear leukocytes is uncommon in this condition[103,104,122,124,130,135,139] as it is in other forms of acute rhabdomyolysis[147]. Vacuolization of muscle fibres may occur[106,121,124,126,130,149]. The nuclei are vesicular, and show prominent nucleoli. Increased sarcoplasmic basophilia has been thought to represent regeneratory activity of the muscle[151], but this concept has been questioned[147,152]; basophilia may actually represent muscle injury. In a few instances muscles were re-examined after resolution of the acute myopathic syndrome or at autopsy[104,106,121,149]; Hed found severe rhabdomyolytic changes in muscles of the trunk and neck, as well as the extremities, in a patient who died 3 weeks after biopsy[104]. By contrast, less severe changes were reported in patients whose muscles were restudied 2 weeks[106], 6 weeks[121], and 18 months[149] after initial biopsy. In these studies the major features were fat accumulation, atrophy, and proliferation of sarcolemmal nuclei.

7.3.2.3 Chronic alcoholic myopathy

The histological features of chronic alcoholic myopathy reflect the response of muscle to injury (Figures 7.4 and 7.5). Atrophy of scattered

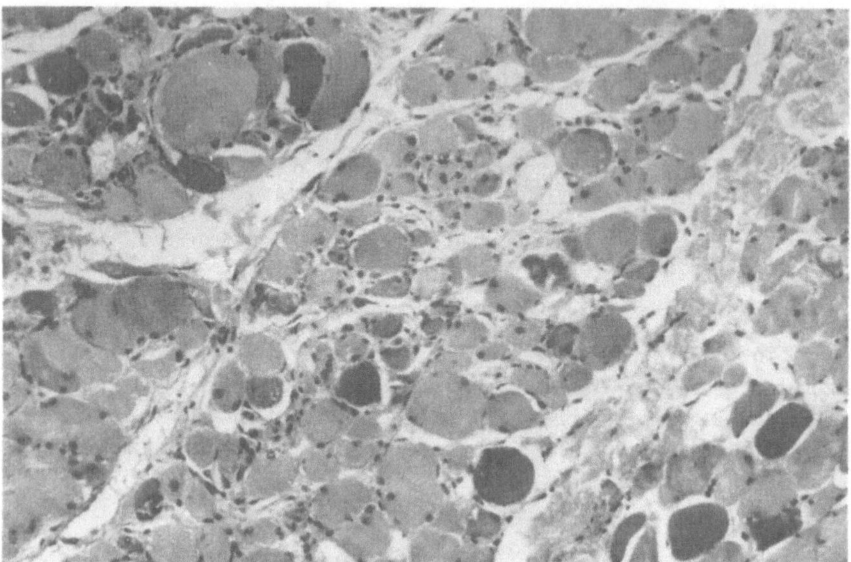

Figure 7.4 Cross-section of muscle biopsy from an alcoholic patient with muscle weakness showing scattered, irregular atrophy of fibres, accumulation of interfibrillar fat, coagulation of many fibres, and focal increase of sarcolemmal nuclei (haematoxylin + eosin × 100)

fibres[104–106,109,117,121,149]; the accumulation of interfibrillar fat[106,119,121,149]; and sarcolemmal nuclear proliferation[109,117,119,121,149] are often seen. Infiltration by macrophages and lymphocytes occurs, but is infrequent[106,117,119], and fibrosis is uncommon in all forms of alcoholic myopathy[144]. In some cases of chronic alcoholic myopathy loss of striations has been described[104,109,119]. Alterations of muscle, at the light microscopic level, are not proportional either to the severity of symptoms or to the degree of muscle weakness. As expected, atrophy is more prevalent in those cases in which weakness has become severe.

7.3.3 Electronmicroscopy

7.3.3.1 Acute alcoholic myopathy

Electronmicroscopic examination of a muscle biopsy obtained during an acute attack in the patient described by Douglas disclosed patchy damage to the cells

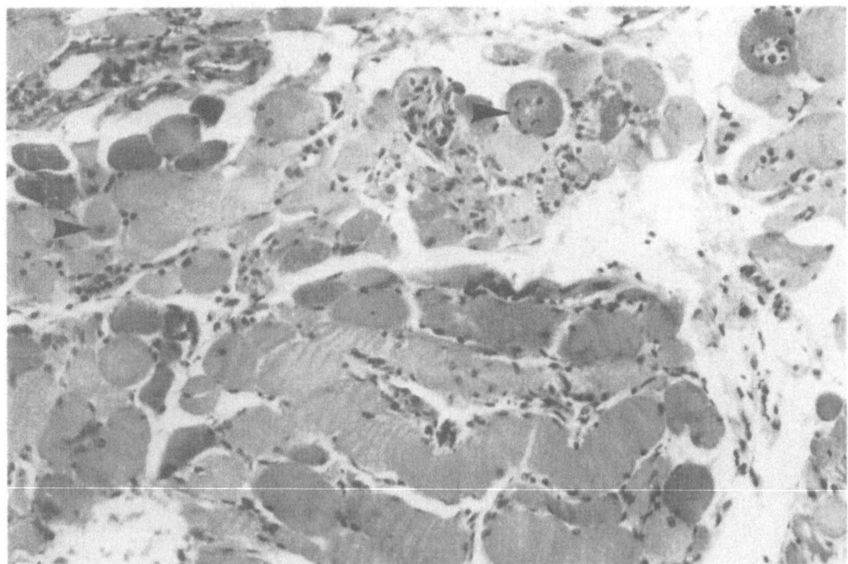

Figure 7.5 Longitudinal and cross-section of muscle biopsy from alcoholic patient with muscle weakness showing loss of striations and coagulative changes of many fibres, with prominent increase in number and size of sarcolemmal nuclei. An occasional internal nucleus is also seen (arrow) (haematoxylin + eosin × 100).

and mitochondria[111] (Figures 7.6 and 7.7). Myofibrils were disordered, entire cells were swollen and a disarray of organelles was noted. Numerous mitochondria were swollen. Endoplasmic reticulum was dilated, and contained fibrillar and granular inclusions. Cell membranes were interrupted, although nuclei and basement membranes remained normal. A second biopsy, 26 days later, while the patient was convalescing, showed only a mild increase in interfibrillar connective tissue. These observations have been confirmed by others[121,124,143]. In addition, changes of the Z, A and I bands have been reported[121,143].

7.3.3.2 Chronic alcoholic myopathy

Klinkerfuss studied five biopsy specimens obtained from chronic alcoholics who displayed weakness, muscle tenderness, and wasting of proximal muscle groups[121]. The myofibrils appeared small, and increased nuclei and intracellular fat droplets were present. Aggregated filaments resembling A band material were seen. Electron-dense mitochondrial inclusions were common, as they were in the study of Fisher *et al.*[153]. These inclusions appeared to arise from the matrix between the inner and outer mitochondrial-limiting membrane, and appeared as rectangles and squares of homogeneous material, or as electron-dense, membrane-bound, rectangular or trapezoidal extensions

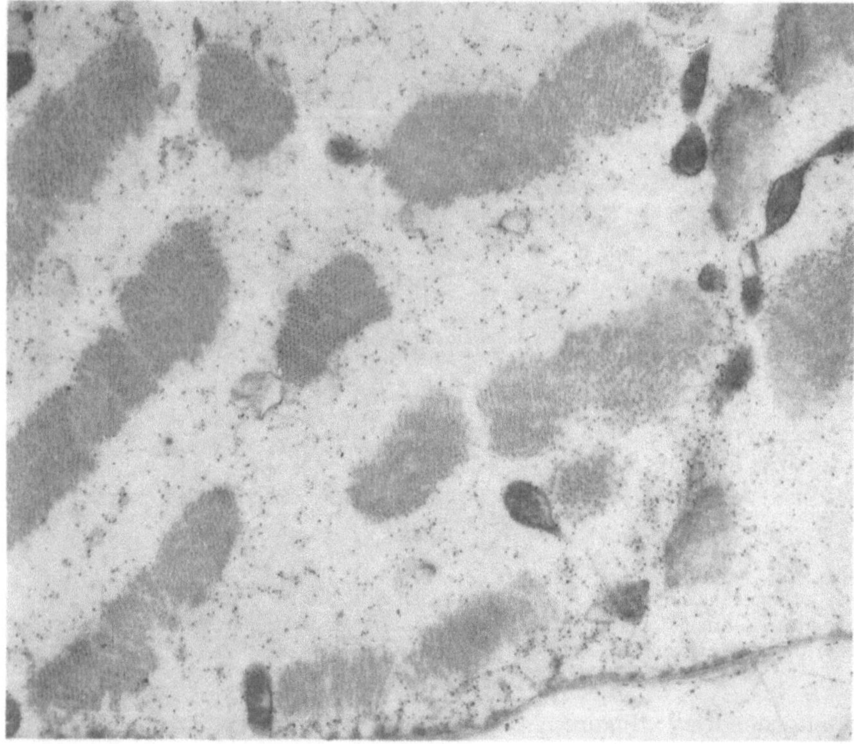

Figure 7.6 Electronmicrograph of obliquely sectioned muscle fibre from patient with acute alcoholic myopathy demonstrates marked separation of fibres (*Ann. Intern. Med.*, **67**, 493 (1967))

from a mitochondrial pole. A third inclusion resembled stacked structures in a laminated form. Although these inclusions were demonstrated in some non-alcoholics, those seen in the alcoholics seemed to have a characteristic pattern[153].

7.3.3.3 Experimental studies

The effects of ethanol have been studied on isolated striated muscle preparations. The active transport of cations is inhibited by ethanol[154–157]. The passive influx of Na^+ may also be reduced[156,158] although Mayer has shown that muscle membrane permeability to sodium is increased after ethanol feeding[159]. The resting membrane potential in rat muscle, following prolonged administration of alcohol, may be quite low[159]. Although early studies suggested that ethanol depressed muscle excitability by depolarization of the muscle fibre membrane[160], Inoue and Frank have shown that alcohol

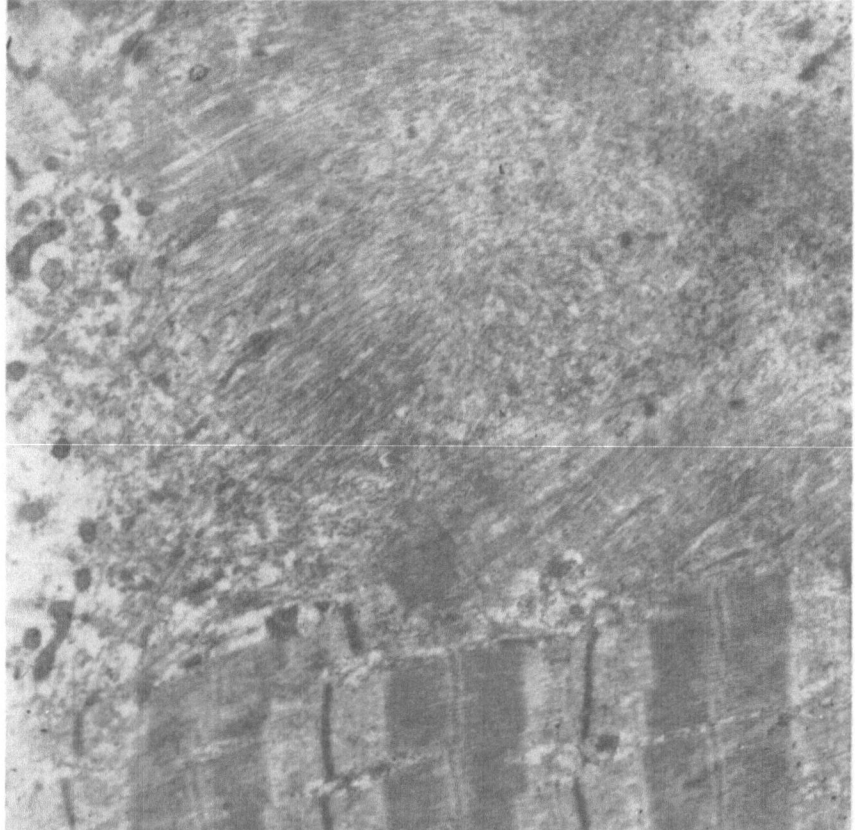

Figure 7.7 Electronmicrograph from patient with chronic alcoholic myopathy. The fibrils are disrupted and disoriented (courtesy Dr G. T. Perkoff, Washington University School of Medicine)

potentiates neuromuscular transmission and does not block by depolarization[161]. Kucera and Smith have suggested that the depressant effects of high concentrations of ethanol could be due to interference with impulse conduction in terminal nerve branches of muscle[162]. This has been confirmed by Etessami[163]. Indeed, a small dose of ethanol may be a stimulant to muscle activity[163], perhaps by increasing the accumulation of catecholamines[164]. Svensson and Waldeck pretreated mice with 4-methyl pyrazole, which inhibits alcohol dehydrogenase[164]. They suggested that the stimulation of motor activity is directly related to alcohol, rather than its metabolite, acetaldehyde. However, it should be noted that pyrazole, itself, is a potent pharmacological agent[165,166]. As it does in the heart, alcohol consumption increases the deposition of fat in striated muscle[167]. Recent studies have shed light on the effects of alcohol on the contractile proteins of skeletal muscle. *In vitro*, both ethanol and acetaldehyde interfere with contractility of isolated actomyosin and inhibit the response to ADP[168].

7.4 SMOOTH MUSCLE

The effects of ethanol on smooth muscle were only recently recognized. Clinical observations of cessation of uterine contractility when ethanol was used for obstetric analgesia suggested a direct inhibitory effect on uterine musculature[169,170]. This theory was challenged by a series of observations on the effects of ethanol on human and animal uterine activity at the onset of labour, during parturition, and during lactation[171–174]. These experiments *in vivo* led Fuchs *et al.* to conclude that ethanol interfered with the release of oxytocin from the neurohypophysis, and that this inhibition of pituitary activity was responsible for diminished myometrial contraction[173]. Mantell and Higgs studied the response of the myometrium to oxytocin, prior to and during infusion of ethanol, in women at term[175]. They confirmed the inhibition of oxytocin released by ethanol but, in addition, concluded that ethanol could further interfere with myometrial activity in pregnancy by non-competitive antagonism of oxytocin at the myometrial level. This interpretation has been questioned[176,177]. Ethanol, in low concentrations, has been shown to depress the activity of isolated human uterine muscle[178,179]. However, diminution of either muscle tonus, or frequency and amplitude of contractions of isolated myometrium, from both pregnant and non-pregnant women, was not induced at ethanol concentrations equivalent to those used therapeutically[180]. In these experiments ethanol did not interfere with the direct effects of oxytocin on the muscle preparations. At high concentrations of ethanol a sustained, but reversible, inhibitory effect on myometrial cells was apparent. The authors concluded that ethanol, at very high concentrations, may interact with, and antagonize, calcium at the level of the cell membrane. These observations were confirmed in studies of spontaneous and electrically induced contractions of isolated strips of myometrium from pregnant and non-pregnant rats[179]. Increased sensitivity of the myometrium to ethanol was noted in preparations from pregnant animals.

Controversy continues with respect to the direct action of ethanol on uterine muscle. Studies of other smooth muscle preparations, however, suggest a direct effect of ethanol on fibre contraction. Longitudinal intestinal smooth muscle, from the guinea-pig, was placed in media of varying concentrations of K^+ and Ca^+, and contraction was studied before and after the addition of ethanol[181]. Indirect antagonism of Ca^+ at the level of the cell membrane was induced by the addition of ethanol. The effects of ethanol could be reversed by high concentrations of calcium in the bathing medium. In later studies, Hurwitz *et al.* suggested that ethanol inhibited acetylcholine-induced contraction of the isolated guinea-pig longitudinal smooth muscle preparation[182]. They demonstrated that this effect could also be reversed by high concentrations of Ca^+. Sunano and Miyazaki demonstrated striking inhibition of both spontaneous and K^+-induced contraction by ethanol[183,184]. The inhibitory effect of ethanol *in vivo* and *in vitro* on the smooth muscle of the digestive tract of rats was shown by Lienard *et al.*[185]. They utilized contrast radiographs in man and demonstrated similar inhibitory effects. Recent studies of intestinal motility in man after alcohol consumption, have indicated inhibition of type I (impending) contractions in the jejunum with augmentation of type III (propulsive) waves in the ileum[186]. These effects on intestinal motility may contribute to the diarrhea seen in some alcoholics.

7.5 SUMMARY

Alcoholic cardiomyopathy is a degenerative disease of the myocardium, which may affect individuals who have ingested excess alcohol for many years. Acute or insidious congestive failure is characteristic, in the absence of coronary artery disease. This disorder is distinct from that seen with thiamine deficiency, and is usually arrested by discontinuing ethanol abuse. Most experimental studies indicate that ethanol exerts a negative ionotropic effect on the heart, which may be complicated by the action of acetaldehyde, its primary metabolite.

Excess ingestion of alcoholic beverages may also lead to clinical syndromes of acute or chronic skeletal muscle injury. Objective evidence of damage to striated muscles may be demonstrable in some alcoholics before the onset of symptoms. Acute alcoholic myopathy characteristically presents with the sudden onset of muscular pain, often accompanied by myoglobinuria, and may lead to death. Some alcoholics exhibit a more gradual development of muscle weakness which may be incapacitating. Experimental studies have shown that both alcohol and acetaldehyde impair certain biochemical functions of muscle.

Alcohol affects smooth muscle *in vivo* and *in vitro* but clinical manifestations from this effect are uncommon.

References

1. Eliaser, M., Jr. and Giansiracusa, F. J. (1956). The heart and alcohol. *Calif. Med.*, **84,** 234
2. Brigden, W. (1957). Uncommon myocardial diseases. *Lancet* **ii,** 1179, 1243

3. Evans, W. (1959). The electrocardiogram of alcoholic cardiomyopathy. *Br. Heart J.*, **21,** 445.
4. Burch, G. E. and Walsh, J. J. (1960). Cardiac insufficiency in chronic alcoholism. *Am. J. Cardiol.*, **6,** 864
5. Wood, G. B. (1855). *A Treatise on the Practice of Medicine, Vol. II,* p. 179. Philadelphia: Lippincott, Gambo and Co.
6. Strumpell, A. (1890). *A Textbook of Medicine for Students and Practitioners,* p. 292. New York: D. Appleton
7. Steel, G. (1893). Heart failure as a result of chronic alcoholism. *Med. Chron.*, **18,** 1
8. Benchimol, A. B. and Schlesinger, P. (1953). Beriberi heart disease. *Am. Heart J.*, **46,** 245
9. Hickie, J. and Hall, G. V. (1960). The cardiomyopathies: a report of fifty cases. *Aust. Ann. Med.*, **9,** 258
10. Massumi, R. A., Rios, J. C., Gooch, A. S., Nutter, D., De Vita, V. T. and Datlow, D. W. (1965). Primary myocardial disease—report of fifty cases and review of the subject. *Circulation,* **31,** 19
11. Dorra, M., Gourgon, R., Coumel, P., Dyan, A., Slama, R. and Bouvrain, Y. (1970). Two cases of cardiac beriberi—notes on the physiopathology of cardiac manifestations in alcoholics. *Presse Med.*, **78,** 875
12. Burch, G. E. and Giles, T. D. (1971). Alcoholic cardiomyopathy. Concept of the disease and its treatment. *Am. J. Med.*, **50,** 141
13. Robin, E. and Goldschlager, N. (1970). Persistence of low cardiac output after relief of high output by thiamine in a case of alcoholic beriberi and cardiac myopathy. *Am. Heart J.*, **80,** 103
14. Riff, D. P., Jain, A. C. and Doyle, J. T. (1969). Acute hemodynamic effect of ethanol on normal human volunteers. *Am. Heart J.*, **78,** 592
15. Regan, T. J., Levinson, G. E., Oldewurtel, H. A., Frank, M. J., Weisse, A. B. and Moschos, C. B. (1969). Ventricular function in noncardiacs with alcoholic fatty liver; role of ethanol in production of cardiomyopathy. *J. Clin. Invest.*, **48,** 397
16. Mitchell, J. H. and Cohen, L. S. (1970). Alcohol and the heart. *Mod. Concepts Cardiovasc. Dis.*, **39, Suppl. 109,** 13
17. Gould, L., Zahir, M., DeMartino, A. and Gomprecht, R. F. (1971). Cardiac effects of a cocktail. *J. Am. Med. Ass.*, **18,** 1799
18. Evans, W. (1961). Alcoholic cardiomyopathy. *Am. Heart J.*, **61,** 556
19. Evans, W. (1964). Alcoholic myocardiopathy. *Prog. Cardiovasc. Dis.*, **7,** 151
20. Pintar, K., Wolanskj, B. M. and Gubbay, E. R. (1965). Alcoholic cardiomyopathy. *Can. Med. Ass. J.*, **93,** 103
21. Kerr, A., Jr. (1967). Myocardopathy, alcohol, and pericardial effusion. *Arch. Intern. Med.*, **119,** 617
22. Auzepy, P., Grosgogeat, Y., Leguillant, F., Manigand, G. and Sarrazin, A. (1969). Alcoholic myocardiopathies. Clinical study. *Presse Med.*, **77,** 1405
23. Ferrero, C. (1970). Alcoholic myocardiopathy. *Ann. Cardiol. Angiol.*, **19,** 47
24. Koide, T., Machida, K., Nakanishi, A., Ozeki, K. and Mashima, S. (1972). Cardiac abnormalities in chronic alcoholism. An evidence suggesting association of myocardial abnormality with chronic alcoholism in 107 Japanese patients admitted to a psychiatric ward. *Jap. Heart J.*, **13,** 418
25. Pavlov, V. M., Vinogradov, A. V., Glukhova, P. A., Makarova, T. E. and Zamurueva, N. K. (1972). Alcoholic cardiopathy. *Ter. Arkh.*, **44,** 15
26. Slany, J. and Mosslacher, H. (1972). Electrocardiographic and vectocardiographic findings in alcoholic myocardiopathies. *Med. Klin.*, **67,** 1429
27. Fernandez, P., Rosenthal, J. E., Cohen, L. S., Hammond, G. and Wolfson, S. (1973). Alcohol-induced Prinzmetal variant angina. *Am. J. Cardiol.*, **32,** 235
28. Regan, T. J., Wu, C. F., Weisse, A. B., Haider, B., Ahmed, S. S., Oldewurtel, H. A. and

Lyons, M. M. (1973). Acute myocardial infarction in toxic cardiomyopathy without coronary obstruction. *Trans. Assoc. Am. Physicians,* **86,** 193
29. McDermott, P. H., Delaney, R. L., Egan, J. D. and Sullivan, J. F. (1966). Myocardosis and cardiac failure in men. *J. Am. Med. Ass.,* **198,** 253
30. Kesteloot, H., Terryn, R., Bosmans, P. and Joossens, J. V. (1966). Alcoholic perimyocardiopathy. *Acta Cardiol.,* **21,** 341
31. Mercier, G. and Patry, G. (1967). Quebec beer-drinkers cardiomyopathy; clinical signs and symptoms. *Can. Med. Ass. J.,* **97,** 884
32. Morin, Y. and Daniel, P. (1967). Quebec beer-drinkers cardiomyopathy: etiological considerations. *Can. Med. Ass. J.,* **97,** 926
33. Edit: (1967). Quebec beer-drinkers cardiomyopathy. *J. Am. Med. Ass.,* **202,** 1145
34. Sanders, M. G. (1970). Alcoholic cardiomyopathy—a critical review. *Q. J. Stud. Alc.,* **31,** 324
35. Wendt, V. E., Wu, C., Balcon, R., Doty, G. and Bing, R. J. (1965). Hemodynamic and metabolic effects of chronic alcoholism in man. *Am. J. Cardiol.,* **15,** 175
36. Wendt, V. E., Ajluni, R., Bruce, T. A., Prasad, A. S. and Bing, R. J. (1966). Acute effects of alcohol on the human myocardium. *Am. J. Cardiol.,* **17,** 804
37. Spodick, D. H., Pigott, V. M. and Chirife, R. (1972). Preclinical cardiac malfunction in chronic alcoholism. Comparison with matched normal controls and with alcoholic cardiomyopathy. *N. Engl. J. Med.,* **287,** 677
38. Asokan, S. K., Frank, M. J. and Withan, A. C. (1972). Cardiomyopathy without cardiomegaly in alcoholics. *Am. Heart J.,* **84,** 13
39. Bridgen, W. and Robinson, J. (1964). Alcoholic heart disease. *Br. Med. J.,* **ii,** 1283
40. Ferrans, V. J., Hibbs, R. G., Weilbaecher, D. G., Black, W. C., Walsh, J. J. and Burch, G. E. (1965). Alcoholic cardiomyopathy—a histochemical study. *Am. Heart J.,* **69,** 748
41. Tobin, J. R. Jr., Driscoll, J. F., Lim, M. T., Sutton, G. C., Szanto, P. B. and Gunnar, R. M. (1967). Primary myocardial disease and alcoholism. The clinical manifestations and course of the disease in a selected population of patients observed for three or more years. *Circulation,* **35,** 754
42. Schenk, E. A. and Cohen, J. (1970). The heart in chronic alcoholism. Clinical and pathologic findings. *Pathol. Microbiol.,* **35,** 96
43. Gould, L. (1970). Cardiac effects of alcohol. *Am. Heart J.,* **79,** 422
44. Bulloch, R. T., Pearce, M. D., Murphy, M. L., Jenkins, B. J. and Davis, J. L. (1972). Myocardial lesions in idiopathic and alcoholic cardiomyopathy. *Am. J. Cardiol.,* **29,**
45. Goch, J. H. (1972). Effect of alcohol abuse on the dynamics of left ventricular contraction. *Pol. Tyg. Lek.,* **27,** 1634
46. Hognestad, J. and Teisberg, P. (1973). Heart pathology in chronic alcoholism. *Acta Pathol. Microbiol. Scand. A.,* **81,** 315
47. DeMakis, J. G., Proskey, A., Rahimtoola, S. H., Jamil, M., Sutton, G. C., Rosen, K. M., Gunnar, R. M. and Tobin, J. R. Jr. (1974). The natural course of alcoholic cardiomyopathy. *Ann. Intern. Med.,* **80,** 293
48. Ferrans, V. J. (1966). Alcoholic cardiomyopathy. *Am. J. Med. Sci.,* **252,** 84
49. Burch, G. E. and Depasquale, N. P. (1969). Alcoholic cardiomyopathy. *Am. J. Cardiol.,* **23,** 723
50. Regan, T. J. (1971). Ethyl alcohol and the heart. *Circulation,* **44,** 957
51. Whereat, A. F. and Perkoff, J. K. (1973). Ethyl alcohol and myocardial metabolism. *Circulation,* **47,** 915
52. Alexander, C. S. (1966). Idiopathic heart disease. I. Analysis of 100 cases, with special reference to chronic alcoholism. *Am. J. Med.,* **41,** 213
53. Deparis, M., Grosgogeat, Y. and Auzepy, P. (1969). Heart in alcoholic liver cirrhosis and alcoholic myocardiopathies. *Presse Med.,* **77,** 1403

54. Lunseth, J. H., Olmstead, E. G. and Abboud, F. (1958). A study of heart disease in one hundred and eight hospitalized patients dying with portal cirrhosis. *Arch. Intern. Med.*, **102,** 405
55. Bonera, E. and Bianchetti, L. (1964). On various aspects of the electrocardiogram of young chronic dysproteinemic alcoholics. *Folia Cardiol.*, **23,** 1
56. Seelig, M. S. (1969). Electrographic patterns of magnesium depletion appearing in alcoholic heart disease. *Ann. N.Y. Acad. Sci.*, **162,** 906
57. Flink, E. B., McCollister, R., Prasad, A. S., Melby, J. C. and Doe, R. P. (1957). Evidences for clinical magnesium deficiency. *Ann. Intern. Med.*, **47,** 956
58. Wener, T., Pintar, K., Simon, M. A., Motola, R., Friedman, R., Mayman, A. and Schucher, R. (1964). The effects of prolonged hypomagnesemia on the cardiovascular system in young dogs. *Am. Heart J.*, **67,** 221
59. Gould, L., Zahir, M., Calder, B. and Lyon, A. F. (1968). Nonobstructive primary myocardial disease. *Am. J. Cardiol.*, **22,** 523
60. Hamby, R. I., Catangay, P., Apiado, O. and Khan, A. H. (1970). Primary myocardial disease. *Am. J. Cardiol.*, **25,** 625
61. Goodwin, J. F. (1970). Congestive and hypertrophic cardiomyopathies. *Lancet*, **i,** 731
62. Gunnar, R. M., Sutton, G. C., Pietras, R. J. and Tobin, J. R., Jr. (1971). Alcoholic cardiomyopathy. *Disease-a-month*, **1,** 30
63. Asokan, S. K. and Frank, M. J. (1971). Improved cardiac performance in alcoholic cardiomyopathy after chelation. *Circulation*, **44 (Suppl. II),** 40
64. Maines, J. E. and Aldinger, E. E. (1967). Myocardial depression accompanying chronic consumption of alcohol. *Am. Heart J.*, **73,** 55
65. Regan, R. J., Koroxenidis, G., Moschos, C. B., Oldewurtel, H. A., Lehan, P. H. and Hellems, H. K. (1966). The acute metabolic and hemodynamic responses of the left ventricle to ethanol. *J. Clin. Invest.*, **45,** 270
66. Pachinger, O. M., Tillmanns, H., Mao., J. C., Fauvel, J-M. and Bing, R. J. (1973). The effect of prolonged administration of ethanol on cardiac metabolism and performance in the dog. *J. Clin. Invest.*, **52,** 2690
67. Grosgogeat, Y., Paillas, J., Auzepy, P., Deparis, M. and Facquet, J. (1971). Alcoholic cardiomyopathies, anatomo-pathologic and electronic microscopy data. *Arch. Mal Coeur.*, **64,** 36
68. Hibbs, R. G., Ferrans, V. J., Black, W. C., Weilbaecher, D. G., Walsh, J. J. and Burch, G. E. (1965). Alcoholic cardiomyopathy. *Am. Heart J.*, **69,** 766
69. Alexander, C. S. (1966). Idiopathic heart disease, II. Electron microscopic examination of myocardial biopsy specimens in alcoholic heart disease. *Am. J. Med.*, **41,** 229
70. Alexander, C. S. (1967). Electron microscopic observations in alcoholic heart disease. *Br. Heart J.*, **29,** 200
71. Mosslacher, H., Slany, J., Hanak, H. and Stockinger, L. (1971). Alcoholic myocardiopathy. Preliminary report on the electronoptic evaluation of myocardium biopsy material. *Z. Kreislaufforsch.*, **60,** 303
72. Suzuki, T. (1967). Electron-microscopic study on alcoholic cardiomyopathy. *Jap. J. Leg. Med.*, **21,** 390
73. Sohal, R. S. and Burch, G. E. (1969). Effects of alcohol ingestion on the intercalated disc in the mouse heart. *Experientia*, **25,** 279
74. Hall, J. L. and Rowlands, D. T., Jr. (1970). Cardiotoxicity of alcohol. An electron microscopic study in the rat. *Am. J. Path.*, **60,** 153
75. Schmalbruch, H. and Dume, T. (1969). Clinically inapparent changes in the human myocardial cell caused by alcoholism. *Arch. Kreislaufforsch.*, **58,** 202
76. Burch, G. E., Colcolough, H. L., Harb, J. M. and Tsui, C. Y. (1971). The effect of ingestion of ethyl alcohol, wine and beer on the myocardium of mice. *Am. J. Cardiol.*, **27,** 522

77. Burch, G. E., Harb, J. M., Colcolough, H. L. and Tsui, C. Y. (1971). The effect of prolonged consumption of beer, wine and ethanol on the myocardium of the mouse. *Johns Hopkins Med. J.*, **129,** 130
78. Ferrans, V. J., Buja, L. M. and Roberts, W. C. (1975). Cardiac morphologic changes produced by ethanol. In M. A. Rothschild, M. Oratz and S. S. Schreiber, eds. *Alcohol and Abnormal Protein Biosynthesis*, p. 158. New York: Pergamon Press
79. Lieber, C. S., Spritz, N. and DeCarli, L. M. (1966). Accumulation of triglycerides in heart and kidney after alcohol ingestion. *J. Clin. Invest.*, **45,** 1041
80. Marciniak, M., Gudbjarnason, S. and Bruce, T. A. (1968). The effect of chronic alcohol administration on enzyme profile and glyceride content of heart muscle, brain and liver. *Proc. Soc. Exp. Biol. Med.*, **128,** 1021
81. Kikuchi, T. and Kako, K. J. (1970). Metabolic effects of ethanol on the rabbit heart. *Circ. Res.*, **26,** 625
82. Mallov, S. and Cerra, F. (1967). Effect of ethanol intoxication and catecholamines on cardiac lipoprotein lipase activity in rats. *J. Pharmacol. Exp. Ther.*, **156,** 426
83. Reitz, R. C., Helsabeck, E. and Mason, D. P. (1973). Effects of chronic alcohol ingestion on the fatty acid composition of the heart. *Lipids,* **8,** 80
84. Lochner, A., Cowley, R. and Brink, A. J. (1969). Effect of ethanol on metabolism and function of perfused rat heart. *Am. Heart J.*, **78,** 770
85. Gailis, L. and Verdy, M. (1971). The effect of ethanol and acetaldehyde on the metabolism and vascular resistance of the perfused heart. *Can. J. Biochem.*, **49,** 227
86. Webb, W. R., Gupta, D. N., Cook, W. A., Sugg, W. L., Bashour, F. A. and Unal, M. O. (1967). Effects of alcohol on myocardial contractility. *Dis. Chest.*, **52,** 602
87. James, T. N. and Bear, E. S. (1967). Effects of ethanol and acetaldehyde on the heart. *Am. Heart J.*, **74,** 243
88. Mendoza, L. C., Hellberg, K., Rickart, A., Tillich, G. and Bing, R. J. (1971). The effect of intravenous ethyl alcohol on the coronary circulation and myocardial contractility of the human and canine heart. *J. Clin. Pharmacol.*, **11,** 165
89. Degerli, I. U. and Webb, W. R. (1963). Alcohol, cardiac function, and coronary flow. *Surgical Forum,* **14,** 252
90. Ganz, V. (1963). The acute effect of alcohol on the circulation and on the oxygen metabolism of the heart. *Am. Heart J.*, **66,** 494
91. Mierzwiak, D. S., Wildenthal, K. and Mitchell, J. H. (1972). Acute effects of ethanol on the left ventricle in dogs. *Arch. Intern. Pharmacodyn. Ther.*, **199,** 43
92. Newman, W. H. and Valicenti, J. F. Jr. (1971). Ventricular function following acute alcohol administration—a strain-gauge analysis of depressed ventricular dynamics. *Am. Heart. J.*, **81,** 61
93. Schreiber, S. S., Briden, K., Oratz, M. and Rothschild, M. A. (1972). Ethanol, acetaldehyde, and myocardial protein synthesis. *J. Clin. Invest.*, **51,** 2820
94. Nakano, T. and Moore, J. E. (1972). Effect of different alcohols on the contractile force in studies of the isolated guinea-pig myocardium. *Eur. J. Pharmacol.*, **20,** 266
95. Fisher, V. T. and Kavaler, F. (1975). The action of ethanol upon contractility of normal ventricular myocardium. In M. A. Rothschild, M. Oratz and S. S. Schreiber, eds. *Alcohol and Abnormal Protein Biosynthesis*, p. 187. New York: Pergamon Press
96. Gimeno, A. L., Gimeno, M. F. and Webb, J. L. (1962). Effect of ethanol on cellular membrane potential and conductivity of isolated rat atrium. *Am. J. Physiol.*, **203,** 194
97. Swartz, M. H., Repke, D. I., Katz, A. M. and Rubin, E. (1974). Effect of ethanol on Ca-binding and Ca-uptake by cardiac microsomes. *Biochem. Pharmacol.*, **23,** 2369
98. Williams, J. W., Tada, M., Katz, A. M. and Rubin, E. (1975). Effects of ethanol and acetaldehyde on the ($Na^+ + K^+$)-activated ATPase activity of cardiac plasma membranes. *Biochem. Pharmacol.*, **24,** 27
99. Jackson, J. (1837). On a peculiar disease resulting from the use of ardent spirits. *Boston Med. Surg. J.*, **11,** 351

100. Huss, M. Cited by Ekbom, K. *et al.*, ref. 106

101. Siemerling, F. (1889). Kasuistische Beitrage zur forensischen Psychiatrie. *Charite Ann.*, **11,** 423

102. Gudden, H. (1896). Klinische und anatomische Beitrage zur Kenntniss der multiplen Alkoholneuritis nebst Bemerkungen under die Regenerationsvorgange in peripheren Nervensystem. *Arch. Psychiatrie Nervenkrankheiten,* **28,** 643

103. Hed, R., Larrson, H. and Fahlgren, H. (1955). Acute myoglobinuria. *Acta Med. Scand.*, **152,** 459

104. Hed, R. (1955). Three cases of non-familiar myoglobinuria. *Acta Med. Scand.* **152 (Suppl. 303),** 86

105. Hed, R., Lundmark, C., Fahlgren, H. and Orell, S. (1962). Acute muscular syndrome in chronic alcoholism. *Acta Med. Scand.*, **171,** 585

106. Ekbom, K., Hed, R., Kirstein, L. and Astrom, K. E. (1964). Muscular affections in chronic alcoholism. *Arch. Neurol.*, **10,** 449

107. Fahlgren, H., Hed, R. and Lundmark, C. (1957). Myonecrosis and myoglobinuria in alcohol and barbiturate intoxication. *Acta Med. Scand.*, **158,** 405

108. Valaritis, T., Pilz, C. G., Oliner, H. and Chomet, B. (1960). Myoglobinuria, myoglobinuric nephrosis and alcoholism. *Arch. Path.*, **70,** 195

109. Perkoff, G. T., Hardy, P. and Velez-Garcia, E. (1966). Reversible acute muscular syndrome in chronic alcoholism. *N. Engl. J. Med.*, **274,** 1277

110. Serratrice, G., Toga, M. and Roux, H. (1966). Proximal muscular syndromes of chronic development occurring in alcoholics (apropos of 14 cases). *Presse Med.*, **74,** 1721

111. Douglas, R. M., Fewings, J. D., Casley-Smith, J. R. and West, R. F. (1966). Recurrent rhabdomyolysis precipitated by alcohol—a case report with physiological and electron microscopic studies of skeletal muscle. *Aust. Ann. Med.*, **15,** 251

112. Brohult, T., Carlson, L. A. and Reichard, H. (1966). Serum enzyme activities, cholesterin and triglycerides in serum after intake of alcohol. *Scand. J. Clin. Lab. Invest.*, **18 (Suppl. 92),** 82

113. Mancall, E. L., McEntee, W. J., Hirschhorn, A. M. and Gonyea, E. F. (1966). Proximal muscular weakness and atrophy in the chronic alcoholics. *Neurology,* **16,** 301

114. Nygren, A. (1966). Serum creatine phosphokinase activity in chronic alcoholism, in connection with acute alcohol intoxication. *Acta Med. Scand.*, **179,** 623

115. Nygren, A. (1967). Serum creatine phosphokinase in chronic alcoholism. *Acta Med. Scand.*, **182,** 383

116. Carlsson, C. (1967). Muscular strength in chronic alcoholics. *Nord. Med.*, **77,** 17

117. Buge, A., Autissier, P., Escourolle, R., Martin, M., Rancurel, G. and Bourdarias, H. (1967). Myoglobinuric myopathy in an alcoholic. *Bull. Soc. Med. Hôp. (Paris)*, **118,** 615

118. Dimberg, R., Hed, R., Kallner, G. and Nygren, A. (1967). Liver–muscle enzyme activities in the serum of alcoholics on a diet poor in carbohydrates. *Acta Med. Scand.*, **181,** 227

119. Faris, A. A., Reyes, M. G. and Abrams, B. M. (1967). Subclinical alcoholic myopathy–electromyographic and biopsy study. *Trans Am. Neurol. Assoc.*, **92,** 102

120. Perkoff, G. T., Dioso, M. M., Bleisch, V. and Klinkerfuss, G. (1967). A spectrum of myopathy associated with alcoholism. I. Clinical and laboratory features. *Ann. Intern. Med.*, **67,** 481

121. Klinkerfuss, G., Bleisch, V., Dioso, M. M. and Perkoff, G. T. (1967). A spectrum of myopathy associated with alcoholism. II. Light and electron microscopic observations. *Ann. Intern. Med.*, **67,** 493

122. Lafair, J. S. and Myerson, R. M. (1968). Alcoholic myopathy. *Arch. Intern. Med.*, **122,** 417

123. Carlsson, C., Dencker, S. J., Grimby, G. and Tichy, J. (1969). Muscle weakness and neurological disorders in alcoholics. *Q. J. Stud. Alc.*, **30,** 585

124. Kahn, L. B. and Meyer, J. S. (1970).Acute myopathy in chronic alcoholism—a study of 22 autopsy cases, with ultrastructural observations. *Am. J. Clin. Path.*, **53,** 516

125. Faris, A. A. and Reyes, M. G. (1971). Reappraisal of alcoholic myopathy. Clinical and biopsy study on chronic alcoholics without muscle weakness or wasting. *J. Neurol. Neurosurg. Psychiatry*, **34**, 86
126. Pittman, J. G. and Decker, J. W. (1971). Acute and chronic myopathy associated with alcoholism. *Neurology*, **21**, 293
127. Nygren, A. and Sundblad, L. (1971). Lactate dehydrogenase isoenzyme patterns in serum and skeletal muscle in intoxicated alcoholics. *Acta Med. Scand.*, **189**, 303
128. Benjafield, J. G. and Rutter, L. F. (1971). Muscle disease in chronic alcoholism. *Lancet*, **i**, 1292
129. Nygren, A. (1971). The ischemic lactic acid response and the muscle LDH-isoenzyme pattern in alcoholics. *Acta Med. Scand.*, **190**, 283
130. Martin, J. B., Craig, J. W., Eckel, R. E. and Munger, (1971). Hypokalemic myopathy in chronic alcoholism. *Neurology*, **21**, 1160
131. Powers, R., Thompson, C. E. and Schroeder, P. E. (1971). Alcoholic myopathy and myoglobinuric nephrosis. *Mich. Med.*, **70**, 1111
132. Carlsson, C., Dencker, S. J., Henricksson, K. G., Magnusson, R., Petersen, I. and Riman, E. (1972). Clinical, histological, and electromyographical studies in chronic alcoholics. *Acta Neurol. Scand.*, **Suppl. 51**, 425
133. Hed, R., Nygren, A. and Sundblad, L. (1972). Muscle and liver serum enzyme activities in healthy volunteers given alcohol on a diet poor in carbohydrates. *Acta Med. Scand.*, **191**, 529
134. Kiessling, K. H., Pilstrom, L., Karlsson, J. and Piehl, K. (1973). Mitochondrial volume in skeletal muscle from young and old physically untrained and trained healthy men and from alcoholics. *Clin. Sci.*, **44**, 547
135. Prasad, P., Tabatznik, B. and Kotler, M. N. (1974). Recurrent acute alcoholic myopathy simulating deep vein thrombosis in association with cardiomyopathy and parasystolic ventricular tachycardia. *Johns Hopkins Med. J.*, **134**, 226
136. Song, S. K. and Rubin, E. (1972). Ethanol produces muscle damage in human volunteers. *Science*, **175**, 327
137. Perkoff, G. T. (1971). Alcoholic myopathy. *Ann. Rev. Med.*, **22**, 125
138. Oh, S. J. (1972). Alcoholic myopathy. A critical review. *Ala. J. Med. Sci.*, **9**, 79
139. Schaposnik, F., Salvioli, M. V., Laguens, R., Neumann, M. and Cacciatore, J. (1969). Phosphocreatinekinase as a sign of muscular damage. *Prensa Med. Argent.*, **56**, 615
140. Flugel, K. A., Purucker, J. and Purucker, M. (1971). Comparative investigations of the muscle potentials in healthy persons and alcoholics. *Electroencephalogr. Clin. Neurophysiol.*, **30**, 261
141. Emery, A. E. H. (1967). The determination of lactate dehydrogenase isoenzymes in normal human muscle and other tissues. *Biochem. J.*, **105**, 599
142. Curran, J. R. and Wetmore, S. J. (1972). Alcoholic myopathy. *Dis. Nerv. Syst.*, **33**, 19
143. O'Brien, E. T. and Goldstraw, P. (1969). Alcoholic myopathy. *Br. Med. J.*, **iv**, 785
144. Schneider, R. (1970). Acute alcoholic myopathy with myoglobinuria. *Southern Med. J.*, **63**, 485
145. Erlenborn, J. W. and Pilz, C. G. (1962). Paroxysmal myoglobinuria. *J. Am. Med. Ass.*, **181**, 95
146. Wu, B. C., Pillay, V. K., Hawker, C. D., Armbruster, K. F., Shapiro, H. S. and Ing, T. S. (1972). Hypercalcaemia in acute renal failure of acute alcoholic rhabdomyolysis. *S. Afr. Med. J.*, **46**, 1631
147. Geller, S. A. (1973). Extreme exertion rhabdomyolysis, a histopathologic study of 31 cases. *Human Path.*, **4**, 241
148. Knochel, J. P., Bilbrey, G. L., Fuller, T. J. and Carter, N. W. (1975). The muscle cell in chronic alcoholism: the possible role of phosphate depletion in alcoholic myopathy. *Ann. N.Y. Acad. Sci.*, **252**, 274

149. Muller, P., Regli, F. and Meyer, M. (1968). Alcoholic myopathy. *Deutsch Med. Wochenschr.*, **93**, 1043
150. Velez-Garcia, E., Hardy, P., Dioso, M. and Perkoff, G. T. (1966). Cysteine-stimulated serum creatine phosphokinase: unexpected results. *J. Lab. Clin. Med.*, **68**, 636
151. Bethlem, J. (1970). *Muscle Pathology*, p. 15. Amsterdam: North-Holland Publishing Co.
152. Baloh, R. *et al.* (1972). Regeneration of human muscle. *Lab. Invest.*, **26**, 319
153. Fisher, E. R., Puntereri, A. J., Jung, Y., Corredor, D. G. and Danowski, T. S. (1971). Alcoholism and other concomitants of mitochondrial inclusions in skeletal muscle. *Am. J. Med. Sci.*, **261**, 85
154. Israel, Y., Kalant, H. and Lawfer, I. (1965). Effects of ethanol on electrolyte transport and electrogenesis in animal tissues. *J. Cell. Comp. Physiol.*, **65**, 127
155. Kalant, H., Mons, W. and Mahon, M. A. (1966). Acute effects of ethanol on tissue electrolytes in the rat. *Can. J. Physiol. Pharmacol.*, **44**, 1
156. Israel, Y. (1970). Cellular effects of alcohol. *Q. J. Stud. Alc.*, **31**, 293
157. Jenny, E. (1970). The uptake and output of calcium ions by sarcoplasmic vesicles of the rabbit skeletal muscle under the influence of ethanol. *Schweiz Arch. Tierheilkd.*, **112**, 436
158. Seeman, P., Kwant, W. O., Goldberg, M. and Chau-Wong, M. (1971). The effect of ethanol and chlorpromazine on the passive membrane permeability to Na^+. *Biochim. Biophys. Acta*, **241**, 349
159. Mayer, R. F. (1973). Recent studies in man and animal of peripheral nerve and muscle dysfunction associated with chronic alcoholism. *Ann. N.Y. Acad. Sci.*, **215**, 370
160. Knutsson, E. (1961). Effects of ethanol on the membrane potential and membrane resistance of frog muscle fibers. *Acta Physiol. Scand.*, **52**, 242
161. Inoue, F. and Frank, G. B. (1967). Effects of ethyl alcohol on excitability and on neuromuscular transmission in frog skeletal muscle. *Br. J. Pharmacol.*, **30**, 186
162. Kucera, J. and Smith, C. M. (1971). Excitation by ethanol of rat muscle spindles. *J. Pharmacol. Exp. Ther.*, **179**, 301
163. Etessami, S. (1972). Effect of ethanol on neuromuscular contraction. *Comp. Gen. Pharmacol.*, **3**, 200
164. Svensson, T. H. and Waldeck, B. (1973). Significance of acetaldehyde in ethanol-induced effects on catecholamine metabolism and motor activity in the mouse. *Psychopharmacologia*, **31**, 229
165. Lieber, C. S., Rubin, E., DeCarli, L. M., Misra, P. S. and Gang, H. (1970). Effects of pyrazole on hepatic function and structure. *Lab. Invest.*, **22**, 615
166. Cederbaum, A. I. and Rubin, E. (1974). Effects of pyrazole, 4-bromopyrazole, and 4-methylpyrazole on mitochondrial function. *Biochem. Pharmacol.*, **23**, 203
167. Beck, W. E., Marchello, J. A. and Ray, D. E. (1971). Effects of some pharmacological agents on bovine intramuscular fat deposition. *J. Anim. Sci.*, **32**, 863
168. Puszkin, S. and Rubin, E. (1975). Effects of ADP on contractility of human muscle actomyosin: inhibition by ethanol and acetaldehyde. *Science*, **188**, 1319
169. Belinkoff, S. and Hall, J. (1950). Intravenous alcohol during labor. *Am. J. Obstet. Gynecol.*, **59**, 429
170. Chapman, E. R. and Williams, P. T., Jr. (1951). Intravenous alcohol as an obstetrical analgesia. *Am. J. Obstet. Gynecol.*, **61**, 676
171. Fuchs, A-R. and Wagner, G. (1963). The effect of ethyl alcohol on the release of oxytocin in rabbits. *Acta Endocrinol.*, **44**, 593
172. Fuchs, A-R. (1966). The inhibitory effect of ethanol on the release of oxytocin during parturition in the rabbit. *J. Endocrinol.*, **35**, 125
173. Fuchs, F., Fuchs, A-R., Poblete, X. F., Jr. and Risk, A. (1967). Effect of alcohol on threatened premature labor. *Am. J. Obstet. Gynecol.*, **99**, 627
174. Wagner, G. and Fuchs, A-R. (1968). Effect of ethanol on uterine activity during suckling in post-partum women. *Acta Endocrinol.*, **58**, 133

175. Mantell, C. D. and Higgins, G. C. (1970). The effect of ethanol on the myometrial response to oxytocin in women at term. *J. Obstet. Gynaecol. Brit. Commonw.*, **77,** 976
176. Coutinho, E. M., Filho, J. A., Xavier, R., Fuchs, A-R. and Fuchs, F. (1970). Effect of ethanol on the response of the non-pregnant human uterus to oxytocin and vasopressin. *J. Obstet. Gynaec. Brit. Commonw.*, **77,** 164
177. Lauersen, N. H., Raghavan, K. S., Wilson, K. H., Fuchs, F. and Niemann, W. H. (1973). Effects of prostaglandin F 2, oxytocin, and ethanol on the uterus of the pregnant baboon. *Am. J. Obstet. Gynecol.*, **115,** 912
178. Beuno-Montano, M., McGaughey, H. S., Harbert, G. M. and Thornton, W. N. Jr. (1966). Drug preservatives and uterine contractility. *Am. J. Obstet. Gynecol.*, **94,** 1
179. Gimeno, M. A., Bedners, A. S., De Vastik, F. J. and Gimeno, A. L. (1971). Effect of ethanol on the motility of isolated rat myometrium. *Arch. Intern. Pharmacodyn. Ther.*, **191,** 213
180. Wilson, K. H., Landesman, R., Fuchs, A-R. and Fuchs, F. (1969). The effect of ethyl alcohol on isolated human myometrium. *Am. J. Obstet. Gynecol.*, **104,** 436
181. Hurwitz, L., Battle, F. and Weiss, G. B. (1962). Action of the calcium antagonists cocaine and ethanol on contraction and potassium efflux of smooth muscle. *J. Gen. Physiol.*, **46,** 315
182. Hurwitz, L., von Hagen, S. and Joines, P. D. (1967). Acetylcholine and calcium on membrane permeability and contraction of intestinal smooth muscle. *J. Gen. Physiol.*, **50,** 1157
183. Sunano, S. and Miyazaki, E. (1969). Effects of ethanol and acetone on action potential and inhibitory potential of guinea-pig taenia coli. *Nature* (*London*), **221,** 380
184. Sunano, S. and Miyazaki, E. (1970). Effects of ethanol and acetone on the electrical and the mechanical activities of the smooth muscle. *Sapporo Med. J.*, **37,** 39
185. Lienard, J., Freville, M., Capron, J. P. and Harichaux, P. (1970). Inhibitory effects of ethanol on the motricity of smooth digestive fibers. *J. Physiol.*, **62 (Suppl. 2),** 294
186. Robles, E. A., Mezey, E., Halsted, C. H. and Schuster, M. (1974). Effect of ethanol on motility of small intestine. *Johns Hopkins Med. J.*, **135,** 17

8
Metabolic Effects of Alcohol on the Blood and Bone Marrow

J. LINDENBAUM

8.1 INTRODUCTION 216
8.2 RED CELLS 216
8.2.1 *Folate deficiency* 216
8.2.1.1 Pathogenesis 217
8.2.2 *Sideroblastic anaemia* 220
8.2.2.1 Pathogenesis 221
8.2.2.2 Biochemical mechanism 223
8.2.3 *Vacuolization of marrow precursor cells* 224
8.2.3.1 Pathogenesis 226
8.2.4 *Haemolytic syndromes and red cell membrane abnormalities* 227
8.2.4.1 Low grade haemolysis of liver disease 227
8.2.4.2 Macrocytosis of liver disease 228
8.2.4.3 Target cells in liver disease 228
8.2.4.4 Acanthocytosis 229
8.2.4.5 Zieve's syndrome 231
8.2.4.6 Stomatocytosis 231
8.2.4.7 Hypophosphataemia and haemolysis 231
8.2.5 *Iron deficiency* 232
8.2.6 *Haemodilution* 232
8.2.7 *Other causes of anaemia in alcoholics* 232
8.3 PLATELETS 232
8.3.1 *Thrombocytopenia* 232
8.3.1.1 Pathogenesis 233
8.3.2 *Abnormal platelet function* 235
8.3.3 *Other causes of thrombocytopenia in alcoholics* 235
8.4 WHITE CELLS 236
8.4.1 *Granulocytopenia* 236
8.4.1.1 Pathogenesis 236
8.4.2 *Impairment of granulocyte mobilization* 238
8.4.3 *Impairment of macrophage function* 239
8.4.4 *Lymphocyte function* 239

8.4.5 *Other factors favouring infection* 239
8.5 SUMMARY 240
References 241

8.1 INTRODUCTION

It has been increasingly recognized that a kaleidoscopic variety of haematological complications may occur in alcoholic patients. Often it has been difficult to disentangle the relative roles of liver disease, infection, malnutrition, and alcohol ingestion in their pathogenesis. Considerable progress has been made in recent years in delineating the importance of ethanol itself as a haematological toxin. Syndromes which were not even recognized 10 years ago, such as alcohol-induced thrombocytopenia or alcohol-induced sideroblastic anaemia, have been well characterized clinically, reproduced experimentally in human volunteers, and at least partially defined in terms of physiological mechanisms. Other haematological derangements have been identified but remain poorly understood. This chapter will review the current state of knowledge of the various disorders of alcoholics affecting red cells, platelets, and white cells.

8.2 RED CELLS

8.2.1 Folate deficiency

Megaloblastic anaemia is commonly encountered in hospitalized malnourished chronic alcoholics[1–15]. This complication is infrequently seen in well-nourished alcoholics in private[16–18] or municipal[12,19] hospitals. The megaloblastic morphological abnormalities have invariably been due to folic acid deficiency[7–13], unless an unrelated associated condition, such as pernicious anaemia[14], is present. Low serum B_{12} concentrations, however, are occasionally seen in patients with severe folate deficiency[8,19]. While almost all of the reported patients with megaloblastic anaemia have had some form of alcoholic liver disease, the correlation of megaloblastic changes with severity of hepatic dysfunction has been poor[9,10], and folate-deficiency megaloblastic anaemia has only very rarely been encountered in cirrhotic patients who are teetotallers[9,11]. The complication develops commonly in imbibers of wine and whisky, which contain little or no folate[20] and is less frequently seen in alcoholics with a preference for beer[9,10], which is rich in folic acid[20]. There is a very strong association between decreased dietary folate intake and the presence of megaloblastosis[8–10,12–14,18]. In some patients, gastrointestinal bleeding[9,11], hypersplenism[9], haemolysis[9,11], and infection[19] may be contributory factors disturbing folate balance. Certain patients, for unknown reasons, appear to be especially prone to recurrent episodes of severe folate deficiency[19]. When marked, the folate depletion state may cause thrombocytopenia and granulocytopenia as well. The megaloblastic marrow changes may sometimes be more striking in the granulocytic series[5,9]. The haematological abnormalities characteristically revert to normal after withdrawal of alcohol and resumption of hospital diet, with or without the supplemental administration of folic acid[4,5,9,14,21,22], and may even do so in patients treated with intravenous fluids only[19].

While the megaloblastic bone marrow changes and the associated morphological findings in the peripheral blood (macro-ovalocytosis and neutrophil hypersegmentation) are almost always accompanied by low serum folate concentrations[7–10,12–15,18,21,22], many alcoholics have low serum folate levels in the absence of morphological evidence of tissue deficiency of the vitamin[8,12,17–19]. Serum folate levels fall early in the course of dietary folate deprivation, and may be subnormal for weeks or months before stores are depleted to the point of causing disturbances in haematopoiesis[23–25]. In addition, in relatively well-nourished alcoholics, high serum ethanol levels may be associated with low serum folate concentrations[18]. Because of the frequent finding of low serum folate levels in alcoholic patients in the absence of morphological evidence of folate deficiency, the serum folate concentration is of limited usefulness as a screening test in the diagnostic workup of anaemia in alcoholics. If marrow and peripheral blood abnormalities indicative of folate depletion are absent in a patient with a low serum folate level, the anaemia is due to some other cause and will not respond to folic acid therapy[9].

8.2.1.1 Pathogenesis

While a decreased dietary folate intake appears to be a necessary factor in the development of folic acid deficiency in alcoholics, it is now well established that ethanol ingestion also plays an important role. This was first demonstrated by the landmark studies of Sullivan and Herbert[26] who administered alcohol along with small doses of folic acid to three patients with untreated megaloblastic anaemia due to folate deficiency. In each case the ingestion of whisky, wine, or ethanol itself prevented the haematological response to folic acid therapy; in addition, if alcohol was added after the marrow had become normoblastic, megaloblastic changes promptly recurred (Figure 8.1). Ethanol also depressed granulocyte and platelet levels. The haematosuppressive effect of alcohol could be overcome with larger doses of folic acid or folinic acid[26]. Subsequently, other investigators were also able to induce megaloblastic marrow abnormalities by the administration of ethanol and a folate-poor diet to human volunteers[13,14,27–29]. In addition, Eichner and Hillman found that when alcohol was given along with a low-folate diet, megaloblastic marrow conversion occurred much more rapidly than when the diet alone was taken[25]. The failure of such morphological changes to occur when alcohol was given with folate supplements to well-nourished volunteers[29,30] indicates that ethanol accelerates the development of megaloblastic erythropoiesis only when folate stores are depleted.

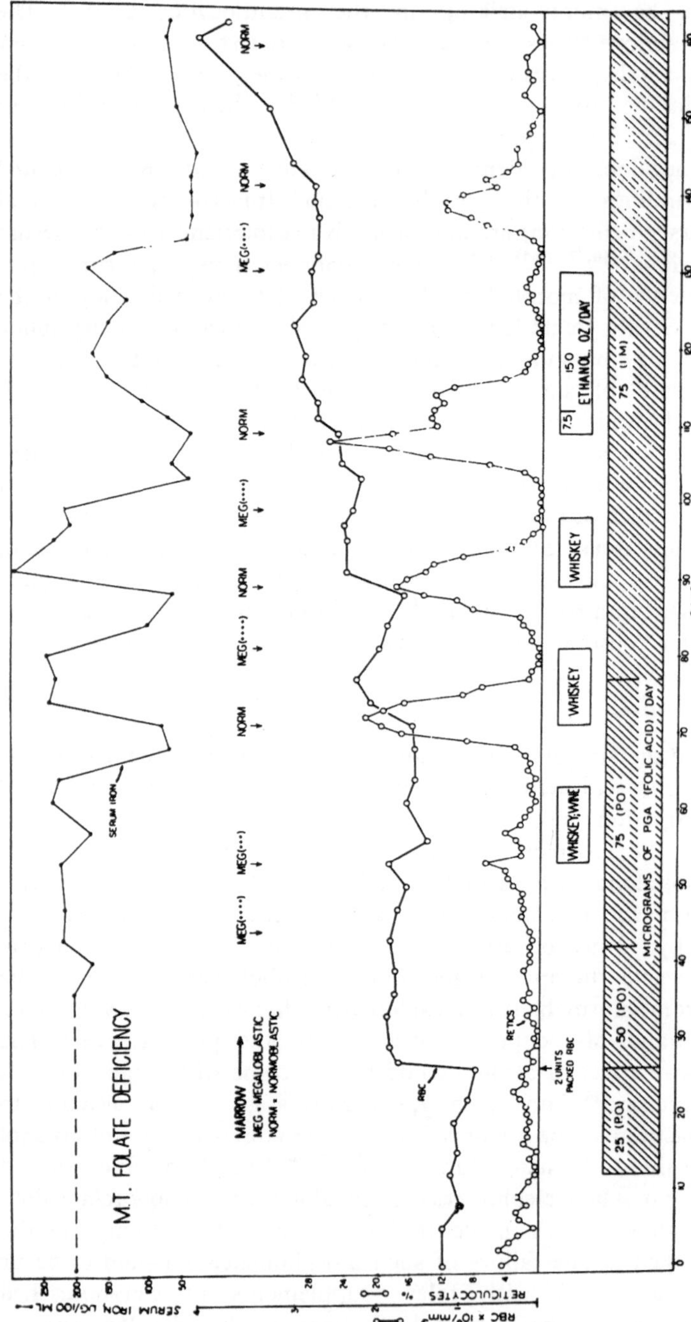

Figure 8.1 Inhibition of bone marrow responses to folic acid therapy by alcohol. In this patient, who was recovering from a folate-deficiency megaloblastic anaemia, reticulocyte responses to 75 mcg doses of folic acid, given orally or parenterally, were reversed by the administration of alcoholic beverages or pure ethanol. The marrow morphology reverted from normoblastic to megaloblastic during each of the four periods of alcohol administration (from Sullivan and Herbert[25])

The manner in which ethanol interferes with folate metabolism has not been established. Malabsorption of folic acid may play a role in some patients with megaloblastic anaemia[9,31]. Impairment of folate absorption in such patients, however, may be the result, rather than the cause, of folate deficiency[31-34]. Furthermore, Sullivan and Herbert showed that alcohol inhibited the haematopoietic response to parenteral (as well as oral) folic acid (Figure 8.1)[26].

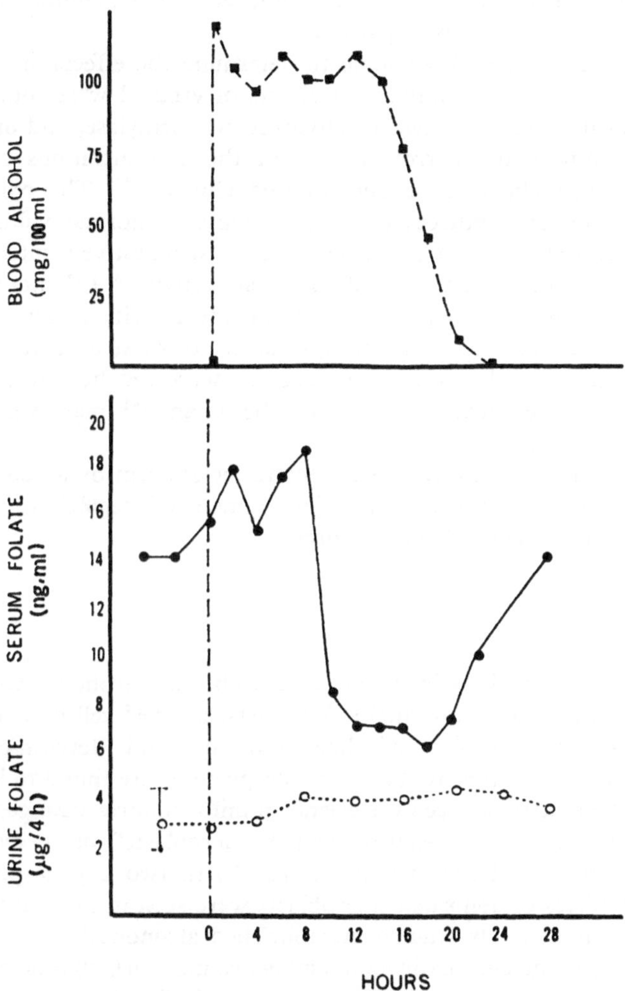

Figure 8.2 Effect of a 13-h intravenous ethanol infusion on serum and urinary folate concentrations in a volunteer subject. During the first 45 min, 40 ml of 10 % ethanol was given, followed by a steady infusion at a rate of 2 ml/min for the remainder of the 13-h period. Serum folate fell abruptly between 8 and 10 h and promptly returned to normal when ethanol was stopped. There was no significant change in urinary folate excretion (from Eichner and Hillman[28])

Eichner and Hillman reported that alcohol administration along with a folate-deficient diet caused a striking fall in serum *L. casei* folate levels within 24 hours (Figure 8.2)[28]. This fall was confirmed in a subsequent study using a radioassay for folate[35] but was not reported by two other groups who gave ethanol with a low folate diet[27,32]. The rapid drop in serum folate was interpreted by Eichner and Hillman to be most likely due to a block in the delivery of storage methylfolate from the liver into the circulation[28]. Later work from the same laboratory with radiolabelled folates in human volunteers was also consistent with this hypothesis[36].

Few other studies have been done to determine the effects of alcohol on folate metabolism. *In vitro* inhibitory effects of ethanol were found on the formate-activating liver enzyme, tetrahydrofolate formylase, and on formate incorporation into bone marrow cells, but the concentrations of ethanol utilized were well above those encountered clinically[37]. The oxidation of [^{14}C]formaldehyde by erythrocytes from patients or normal volunteers ingesting alcohol was reported to be decreased and tentatively interpreted as consistent with an inhibition of tetrahydrofolate activity[38]. Ethanol and folate have been found to have opposite effects on the activity of several jejunal glycolytic enzymes in man[39], but the significance of these observations is uncertain. In patients with severe liver disease, decreased hepatic avidity for folate[40] and increased urinary losses of the vitamin[41] may contribute to negative folate balance.

In summary, alcohol interferes with folate metabolism by a poorly understood mechanism, and accelerates the development of megaloblastic anaemia in individuals with depleted folate stores.

8.2.2 Sideroblastic anaemia

Bone marrow examinations in malnourished chronic alcoholics admitted to hospital frequently show abnormal sideroblasts, i.e., red cell precursors containing increased numbers of haemosiderin- and ferritin-containing granules[13,14]. Ultrastructurally, the iron-rich proteins are found to be heavily deposited in the matrix between the cristae of mitochondria arranged in a ring surrounding the nucleus (so-called 'ringed sideroblasts') or in cytoplasmic bodies, which may be lysosomal in nature[42,43]. In two city hospital series, significant numbers of abnormal sideroblasts were seen in the marrows of 55 and 31 % of consecutively studied malnourished alcoholics[13,14]. The percentage of involved polychromatic and orthochromic normoblasts has varied widely[13,14,44]. The red cells in the peripheral blood of such patients are often, but not always, hypochromic and microcytic[13,14,19]. When the sideroblastic changes appear to be primarily responsible for anaemia, haemosiderin-containing erythrocytes ('siderocytes' or 'Pappenheimer bodies') can usually be detected in smears of peripheral blood[19]. While the majority of patients with sideroblastic abnormalities also have megaloblastic changes and other evidence of folate depletion[13,14,19], in some patients the marrow is entirely normoblastic, the peripheral blood shows no evidence of folate deficiency, and serum and red cell folate values are normal[19,42,42a]. The sideroblasts characteristically disappear rapidly from the marrow during the first week in hospital, but may persist for as long as 12 days[13,14,19].

Serum iron concentrations may or may not be elevated in patients with sideroblastic marrows[13,14]. One of the factors affecting the detection of hyperferraemia is the period elapsing between cessation of alcohol ingestion and the time the serum is obtained for iron determination. Serum iron levels fall abruptly after alcohol withdrawal, even in those patients with normal values on admission to hospital[13,14,17,45]. In many instances, the fall in iron concentration reflects improvement in iron utilization by the previously megaloblastic or sideroblastic marrow[14] but the decline in serum iron may be seen in the absence of these marrow abnormalities[26,30,45].

Factors which may decrease the likelihood of finding abnormal sideroblasts in a given alcoholic patient may include concomitant iron deficiency[13,14,18], decreased numbers of late normoblasts in marrows showing severely ineffective megaloblastic erythropoiesis[14], and (as will be discussed below) the presence of an adequate diet.

8.2.2.1 Pathogenesis

Florid sideroblastic changes have only been encountered in alcoholic patients who are also malnourished[13,14,19]. Better-nourished alcoholics may show no changes or less impressive accumulations of iron in the cytoplasm of marrow normoblasts[17,45]. These clinical observations suggest that a nutritional factor is important in the pathogenesis of sideroblastic anaemia in alcoholics.

This factor is most likely to be pyridoxine deficiency. Since iron is incorporated into haem in the final (mitochondrial) step in haem synthesis, the accumulation of non-haem iron in the mitochondria of developing red cells in sideroblastic anaemias may reflect a disorder of haem synthesis[46]. Pyridoxal phosphate is required as a coenzyme in an earlier (also mitochondrial) step in haem synthesis, the formation of d-amino levulinic acid (d-ALA) from glycine and succinate[46]. Non-alcoholic patients with sideroblastic anaemias often respond to pyridoxine therapy[42,46]. Alcoholics frequently have decreased serum[47–50], whole blood[49], and hepatic[47,51] levels of pyridoxal coenzymes. Furthermore, alcoholics with sideroblastic anaemia have lower serum and whole blood pyridoxal phosphate concentrations than alcoholics with anaemia due to other causes (Figure 8.3)[49].

Sideroblastic marrow changes have recently been produced by the experimental chronic administration of ethanol to human volunteers. When alcohol was given with a diet low in pyridoxine (and folate) content, sideroblastic changes developed after several weeks in one subject studied by Hines[13], two of three studied by Hines and Cowan[27], and one of two by

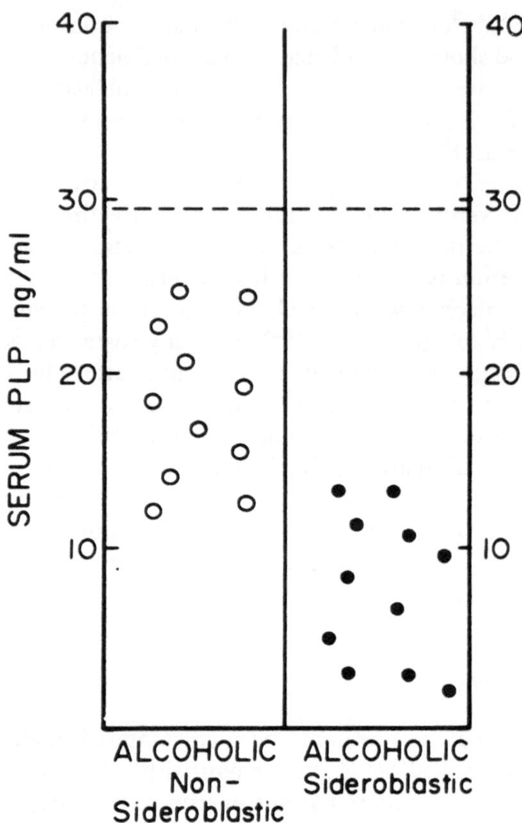

Figure 8.3 Serum pyridoxal phosphate (PLP) concentrations in a group of alcoholic patients who did or did not have sideroblastic bone marrow abnormalities on admission to the hospital (from Hines[49])

Eichner and Hillman[14]. The changes reverted to normal after pyridoxal phosphate therapy despite continued ethanol administration[13,27]. Evidence of deficiency of pyridoxal coenzymes, as measured by serum B_6 levels[27] or increased urinary excretion of xanthurenic and kynurenic acids[14] was also documented in these subjects. In contrast, sideroblastic abnormalities did not develop when alcohol was given for comparable periods with an adequate diet as well as pyridoxine supplements to nine subjects by Lindenbaum and Lieber[30] or to three subjects by Eichner and Hillman[14]. Nor were they seen in the three subjects of Cowan who received ethanol with a nutritious diet without pyridoxine supplementation[29]. An exception was the volunteer described by Hines, who developed sideroblastic changes during the second month of experimental alcohol ingestion despite daily parenteral injections of pyridoxine[49]. Larger doses of ethanol were used in this subject than in the previously mentioned experiments where sideroblastic changes were not noted[14,29,30].

In general, then, both the clinical and experimental evidence indicates that alcohol ingestion will induce sideroblastic marrow changes in the presence of concomitant nutritional deficiency of pyridoxine, which is analogous to the production of megaloblastic anaemia in the setting of combined ethanol administration and dietary folate deficiency. Since associated folate deficiency has usually been present both clinically and experimentally when the sideroblastic changes have been noted, it has been suggested that folate depletion may be a necessary precondition for their development[14]. This appears to be unlikely for several reasons. As mentioned above, some patients present with a pure sideroblastic anaemia, without evidence of folate depletion[19,42,42a]. Also, sideroblastic changes induced experimentally by alcohol do not respond to folic acid administration[27] and may develop despite generous prophylactic folate supplementation[49].

8.2.2.2 Biochemical mechanism

A possible mechanism whereby alcohol interferes with pyridoxine metabolism is indicated by the recent work of Lumeng and Li[50]. These workers found that the activity of two enzymes involved in pyridoxine metabolism, pyridoxal kinase and pyridoxine phosphate oxidase, were normal in intact erythrocytes from alcoholic patients with low serum pyridoxal phosphate concentrations. However, acetaldehyde (but not ethanol) impaired the net formation of pyridoxal phosphate in human red cells *in vitro* (Figure 8.4) by causing the accelerated degradation of phosphorylated B_6 compounds[50]. This action of acetaldehyde was subsequently studied in rat hepatocyte preparations and reported to be due to displacement of pyridoxal phosphate from cytosolic binding proteins, thereby rendering it susceptible to hydrolysis by B_6-phosphate phosphatase[52]. The preliminary report of Hines, who found decreased erythrocyte pyridoxal phosphokinase activity after alcohol ingestion, is at apparent variance with this work[49]; the discordance may be due to methodological differences[50].

If it seems likely, then, that alcohol causes sideroblastic anaemia via an impairment of B_6 metabolism, it has not been demonstrated that this is indeed related to a block in haem synthesis at the B_6-dependent step of d-ALA synthesis. Other disturbances in the haem synthetic pathway may be present. Ali and Sweeney reported elevated red cell coproporphyrin and protoporphyrin levels in eleven alcoholic patients with ringed sideroblasts[44] and Krasner and colleagues found decreased ALA dehydratase activity in the serum of alcoholics[53]. It is also possible that depletion of B_6 coenzymes interferes primarily with steps in globin synthesis, with a secondary effect on haem synthesis. The possible importance of alcohol-induced mitochondrial damage, which has been well documented in other organs[54], in red cell precursors also requires further evaluation.

Whether the hypomagnesaemia and hypokalaemia commonly seen in patients with ringed sideroblasts are factors in pathogenesis remains

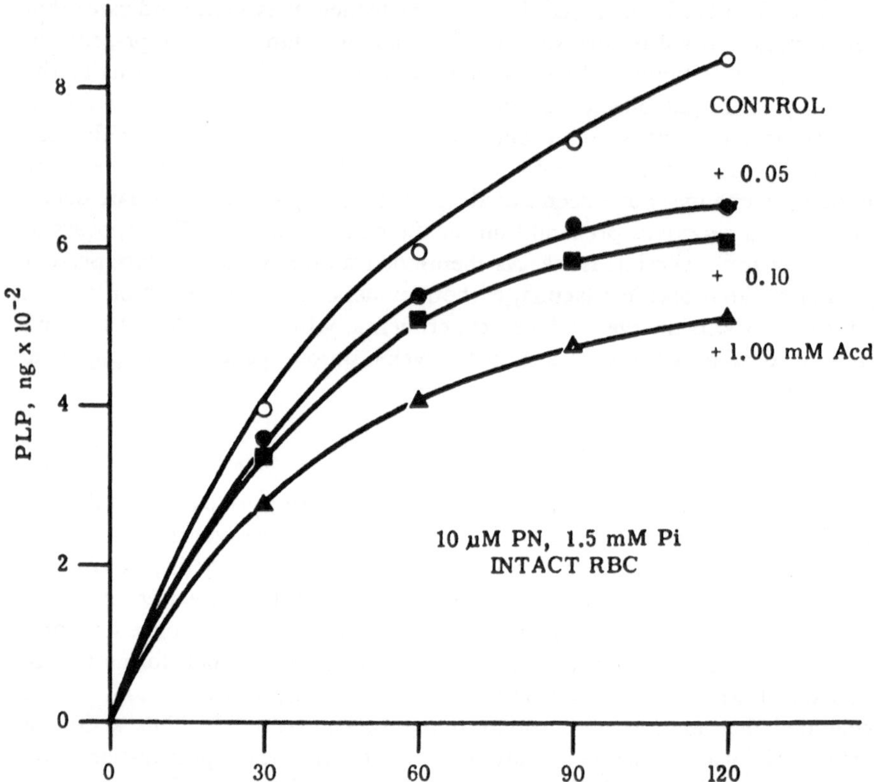

Figure 8.4 Effect of 0.05, 0.10, and 1.00 mM acetaldehyde concentrations on the net synthesis of pyridoxine (PN) by intact human red blood cells in medium containing 1.5 mM inorganic phosphate (Pi). Acetaldehyde produced a dose-related 30–50 % inhibition of net PLP synthesis. Ethanol in concentrations up to 70 mM had no effect. In other experiments, the effect of acetaldehyde on net synthesis was shown to be due to accelerated breakdown of PLP (from Lumeng and Li[50])

speculative[13,27]. The same can be said for the possible role in the development of hepatic haemosiderosis and haemochromatosis contributed by alcohol-induced interference with iron incorporation into red cells in sideroblastic and megaloblastic states[17,26,55].

In summary, alcohol administration, usually in association with a diet lacking in vitamin B_6, results in sideroblastic bone marrow abnormalities, possibly due to an acetaldehyde-induced acceleration of the hydrolysis of pyridoxal phosphate.

8.2.3 Vacuolization of marrow precursor cells

A third effect of alcohol on erythrocytes, apparently unrelated to the megaloblastic and sideroblastic abnormalities, is the induction of vacuolization

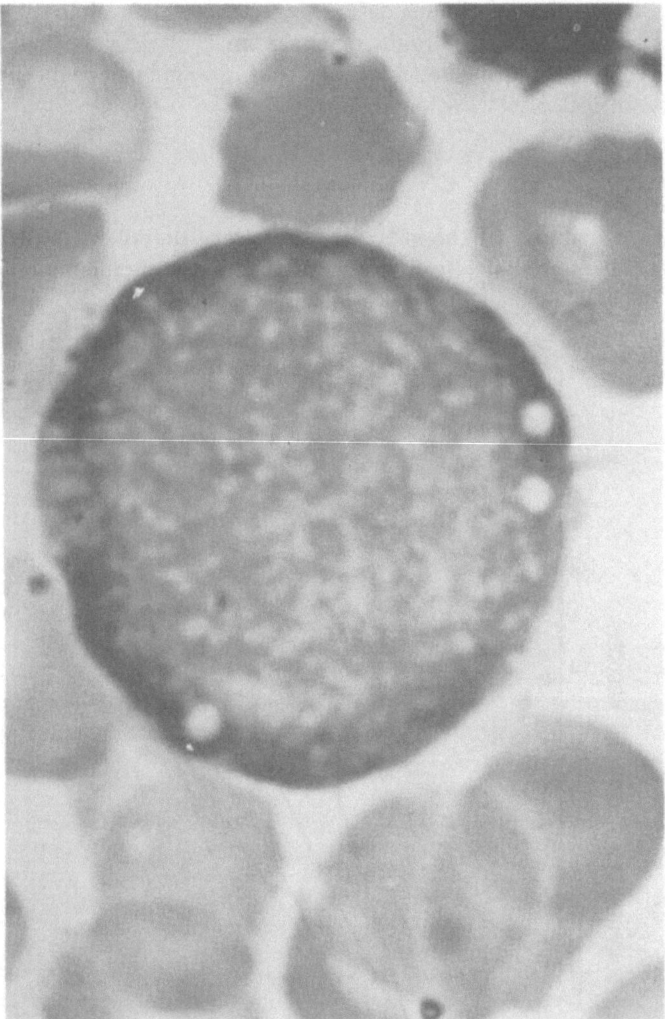

Figure 8.5 Vacuolated pronormoblast from the bone marrow of a human volunteer after 17 days of administration of ethanol as 60 % of total caloric intake while adequate protein ingestion was maintained and vitamin supplements were given (from Lindenbaum and Lieber[30])

(Figure 8.5) in bone marrow red cell precursors. The presence of vacuoles in developing erythrocytes, first described by McCurdy and colleagues[56], is a characteristic finding in the majority of recently intoxicated patients[12,14,17,45,56]. Vacuolization may also be present in white cell precursors, though less frequently, unless an associated infection is present. Within a week of admission to hospital and withdrawal of alcohol (and often within 24 hours) the vacuoles are no longer demonstrable. Vacuolization occurs independently of megaloblastic change, folate deficiency, sideroblastic change, or thrombocytopenia, and is unrelated to nutritional status[12,13,17,45,57]. Similar vacuoles have also been reported in the marrow cells of infants born to mothers receiving intravenous alcohol therapeutically[58].

8.2.3.1 Pathogenesis

The rapid reversibility of the vacuolization after ethanol withdrawal and its morphological resemblance to that seen after chloramphenicol administration

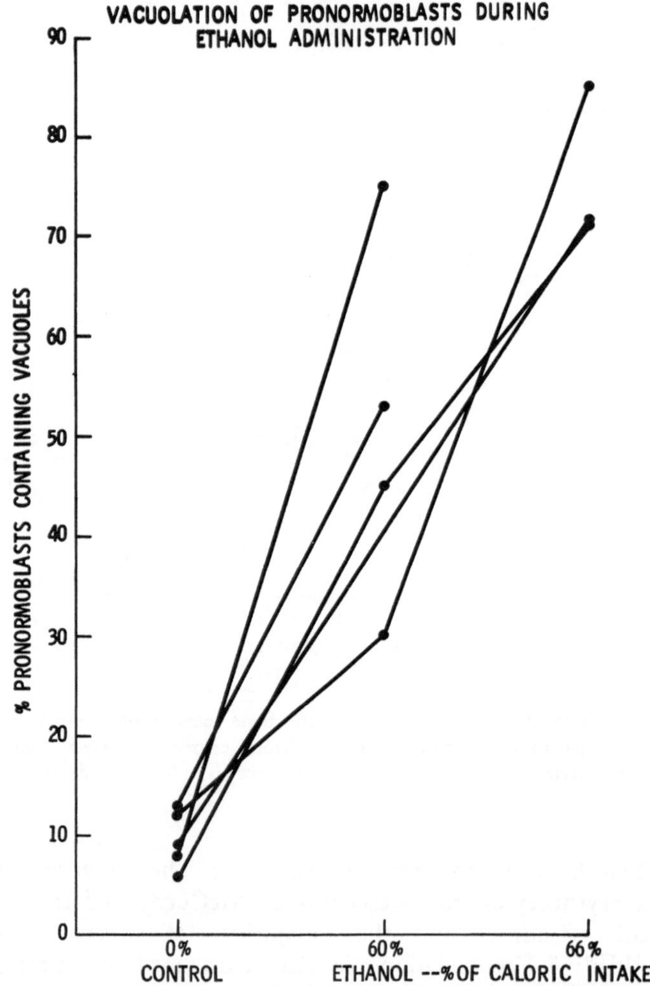

Figure 8.6 Increases in percentage of vacuolated marrow pronormoblasts in five human subjects receiving ethanol for 17–63 days as 60 or 66 % of total caloric intake; '0 %' values are from pre-ethanol marrow aspirates (modified from Lindenbaum and Lieber[30])

suggested a possible toxic depression of erythropoiesis by alcohol[12,56]. The experimental administration of ethanol, substituted isocalorically for carbohydrate, along with excellent protein and vitamin intake, including folate supplementation, resulted in vacuolization of marrow red and white cell precursors in well-nourished human volunteers (Figures 8.5 and 8.6)[30]. The effect was dose-related[30]. Vacuole formation in promyelocytes was less striking than that in pronormoblasts and was only seen with relatively large doses of ethanol. The vacuolization cleared rapidly after cessation of alcohol. The nature of the vacuoles was not established. They did not stain with histochemical reactions for fat, mucopolysaccharides, DNA, RNA, peroxidase, or acid and alkaline phosphatases[30]. Ultrastructurally, vacuolated red cell precursors in the bone marrow of intoxicated patients showed marked membrane convolutions adjacent to the vacuoles which lacked organelles or organized structure, suggesting an effect of alcohol on the cell membrane[59].

The functional significance of the vacuolization is unknown. When it was produced experimentally, there was no associated fall in haematocrit, reticulocyte count, or granulocyte count, nor was there impairment of the incoporation of radioactive iron into circulating erythrocytes[30]. In addition, the vacuoles have frequently been seen clinically in intoxicated patients who were not anaemic[12,17,45,56].

The relationship of the vacuolization to changes in serum osmolality related to ethanol ingestion requires further study, since similar vacuoles have recently been reported in a diabetic patient with hyperosmolar coma[60]. It is uncertain whether alcohol-induced vacuolization is related to the reticulocytosis seen in many non-folate-deficient alcoholic patients after cessation of drinking[4,61]. The elevated reticulocyte count seen after ethanol withdrawal may cause confusion with a haemolytic state[14].

8.2.4 Haemolytic syndromes and red cell membrane abnormalities

8.2.4.1 Low grade haemolysis of liver disease

A variety of haemolytic syndromes have been described in patients with alcoholic liver disease. It has been suggested frequently that an abnormality in red cell morphology or in plasma lipid concentration is related to the presence of haemolysis. Critical evaluation of such inferences requires recognition of the fact that a shortened red cell life span has been reported in many studies in one-third to three-quarters of patients with alcoholic and non-alcoholic cirrhosis[62]. The degree of shortening of erythrocyte survival has varied from mild to moderate[62]. Often, no anaemia, or only mild anaemia, is present because of adequate compensatory production of red cells by the bone marrow[63]. The mechanisms underlying the usually low-grade chronic haemolytic state are uncertain. Coombs' tests are usually negative and the haemolysis is not altered by steroid therapy[4]. Since normal donor cells have a shortened life span in the cirrhotic patient, an extracorpuscular factor is present[4]. The frequently associated lowering of the serum iron and iron-binding capacity[4,64] are reminiscent of the anaemia of chronic inflammatory and neoplastic conditions, where there is also a modest impairment of erythrocyte survival[65]. Increased splenic uptake of radioactively labelled red cells has been demonstrated in many cirrhotics, and probably plays a role in some anaemic patients[4,62,66] but not in others[64,67].

8.2.4.2 Macrocytosis of liver disease

Abnormalities of red cell morphology, surface area, and lipid content have been repeatedly described in patients with alcoholic and non-alcoholic liver disease. Macrocytic red cells are observed in Wright-stained peripheral blood smears in most patients with alcoholic cirrhosis and other severe forms of liver disease[68–71]. This 'macrocytosis of liver disease' has multiple etiologies. In some patients, the presence of morphologically large cells is associated with an increased mean cell *volume* (so-called 'thick' or 'volume' macrocytosis[68,72]). In these patients either reticulocytosis or folic acid deficiency frequently appear to be responsible for the presence of large cells[69,72]. Recently volume macrocytosis of unknown cause has been reported in some alcoholics in the absence of severe liver disease, folate deficiency, or reticulocytosis[73,74]. In the majority of cirrhotic patients, however, the macrocytosis is not associated with an increased cell volume[68,75]; instead, mean cell *diameter* is increased ('thin' macrocytosis, 'macroplania') without an increase in cell volume. Such flattened cells have an increased surface membrane area associated with increased membrane cholesterol and phospholipid content[75,76], and are resistant to osmotic lysis[68,75]. This 'thin' macrocytosis does not correlate with the presence or absence of anaemia, reticulocytosis, or nutritional deficiency[68]. It is said not to occur in patients with fatty liver in the absence of more severe hepatic disease[68]. Normal erythrocytes transfused into the circulation of patients with cirrhosis acquire the increased osmotic resistance of the recipient's cells[75].

8.2.4.3 Target cells in liver disease

The presence of target cells in the blood smears of some patients with severe hepatic disease, usually with an obstructive component, appears to be an exaggerated form of the thin macrocytosis[70,75,77]. The target cells of patients with liver disease similarly have an increased surface:volume ratio, elevations in both the cholesterol and phospholipid content of the cell membrane[72,78], and increased osmotic resistance[79]. The target cell abnormality also does not correlate with the presence of anaemia[70,77]. The target forms disappear when jaundice subsides[78]. Target erythrocytes from patients with biliary obstruction rapidly lose their osmotic resistance when transfused into normal subjects[79];

this also occurs *in vitro* when the cells are incubated in normal serum[79]. The reverse is true when normal cells are transfused into patients with obstructive jaundice, or incubated *in vitro* with jaundiced sera. The changes in *in vitro* osmotic fragility can be correlated with increases in erythrocyte surface area and lipid content[79].

8.2.4.4 Acanthocytosis

Another abnormality of the red cell membrane encountered in patients with alcoholic liver disease is the presence of irregularly spiculated and contracted erythrocytes (Figure 8.7), resembling those seen in congenital abetalipoproteinaemia ('acanthocytes' or 'spur cells'). In contrast to the thin macrocytosis and target cell phenomena, acanthocytosis has characteristically been observed in patients with brisk haemolytic anemia. Almost all the reported

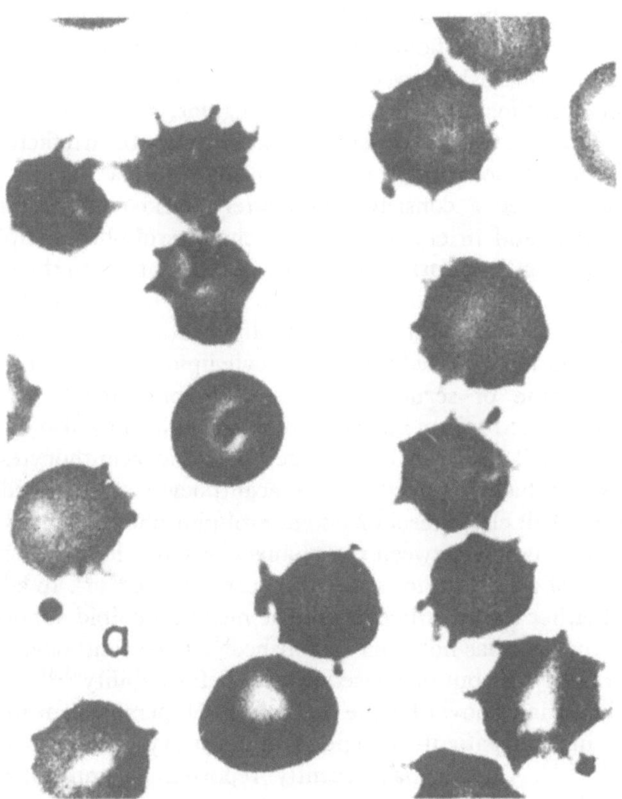

Figure 8.7 Irregularly spiculated red blood cells ('acanthocytes' or 'spur cells') from the peripheral blood smear of a patient with alcoholic cirrhosis and a severe haemolytic anaemia (Wright's stain) (from Cooper *et al.*[87])

cases have been in patients with advanced alcoholic cirrhosis, who had hyperbilirubinaemia, ascites, splenomegaly, and a generally poor prognosis[77,80–87]. A few patients have been reported, however, in whom acanthocytosis was associated with severe, non-alcoholic liver disease, including cardiac cirrhosis[82], acute yellow atrophy secondary to vital hepatitis[85], neonatal liver disease[88,89], and metastatic carcinoid tumour[90]. A marked shortening of the survival of autologous red cells has been demonstrated in many of these patients, often but not always associated with increased splenic sequestration[80–84,86]. When transfused into normal recipients, the patients' erythrocytes have had a shortened survival, while normal donor cells transfused into the patients also survive poorly[80,81,83,84], and have been reported to acquire membrane spiculation[91]. The red cells of a patient with acanthocytosis survived normally when transfused into an asplenic recipient[84].

The pathogenesis of acanthocytosis in patients with liver disease remains obscure despite numerous investigations. Studies in which separated cells or plasma from patients and normal controls have been incubated together have yielded conflicting results as to whether the acanthocytosis is reversible or inducible *in vitro*[80–84,86,87,90]. Some of the reported discrepancies appear to be due to failure to distinguish between the irregular spiculation and distortion of cell outline of acanthocytes and the more regular, superficial scalloping of crenated cells ('burr' cells, 'echinocytes')[92] which may be artefactual and can be induced by incubation of red cells in normal plasma[84,87,92].

Cooper has reported a consistent and often marked increase in red cell cholesterol content and in erythrocyte-free cholesterol/phospholipid ratio in patients with the acanthocytosis of liver disease (in contrast to the slight elevation of this ratio in patients with target cells)[77,83,87]. He has also shown a good correlation between free cholesterol/phospholipid ratios in red cells and serum of these patients and has related the erythrocyte lipid abnormalities to the free cholesterol saturation of serum low-density lipoproteins[77,87]. It has been speculated that elevated serum bile acid concentrations may also contribute to the increased red cell lipids in both target cells and acanthocytes[77,79,83,87].

Others, however, have reported cases of acanthocytosis associated with liver disease where red cell cholesterol or cholesterol/phospholipid ratios were normal[80,81,84,90]. Dissociation between the changes in red cell cholesterol content and the presence of acanthocytosis has also been reported[85,87]. In addition, the relationship of either the acanthocytes or the membrane lipid abnormalities to the haemolytic process has not been established[93]. The acanthocytes have normal osmotic fragility[83,87] but decreased *in vitro* deformability[85,87,90]. The latter might result in their removal by the spleen[83,85]. Hypersplenism may play an important role in some patients, independent of the erythrocyte membrane abnormalities[80–82,87,93]. Cooper has recently reported an interesting case in which the acanthocytes were no longer seen following splenectomy, suggesting that splenic 'conditioning' may play a role in the genesis of the morphological abnormality[87].

8.2.4.5 Zieve's syndrome

In 1958 Zieve reported a series of 20 alcoholic patients with hypercholesterolaemia, transient hyperbilirubinaemia, acute fatty liver, and a mild anaemia which was interpreted as haemolytic[94]. The constellation of alcoholic liver disease, hyperlipaemia, and haemolysis was felt to represent a distinct syndrome, and it was speculated that the hyperlipaemia in some way caused the haemolysis[94]. Subsequently, additional, more or less similar cases have been reported[95–100]. The problem has recently been reviewed critically by Eichner[101]. The evidence that acute haemolytic anaemia was actually present in many of the reported cases is equivocal; many may have been recovering from marrow failure or have had chronic low grade haemolysis associated with liver disease with a fall in haematocrit related to changes in hydration[101]. Even when haemolysis was present, a causal relationship with elevations in serum lipids has not been demonstrated[96,97,101], and the usefulness of the concept of such a syndrome is questionable.

8.2.4.6 Stomatocytosis

Douglass and Twomey recently reported four alcoholic patients with transient stomatocytosis[102]. Stomatocytes (red cells with a central slit or mouth-like zone of pallor on Wright's stain) have previously been reported in association with rare congenital haemolytic anaemias[103,104]. The four alcoholic patients had mild to moderate hepatic dysfunction associated with fatty liver[102]. Varying degrees of anaemia and shortening of red cell survival were documented but appeared to be unrelated to the numbers of stomatocytes seen. There was no evidence of increased splenic sequestration. The stomatocytosis recurred in two patients after discharge from hospital and resumption of heavy drinking[102]. The same workers also found increased numbers of stomatocytes in 11 of 40 unselected patients with acute alcoholism[102]. Two alcoholics with stomatocytosis are mentioned in a recent French study[105]. We have encountered transient stomatocytosis and haemolytic anaemia in an alcoholic patient with fatty liver as well as in a non-alcoholic man with viral hepatitis[19]. The pathogenesis of the abnormality in red cell morphology in such patients has not yet been elucidated, nor has a definite relationship between the presence of stomatocytes and haemolytic anaemia been shown.

8.2.4.7 Hypophosphataemia and haemolysis

Jacob and Amsden recently reported an alcoholic patient with pancreatitis, ketoacidosis, mild cirrhosis, and profound hypophosphataemia (serum P = 0.1 mg/100 ml). A brisk acute haemolytic anaemia with spherocytes on blood smear was documented[106]. Markedly diminished levels of erythrocyte ATP and decreased *in vitro* filterability of the patient's red cells were present at the time of hypophosphataemia. These authors speculated that lack of ATP secondary to phosphate depletion resulted in rigidity of the red cell membrane leading to haemolysis[106]. Two other patients with haemolytic episodes associated with severe hypophosphataemia (and less profoundly depressed red cell ATP levels) have subsequently been reported[107,108]. Alterations in red cell glycolytic intermediates and increased erythrocyte phospholipid levels were found in one of them[107]. As Kloch and co-workers[107] indicate, the interpretation of the cause of haemolytic episodes in alcoholic patients requires great caution; nonetheless, the possibility that hypophosphataemia and haemolysis are related is intriguing and worthy of further investigation. The reasons for the not uncommon development of phosphate depletion in alcoholics[108] have not been determined.

8.2.5 Iron deficiency

Iron deficiency anaemia, usually the result of gastrointestinal blood loss, has been a common finding in several published series of alcoholic patients[18,64,109]. Accumulation of iron in the serum and bone marrow stores due to ineffective erythropoiesis secondary to folate deficiency may sometimes mask the presence of associated iron deficiency. The latter may become apparent only after alcohol withdrawal and correction of the megaloblastic state[18].

8.2.6 Haemodilution

In patients with cirrhosis, expansion of the plasma volume is a common finding[110–112]. This may result in an apparent anaemia, with haematocrit values as low as 28 % in the face of a normal red cell mass[63,109,113,114].

8.2.7 Other causes of anaemia in alcoholics

Other possible factors causing anaemia in alcoholic patients include the presence of chronic infection, hypoproliferative anaemia secondary to fatty liver[14], and marrow failure due to unidentified factors associated with cirrhosis[64]. In addition, the importance of nutritional deficiency states such as protein and riboflavin deficiency, which have been reported to cause anaemia in non-alcoholic patients[115,116], has not been fully explored in alcoholics.

8.3 PLATELETS

8.3.1 Thrombocytopenia

In 1968, two groups of investigators reported an association between alcohol intoxication and thrombocytopenia[57,117]. This has subsequently been confirmed[14,15,105,118,119,120]. The incidence of thrombocytopenia has been found to be 14[57], 18[120], 32[119], 35[14], 44[105], and 81 %[15] of acutely ill hospitalized alcoholics. Three % of a group of 112 chronic alcoholics of varying socioeconomic backgrounds not requiring emergency admission to hospital had low platelet counts[18]. It is probable that the decrease in circulating platelets associated with alcoholism is the commonest cause of thrombocytopenia in the United States[121].

In the majority of cases, the thrombocytopenia is not associated with folate deficiency[57,105,117], infection[15,57,105,117], hypersplenism[15,57,105,117], or disseminated intravascular coagulation[15,105,117]. There has been no correlation with the presence of anaemia[14,15,105,119] or abnormalities of liver function[15,57,105,119]. Haemorrhagic manifestations are often absent, but may be severe in occasional cases[15,57,105,117]. In some patients there is an associated granulocytopenia[14,18,57,105,117,120]. The platelet count may not change for 1–3 days after admission, may even show a fall, or may begin to rise immediately[15,105]; in any case a rapid return to or towards normal occurs within a week of alcohol withdrawal[15,57,105,119]. Failure of the platelet count to rise within 5–7 days indicates the presence of some other underlying disorder affecting platelets[61]. After the platelet count returns to normal, a rebound thrombocytosis, which may approach levels of 1 000 000 cells/μl, characteristically occurs 5–19 days after admission to hospital, usually during the second week[15,57,105,118]. Thrombocytosis after alcohol withdrawal also occurs in the majority of alcoholics whose platelet counts are normal at the time of admission[15,57].

8.3.1.1 Pathogenesis

The clinical observations of thrombocytopenia in the absence of associated folate deficiency, and its recurrence after short periods of binge-drinking soon after leaving the hospital in patients who were well-nourished at the time of discharge, suggested that alcohol intoxication itself was the cause of the thrombocytopenia[57]. This hypothesis was subsequently confirmed by several groups who induced thrombocytopenia experimentally in human subjects by the administration of ethanol or whisky for 10 days or more[15,29,30,122–124]. Ethanol caused a depression in circulating platelets despite the concomitant administration of a nutritious diet and vitamin supplements including large doses of folic acid (Figure 8.8)[30].

The exact mechanisms whereby alcohol induces thrombocytopenia have not been fully elucidated. An increase in platelet size occurs during recovery from thrombocytopenia in alcoholics[125], suggesting increased production of platelets by the bone marrow after alcohol withdrawal. Megakaryocyte numbers have appeared to be normal or increased at the time of thrombocytopenia in such patients[57,105,117,119], with occasional exceptions[105,119]. However, it is well recognized that estimation of megakaryocyte numbers from smears of aspirated marrow samples may give a misleading impression as to the total

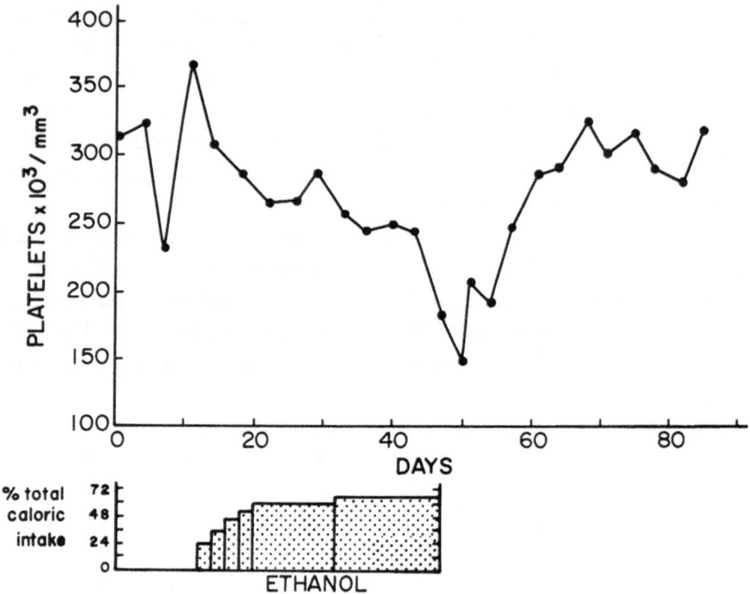

Figure 8.8 Ethanol-induced depression of the platelet count of a volunteer subject who ingested alcohol for 35 days. Folic acid, 1200 μg, was given daily throughout the study (from Lindenbaum and Lieber[30])

megakaryocyte mass. Cowan induced thrombocytopenia experimentally in two subjects by the administration of alcohol along with a standard hospital diet and large doses of folic acid[29]. Marrow megakaryocyte numbers, as calculated from biopsy specimens which were correlated with quantitative studies of erythropoiesis, were increased 1.4 and 1.9-fold over normal, while the lifespan of [^{51}Cr]tagged autologous platelets was significantly decreased by alcohol ingestion. In these experiments, the induction of thrombocytopenia by ethanol thus appeared to result from a combination of decreased platelet survival and ineffective thrombocytopoiesis (i.e., decreased production of platelets despite a normal to increased marrow megakaryocyte mass)[29]. A shortened platelet lifespan has also been reported when thrombocytopenia was produced by alcohol given with a folate deficient diet[26,29] and in a thrombocytopenic patient studied shortly after admission to hospital[117]. In one experimental subject studied by Sullivan, however, platelet lifespan was reported to be normal and marrow megakaryocyte numbers, as estimated from aspirates rather than biopsy specimens, were reduced[122].

Available data suggests that the thrombocytopenic response to chronic alcohol ingestion may be dose-related[29,30,122]. In addition, poorly defined host factors may determine the likelihood of occurrence of this complication, since certain patients develop it repeatedly[57,105,117] while other heavy drinkers appear to escape it[61]. Also, in experimental studies the same alcohol dosage regimen will cause thrombocytopenia in some subjects but not in others[29,30].

An acute effect of ethanol on the platelet count has also been reported. A transient depression of circulating platelets was demonstrated in three subjects after oral[123], and in one subject after intravenous[126], ethanol administration. However, no effect of intravenous ethanol was demonstrable in another subject studied by the same investigators[126], or in two other studies[29,105].

8.3.2 Abnormal platelet function

Haut and Cowan have recently reported significant impairment in platelet function after the chronic administration of large quantities of ethanol with hospital diet and folate supplements[124]. The alterations included prolongation of the bleeding time, impairment of both primary and secondary aggregation induced by adenosine diphosphate and epinephrine, prolongation of the lag period and diminution in the rate and extent of collagen-induced aggregation, decreased platelet factor 3 availability, and subnormal release of adenine nucleotides. The abnormalities of platelet function were more severe in subjects who developed thrombocytopenia, but were also found in the presence of a normal platelet count. They could only be partially reproduced by the acute intravenous administration of ethanol, by the addition of ethanol to normal platelets *in vitro*, or by the addition of plasma from subjects ingesting alcohol to normal platelets *in vitro*. These findings suggested that alcohol damages platelets, perhaps by an effect on the cell membrane, and may be related to the shortening of the platelet lifespan, as well as megakaryocyte dysfunction[124]. *In vitro* studies with other agents which affect plasma osmolality suggested that ethanol-induced hyperosmolality may contribute to impairment in platelet function[127]. The carbohydrate metabolism of resting platelets obtained from subjects with alcohol-induced thrombocytopenia was normal, but abnormalities of $^{14}CO_2$ production were reported after the addition of aggregating agents *in vitro*[128].

8.3.3 Other causes of thrombocytopenia in alcoholics

In addition to alcohol-induced thrombocytopenia, several other entities frequently need to be considered in the differential diagnosis of a low platelet count in the alcoholic patient. These include: severe folate deficiency[26], hypersplenism[129], gram-negative or gram-positive septicaemia[130], and disseminated intravascular coagulation associated with shock, sepsis, or cirrhosis[131]. In patients with megaloblastic states, the severity of thrombocytopenia can be related to the degree of anaemia[132]. The presence of significant thrombocytopenia in a patient with mild or no anaemia suggests that folate deficiency, even if present, is not the primary cause of the low platelet count.

8.4 WHITE CELLS

Early in the century Welch, Osler, and others observed that alcoholics had a greatly increased liability to infections, particularly pneumonias, and a greater mortality rate when infected[133–135]. Probably many factors are responsible for the decreased resistance of alcoholics to infections. Several disorders involving impairment of white blood cell function may be contributory.

8.4.1 Granulocytopenia

That a paradoxical granulocytopenia may occur in alcoholics with severe bacterial infections has long been recognized[136]. McFarland and Libre reported 12 episodes of neutropenia associated with infection (usually bacterial pneumonia) in 10 chronic alcoholics[137]. The granulocytopenia was characteristically transient; if the patient survived, the white cell count began to rise within 2–4 days of admission, often with a subsequent 'rebound' leukocytosis. In such cases, there is frequently an associated thrombocytopenia[105,137]. In normal individuals most of the granulocytes in the body are present in a reserve 'compartment' in the bone marrow[138]. In infected alcoholic patients with granulocytopenia, bone marrow morphological examination has shown normal to decreased cellularity with decreased numbers of granulocytes[19,137]. In some patients, megaloblastic changes consistent with folate deficiency may be present[14,137] while in others there is no morphological or biochemical evidence of folic acid deficiency[19,137]. The bone marrow findings rapidly return to normal during the first week in hospital[19,137].

Episodes of granulocytopenia have also been reported in association with alcohol intoxication in the absence of infection[18,57,105,120]. The incidence of leukopenia in two series of non-infected alcoholic patients was reported to be 3.6[18] and 8.5 %[120]. In both series the degree of leukopenia was usually mild. There has been a high incidence of associated thrombocytopenia[18,57,120]. The granulocytopenia has returned to normal within a few days of admission to hospital[57,120]. Only mild hepatic disease, without splenomegaly, has been noted. The bone marrow is characteristically normoblastic, red cell folate levels have been normal, and serum folate concentrations low, normal, or high[57,120]. Recurrent granulocytopenia is one patient was not prevented by prophylactic folic acid therapy[120]. Marrow granulocute reserves, as estimated morphologically, and by the increment in peripheral granulocyte count noted after endotoxin administration (Figure 8.9), were depleted in alcoholic patients with and without leukopenia[120,137]. The marrow reserves returned to normal after a short period of hospitalization and alcohol withdrawal[120,137].

8.4.1.1 Pathogenesis

The pathogenesis of the decreased marrow granulocyte reserves in alcoholic patients has not been established. Folate deficiency may play a contributory

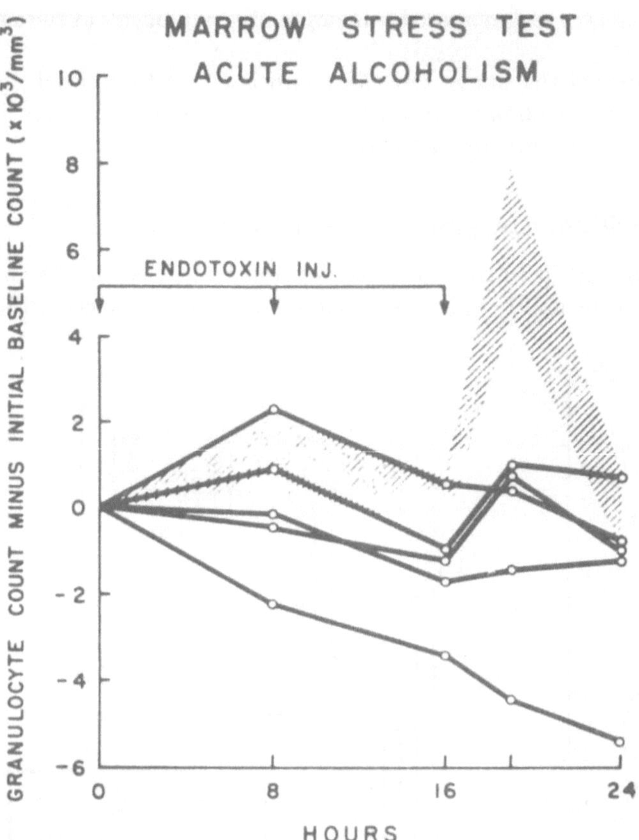

Figure 8.9 Decreased bone marrow neutrophil reserves, as evidenced by subnormal increments in the peripheral blood granulocyte count after several injections of endotoxin in five chronic alcoholics, as compared to normal controls (shaded area) (from McFarland and Libre[137])

role in some patients but is probably not the main cause of the granulocytopenia[57,120]. Unrecognized host factors may be important, in view of the tendency of certain patients to develop recurrent leukopenia with each bout of intoxication[57,120]. The possible role of copper deficiency, recently documented as a cause of granulocytopenia in malnourished non-alcoholic patients[139], requires evaluation. The addition of ethanol *in vitro* has been reported to inhibit the growth of granulocyte colonies derived from human bone marrow[140]. Experimental chronic alcohol administration to dogs has been reported to cause a mild granulocytopenia with decreased marrow cellularity[141]. In experiments in human volunteers, however, ethanol administration has not been reported to cause leukopenia[30] except in the presence of severe folate deficiency[26].

In infected alcoholic patients with granulocytopenia, the decrease in circulating neutrophils is probably due to a combination of decreased marrow white cell reserves and increased utilization of granulocytes at the site of infection.

In addition to the above described entities, the differential diagnosis of neutropenia in alcoholics will include severe folate deficiency as well as hypersplenism in patients with cirrhosis.

8.4.2 Impairment of granulocyte mobilization

An important factor in the decreased resistance to infection may be an effect of ethanol on the ability of leukocytes to migrate into a focus of inflammation.

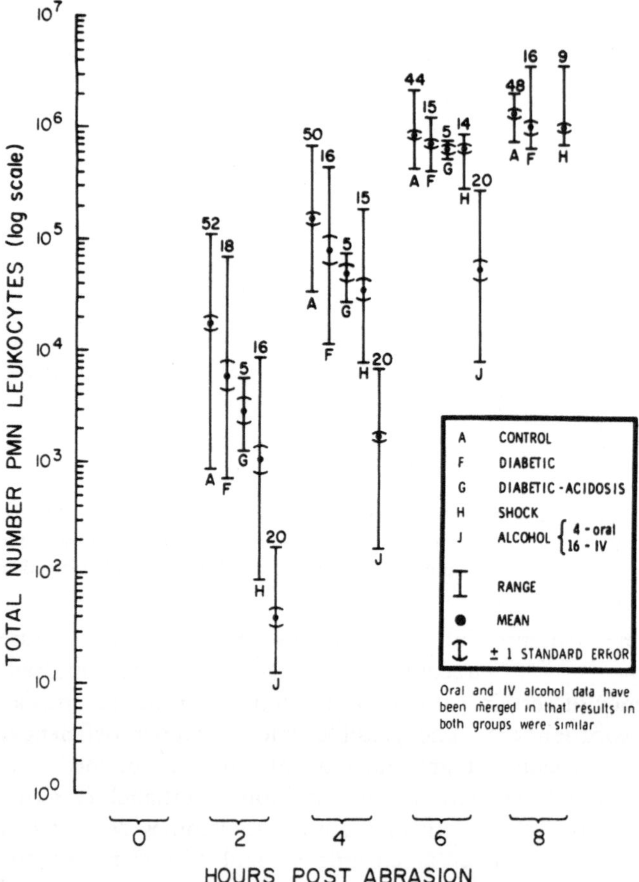

Figure 8.10 Effect of moderate doses of alcohol (50–75 ml of 94 % alcohol given intravenously as a 10 % solution or orally as a 20 % solution over a 20–30 min period) on leukocyte mobilization into areas of experimentally traumatized skin over an 8-h period in 20 non-alcoholic volunteers (group J). Other groups studied included normal controls (A), patients with diabetes in control (F) or in acidosis (G), and patients in terminal shock (H). The numbers above the bars indicate number of patients studied (from Brayton *et al.*[143])

Alcohol intoxication in rabbits was shown to markedly inhibit the emigration of leukocytes to sites of experimental pneumococcal infection[142]. This effect was observed in severely intoxicated, stuporous animals[142]. The acute administration of relatively much smaller doses of ethanol to nutritionally normal human volunteers produced a profound depression in the rate of leukocyte mobilization into areas of traumatized skin (Figure 8.10), without affecting phagocytosis or intracellular killing of staphylococci[143]. Alcohol in low concentrations also decreases leukocyte mobility *in vitro*[144]. The mechanism of this effect has not been determined.

The serum of patients with advanced cirrhosis may have a markedly reduced capacity to stimulate chemotaxis[145]. In concentrations encountered clinically, ethanol did not impair leukocyte chemotaxis *in vitro*[146]. Severe hypophosphataemia has been reported to result in impaired neutrophil function[147].

8.4.3 Impairment of macrophage function

Intoxicated animals show decreased clearance of bacteria from the lungs[135,148] and peritoneal cavity[149]. Decreased mobilization of alveolar macrophages may play a major role in the impaired pulmonary bacterial clearance[150]. Ethanol-treated rats also show decreased clearance of intravenously injected microaggregated albumin by the reticuloendothelial system[151]. These studies in animals suggest that alcohol has a profound effect on the clearance mechanisms of the monocyte–macrophage system, an important line of defence against micro-organisms.

Patients with alcoholic and non-alcoholic cirrhosis have high titres of antibodies to the normal enteric flora, and it has been suggested that this is due to decreased clearance function by hepatic Kupfer cells, or to shunting of blood around the liver[152,153].

8.4.4 Lymphocyte function

The addition of ethanol *in vitro* has been reported to inhibit lymphocyte transformation[140]. Impaired development of dermal delayed hypersensitivity reactions to dinitrochlorobenzene has been reported in patients with alcoholic liver disease[154] and the plasma of cirrhotic patients has been found to inhibit lymphocyte transformation[155].

8.4.5 Other factors favouring infection

Other factors probably contribute to the decreased resistance of alcoholics to infection. These include depression of the cough reflex by ethanol[156], impairment of reflex closure of the glottis[135], and associated cigarette smoking[135]. Folate deficiency in animals predisposes to infection[157].

8.5 SUMMARY

Our current understanding of the roles of ethanol ingestion, nutritional factors, and liver disease in the development of haematological complications in alcoholics is summarized in Table 8.1 and in the following paragraphs.

Table 8.1 Haematological abnormalities in alcoholics

	Direct relationship with		
Haematological finding	*Ethanol ingestion*	*Nutritional deficiency*	*Liver disease*
Megaloblastic pancytopenia	+	+	0
Sideroblastic anaemia	+	+	0
Vacuolization of marrow cells	+	0	0
'Flat' macrocytosis	0	0	+
Target cells	0	0	+
Acanthocytosis	0	0	+
Stomatocytosis	?	0	?
Low-grade chronic haemolysis	0	0	+
Hypervolaemia	0	0	+
Anaemia of chronic disease	0	0	+
Thrombocytopenia	+	+	+
Abnormal platelet function	+	0	+
Hypersplenism	0	0	+
Granulocytopenia	?	?	+
Decreased mobilization of phagocytes	+	0	0

(1) Megaloblastic pancytopenia due to folic acid deficiency is common in alcoholics and is caused by a combination of nutritional deficiency and a poorly understood effect of ethanol on folate metabolism.

(2) Sideroblastic anaemia is also commonly seen in malnourished alcoholics and is possibly due to a defect in haem synthesis secondary to depletion of pyridoxal phosphate. The latter appears to be the result of a combination of nutritional deficiency and accelerated hydrolysis of B_6 phosphate caused by acetaldehyde.

(3) Vacuolization of marrow red and white cell precursors is caused by ethanol administration in the absence of nutritional deficiency and is often not accompanied by other evidence of depression of haematopoiesis.

(4) Abnormalities of red cell morphology and increased erythrocyte membrane lipid concentrations occur frequently in patients with advanced alcoholic liver disease. The commonly seen 'thin' macrocytes and target cells are unrelated to any haemolytic process; in contrast, acanthocytosis in alcoholics has only been noted in the presence of brisk haemolysis and severe cirrhosis. Stomatocytosis is an occasional complication of uncertain significance. Red cell rigidity and haemolysis occurs in profoundly hypophosphataemic patients.

(5) Low-grade chronic haemolysis, plasma volume expansion, iron deficiency secondary to gastrointestinal bleeding, and the anaemia of chronic

disease related to infection or hepatic inflammation are other common factors contributing to low haematocrit levels.

(6) Thrombocytopenia is very frequently encountered. Alcohol causes thrombocytopenia in the absence of nutritional deficiency, due to a combination of decreased platelet survival and ineffective thrombocytopoiesis. Ethanol administration also impairs platelet function.

(7) Granulocytopenia may occur in infected patients and with intoxication in the absence of infection. The role of ethanol in the decreased marrow neutrophil reserves seen in such individuals is not established. Alcohol administration interferes with the mobilization of granulocytes and with the clearing function of the macrophage–monocyte system. Other factors also contribute to the decreased resistance of alcoholics to infection.

References

1. Jarrold, T. and Vilter, R. W. (1949). Hematologic observations in patients with chronic hepatic insufficiency: sternal bone marrow morphology and bone marrow plasmacytosis. *J. Clin. Invest.*, **28**, 286
2. Movitt, E. R. (1949). Megaloblastic bone marrow in liver disease. *Am. J. Med.*, **7**, 145
3. Movitt, E. R. (1950). Megaloblastic erythropoiesis in patients with cirrhosis of the liver. *Blood*, **5**, 468
4. Jandl, J. H. (1955). Anemia of liver disease: observations on its mechanism. *J. Clin. Invest.*, **34**, 390
5. Jandl, J. H. and Lear, A. A. (1956). The metabolism of folic acid in cirrhosis. *Ann. Intern. Med.*, **45**, 1027
6. Krasnow, S., Walsh, J. R., Zimmerman, H. and Heller, P. (1957). Megaloblastic anemia in 'alcoholic' cirrhosis. *Arch. Intern. Med.*, **100**, 870
7. Herbert, V., Baker, H., Frank, O., Pasher, I., Sobotka, H. and Wasserman, L. R. (1960). The measurement of folic acid activity in serum: a diagnostic acid in the differentiation of the megaloblastic anemias. *Blood*, **15**, 228
8. Herbert, V., Zalusky, R. and Davidson, C. S. (1963). Correlation of folate deficiency with alcoholism and associated macrocytosis, anemia, and liver disease. *Ann. Intern. Med.*, **58**, 977
9. Klipstein, F. A. and Lindenbaum, J. (1965). Folate deficiency in chronic liver disease. *Blood*, **25**, 443
10. Deller, D. J., Kimber, C. L. and Ibbotson, R. N. (1965). Folic acid deficiency in cirrhosis of the liver. *Am. J. Dig. Dis.*, **10**, 35
11. Kimber, C. L., Deller, D. J. and Lander, H. (1965). Megaloblastic and transitional megaloblastic anemia associated with chronic liver disease. *Am. J. Med.*, **38**, 767
12. Jarrold, T., Will, J. J., Davies, A. R., Duffy, P. H. and Bramschreiber, B. L. (1967). Bone marrow-erythroid morphology in alcoholic patients. *Am. J. Clin. Nutr.*, **20**, 716
13. Hines, J. D. (1969). Reversible megaloblastic and sideroblastic marrow abnormalities in alcoholic patients. *Br. J. Haematol.*, **16**, 87
14. Eichner, E. R. and Hillman, R. S. (1971). The evolution of anemia in alcoholic patients. *Am. J. Med.*, **50**, 218
15. Cowan, D. H. and Hines, J. D. (1971). Thrombocytopenia of severe alcoholism. *Ann. Intern. Med.*, **74**, 37
16. Williams, I. R. and Girdwood, R. H. (1970). The folate status of alcoholics. *Scot. Med. J.*, **15**, 285
17. Hourihane, C. O. and Weir, D. G. (1970). Suppression of erythropoiesis by alcohol. *Br. Med. J.*, **i**, 86

18. Eichner, E. R., Buchanan, B., Smith, J. W. and Hillman, R. S. (1972). Variations in the hematologic and medical status of alcoholics. *Am. J. Med.*, **263,** 35
19. Lindenbaum, J. Unpublished observations
20. Herbert, V. (1963). A palatable diet for producing experimental folate deficiency in man. *Am. J. Clin. Nutr.*, **12,** 17
21. Herbert, V. (1962). The diagnosis and treatment of folic acid deficiency. *Med. Clin. N. Am.*, **46,** 1365
22. Herbert, V. (1963). Current concepts in therapy: megaloblastic anemia. *N. Engl. J. Med.*, **268,** 201
23. Herbert, V. (1962). Experimental nutritional folate deficiency in man. *Trans. Ass. Am. Phys.*, **75,** 307
24. Herbert, V. (1962). Minimal daily adult folate requirement. *Arch. Intern. Med.*, **110,** 649
25. Eichner, E. R., Pierce, H. I. and Hillman, R. S. (1971). Folate balance in dietary-induced megaloblastic anemia. *N. Engl. J. Med.*, **284,** 933
26. Sullivan, L. W. and Herbert, V. (1964). Suppression of hematopoiesis by ethanol. *J. Clin. Invest.*, **43,** 2048
27. Hines, J. D. and Cowan, D. H. (1970). Studies on the pathogenesis of alcohol-induced sideroblastic bone-marrow abnormalities. *N. Engl. J. Med.*, **283,** 441
28. Eichner, E. R. and Hillman, R. S. (1973). Effect of alcohol on serum folate level. *J. Clin. Invest.*, **52,** 584
29. Cowan, D. H. (1973). Thrombokinetic studies in alcohol-related thrombocytopenia. *J. Lab. Clin. Med.*, **81,** 64
30. Lindenbaum, J. and Lieber, C. S. (1969). Hematologic effects of alcohol in man in the absence of nutritional deficiency. *N. Engl. J. Med.*, **281,** 333
31. Halsted, C. H., Robles, E. A. and Mezey, E. (1971). Decreased jejunal uptake of labeled folic acid (^{3}H-PGA) in alcoholic patients: roles of alcohol and nutrition. *N. Engl. J. Med.*, **285,** 701
32. Halsted, C. H., Robles, E. A. and Mezey, E. (1973). Intestinal malabsorption in folate-deficient alcoholics. *Gastroenterology*, **64,** 526
33. Hermos, J. A., Adams, W. H., Liu, Y. K., Sullivan, L. W. and Trier, J. S. (1972). Mucosa of the small intestine in folate-deficient alcoholics. *Ann. Intern. Med.*, **76,** 957
34. Lindenbaum, J. and Pezzimenti, J. F. (1972). Effects of B_{12} and folate deficiency on small intestinal function. *Clin. Res.*, **20,** 871
35. Paine, C. J., Eichner, E. R. and Dickson, V. (1973). Concordance of radioassay and microbiological assay in the study of the ethanol-induced fall in serum folate level. *Am. J. Med. Sci.*, **266,** 135
36. Lane, F., Goff, P., McGuffin, R. and Hillman, R. (1973). The influence of ethanol on folate metabolism. *Blood*, **42,** 998
37. Bertino, J. R., Ward, J., Sartorelli, A. C. and Silber, R. (1965). An effect of ethanol on folate metabolism. *J. Clin. Invest.*, **44,** 1028
38. Trau, N., Laplante, M. and Lebel, E. (1972). Abnormal oxidation of [^{14}C]formaldehyde to $^{14}CO_2$ in erythrocytes of alcoholics and nonalcoholics after consumption of alcoholic beverages. *J. Nucl. Med.*, **13,** 677
39. Greene, H. L., Stifel, F. B., Herman, R. H., Herman, Y. F. and Rosensweig, N. S. (1974). Ethanol-induced inhibition of human intestinal enzyme activities: reversal by folic acid. *Gastroenterology*, **67,** 434
40. Cherrick, G. R., Baker, H., Frank, O. and Leevy, C. M. (1965). Observations on hepatic avidity for folate in Laennec's cirrhosis. *J. Lab. Clin. Med.*, **66,** 6
41. Retief, E. P. and Huskisson, Y. J. (1969). Serum and urinary folate in liver disease. *Br. Med. J.*, **ii,** 150
42. Hines, J. D. and Grasso, J. A. (1970). The sideroblastic anemias. *Sem. Hematol.*, **7,** 86
42a. Hines, J. D. and Cowan, D. H. (1974). Anemia in alcoholism. In N. V. Dimitrov and J. H. Nodine, eds. *Drugs and Hematologic Reactions*, p. 141. New York: Grune and Stratton

43. Grasso, J. A. and Hines, J. D. (1969). A comparative electron microscopic study of refractory and alcoholic sideroblastic anemia. *Br. J. Haematol.*, **17**, 34
44. Ali, M. A. M. and Sweeney, G. (1974). Erythrocyte coproporphyrin and protoporphyrin in ethanol-induced sideroblastic erythropoiesis. *Blood*, **43**, 291
45. Waters, A. H., Morley, A. A. and Rankin, J. G. (1966). Effect of alcohol on haemopoiesis. *Br. Med. J.*, **ii**, 1565
46. Aoki, Y., Urata, G., Wada, O. and Takaku, F. (1974). Measurement of δ-aminolevulinic acid synthetase activity in human erythroblasts. *J. Clin. Invest.*, **53**, 1326
47. Leevy, C. M., Baker, H., tenHove, W., Frank, O. and Cherrick, G. R. (1965). B-complex vitamins in liver disease of the alcoholic. *Am. J. Clin. Nutr.*, **16**, 339
48. Hines, J. D. and Love, D. S. (1969). Determination of serum and blood pyridoxal phosphate concentrations with purified rabbit skeletal muscle apophosphorylase b. *J. Lab. Clin. Med.*, **73**, 343
49. Hines, J. D. (1973). Alcohol-induced abnormalities in the metabolism of vitamin B_6 in humans. *Proc. First Ann. Alcoholism Conf. of NIAAA*, Washington, D.C., p. 6.
50. Lumeng, L. and Li, T. (1974). Vitamin B_6 metabolism in chronic alcohol abuse. *J. Clin. Invest.*, **53**, 693
51. Frank, O., Luisada-Opper, A., Sorrell, M. F., Thomson, A. D. and Baker, H. (1971). Vitamin deficits in severe alcoholic fatty liver of man calculated from multiple reference units. *Exper. Molec. Pathol.*, **15**, 191
52. Veitch, R. L., Lumeng, L. and Li, T. K. (1974). The effect of ethanol and acetaldehyde on vitamin B_6 metabolism in liver. *Gastroenterology*, **66**, 868
53. Krasner, N., Moore, M. R., Thompson, G. G., McIntosh, W. and Goldberg, A. (1974). Depression of erythrocyte δ-aminolaevulinic acid dehydratase activity in alcoholics. *Clin. Sci. Molec. Med.*, **46**, 415
54. Rubin, E., Beattie, D. S., Toth, A. and Lieber, C. S. (1972). Structural and functional effects of ethanol on hepatic mitochondria. *Fed. Proc.*, **31**, 131
55. Neame, P. B. and Beck, I. (1970). Recurrent alcoholic sideroblastosis and hepatic hemosiderosis. *N. Engl. J. Med.*, **283**, 1173
56. McCurdy, P. R., Pierce, L. E. and Rath, C. E. (1962). Abnormal bone marrow morphology in acute alcoholism. *N. Engl. J. Med.*, **266**, 505
57. Lindenbaum, J. and Hargrove, R. L. (1968). Thrombocytopenia in alcoholics. *Ann. Intern. Med.*, **68**, 526
58. Lopez, R. and Montoya, M. F. (1971). Abnormal bone marrow morphology in the premature infant associated with maternal alcohol infusion. *J. Pediat.*, **79**, 1008
59. Yeung, K. Y., Klug, P. P., Brower, M. and Lessin, L. S. (1973). Mechanism of alcohol-induced vacuolization in human bone marrow cells. *Blood*, **42**, 998
60. Lehane, D. E. (1974). Vacuolated erythroblasts in hyperosmolar coma. *Arch. Intern. Med.*, **134**, 763
61. Lindenbaum, J. (1974). Hematologic effects of alcohol. In B. Kissin and H. Begleiter, eds. *The Biology of Alcoholism, Volume 3, Clinical Pathology*, p. 461. New York: Plenum Press
62. Subhiyah, B. W. and Al-Hindawi, A. Y. (1967). Red cell survival and splenic accumulation of radiochromium in liver cirrhosis with splenomegaly. *Br. J. Haematol.*, **13**, 773
63. Hall, C. A. (1960). Erythrocyte dynamics in liver disease. *Am. J. Med.*, **28**, 541
64. Kimber, C., Deller, D. J., Ibbotson, R. N. and Lander, H. (1965). The mechanism of anemia in chronic liver disease. *Q. J. Med.*, **34**, 33
65. Cartwright, G. E. (1966). Anemia of chronic disorders. *Semin. Hematol.*, **3**, 351
66. Felsher, B. F., Redeker, A. G. and Reynolds, T. B. (1968). Indirect reacting hyperbilirubinemia in cirrhosis: its relation to red cell survival. *Am. J. Dig. Dis.*, **13**, 598
67. Hume, R., Williamson, J. M. and Whitelaw, J. W. (1970). Red cell survival in biliary cirrhosis. *J. Clin. Pathol.*, **23**, 297
68. Bingham, J. (1958). The macrocytosis of hepatic disease. I. Thin macrocytosis. *Blood*, **14**, 694

69. Bingham, J. (1960). The macrocytosis of hepatic disease. II. Thick macrocytosis. *Blood,* **15,** 244

70. Bingham, J. R. (1961). The macrocytosis of hepatic disease: thin, thick and target macrocytosis. *Can. Med. Ass. J.,* **85,** 178

71. Berman, L., Axelrod, A. R., Horan, T. N., Jacobson, S. D., Sharp, E. A. and VonderHeide, E. C. (1949). The blood and bone marrow in patients with cirrhosis of the liver. *Blood,* **4,** 511

72. Kilbridge, T. M. and Heller, P. (1969). Determinants of erythrocyte size in chronic liver disease. *Blood,* **34,** 739

73. Wu, A., Chanarin, I. and Levi, A. J. (1974). Macrocytosis of chronic alcoholism. *Lancet,* **i,** 829

74. Unger, K. W. and Johnson, D., Jr. (1974). Red blood cell mean corpuscular volume: a potential indicator of alcohol usage in a working population. *Med. Sci.,* **267,** 281

75. Werre, J. M., Helleman, P. W., Verloop, M. C. and de Gier, J. (1970). Causes of macroplania of erythrocytes in diseases of the liver and biliary tract with special reference to leptocytosis. *Br. J. Haematol.,* **19,** 223

76. Neerhout, R. C. (1968). Abnormalities of erythrocyte stromal lipids in hepatic disease. *J. Lab. Clin. Med.,* **71,** 438

77. Cooper, R. A., Diloy-Puray, M., Lando, P. and Greenberg, M. S. (1972). An analysis of lipoproteins, bile acids, and red cell membranes associated with target cells and spur cells in patients with liver disease. *J. Clin. Invest.,* **51,** 3182

78. Neerhout, R. C. (1968). Reversibility of the erythrocyte lipid abnormalities in hepatic disease. *J. Pediat.,* **73,** 364

79. Cooper, R. A. and Jandl, J. H. (1968). Bile salts and cholesterol in the pathogenesis of target cells in obstructive jaundice. *J. Clin. Invest.,* **47,** 809

80. Smith, J. A., Lonergan, E. T. and Sterling, K. (1965). Spur-cell anemia: hemolytic anemia with red cells resembling acanthocytes in alcoholic cirrhosis. *N. Engl. J. Med.,* **271,** 396

81. Silber, R., Amorosi, E., Lhowe, J. and Kayden, H. J. (1966). Spur-shaped erythrocytes in Laennec's cirrhosis. *N. Engl. J. Med.,* **275,** 639

82. Grahn, E. P., Dietz, A. A., Stefani, S. S. and Donnelly, W. J. (1968). Burr cells, hemolytic anemia and cirrhosis. *Am. J. Med.,* **45,** 78

83. Cooper, R. A. (1969). Anemia with spur cells: a red cell defect acquired in serum and modified in the circulation. *J. Clin. Invest.,* **48,** 1820

84. Douglass, C. G., McCall, M. S. and Frenkel, E. P. (1968). The acanthocyte in cirrhosis with hemolytic anemia. *Ann. Intern. Med.,* **68,** 390

85. McBride, J. A. and Jacob, H. S. (1970). Abnormal kinetics of red cell membrane cholesterol in acanthocytes: studies in genetic and experimental abetalipoproteinaemia and in spur cell anaemia. *Br. J. Haematol.,* **18,** 383

86. Martinez-Maldonado, M. (1968). Role of lipoproteins in the formation of spur cell anaemia. *J. Clin. Path.,* **21,** 620

87. Cooper, R. A., Kimball, D. B. and Durocher, J. R. (1974). Role of the spleen in membrane conditioning and hemolysis of spur cells in liver disease. *N. Engl. J. Med.,* **290,** 1279

88. Tchernia, G., Navarro, J., Becart, R. and Casasoprana, A. (1968). Anémie hémolytique avec acanthocytose et dyslipidémie au cours de deux hépatites néonates. *Arch. Franc. Pédiat.,* **25,** 729

89. Marie, J., Fleury, F., Hennequet, A., Cloup, M. and Watchi, J.-M. (1967). Ictère grave cirrhogène avec acanthocytose chez le nourrisson. *Arch. Franc. Pédiat.,* **24,** 585

90. Keller, J. W., Majerus, P. W. and Finke, E. H. (1971). An unusual type of spiculated erythrocyte in metastatic liver disease and hemolytic anemia. *Ann. Intern. Med.,* **74,** 732

91. Turpin, F., Vaugier, G., Bécart-Nichel, R. and Binet, J. L. (1971). Acanthocytose dans un cas de cirrhose alcoolique avec anémie. Transformation en acanthocytes de globules rouges transfusés. *Nouvelle Rev. Franc. Hématol.,* **11,** 791

92. Brecher, G. and Bessis, M. (1972). Present status of spiculed red cells and their relationship to the discocyte–echinocyte transformation: a critical review. *Blood,* **40,** 333

93. Shohet, S. B. (1974). 'Acanthocytogenesis'—or how the red cell won its spurs. *N. Engl. J. Med.*, **290,** 1316
94. Zieve, L. (1958). Jaundice, hyperlipemia and hemolytic anemia: a heretofore unrecognized syndrome associated with alcoholic fatty liver and cirrhosis. *Ann. Intern. Med.*, **48,** 471
95. Kessel, L. (1962). Acute transient hyperlipemia due to hepatopancreatic damage in chronic alcoholics (Zieve's syndrome). *Am. J. Med.*, **32,** 747
96. Blass, J. P. and Dean, H. M. (1966). The relation of hyperlipemia to hemolytic anemia in an alcoholic patient. *Am. J. Med.*, **40,** 283
97. Balcerzak, S. P., Westerman, M. P. and Heinle, E. W. (1968). Mechanism of anemia in Zieve's syndrome. *Am. J. Med.*, **225,** 277
98. Gadrat, J., Douste-Blazy, L., Ribet, A., Pascal, J. P. and Frexinos, J. (1967). Syndrome de Zieve associé a une pancréatite calcifiante. *Presse Med.*, **75,** 789
99. Albahary, C., Auffret, M. and Le Gland, J. L. (1968). Syndrome de Zieve, hyperlipidémie alcoolique et anémie hémolytique. *Presse Med.*, **76,** 371
100. Zieve, L. (1966). Hemolytic anemia in liver disease. *Medicine*, **45,** 497
101. Eichner, E. R. (1973). The hematologic disorders of alcoholism. *Am. J. Med.*, **54,** 621
102. Douglass, C. C. and Twomey, J. J. (1970). Transient stomatocytosis with hemolysis: a previously unrecognized complication of alcoholism. *Ann. Intern. Med.*, **72,** 159
103. Zarkowsky, H. S., Oski, F. A., Sha'afi, R. *et al.* (1968). Congenital hemolytic anemia with high sodium, low potassium red cells. I. Studies of membrane permeability. *N. Engl. J. Med.*, **278,** 573
104. Oski, F. A., Naiman, J. L., Blum, S. F. *et al.* (1969). Congenital hemolytic anemia with high-sodium, low-potassium red cells. *N. Engl. J. Med.*, **280,** 909
105. Coste, T., Gouffier, C. E. and Paraf, A. (1972). Les troubles hématologiques de l'alcoolisme aigu. *Sem. Hôp. Paris*, **48,** 2427
106. Jacob, H. S. and Amsden, T. (1971). Acute hemolytic anemia with rigid red cells in hypophosphatemia. *N. Engl. J. Med.*, **285,** 1446
107. Klock, J. C., Williams, H. E. and Mentzer, W. C. (1974). Hemolytic anemia and somatic cell dysfunction in severe hypophosphatemia. *Arch. Intern. Med.*, **134,** 360
108. Territo, M. C. and Tanaka, K. R. (1974). Hypophosphatemia in chronic alcoholism. *Arch. Intern. Med.*, **134,** 445
109. Sheehy, R. W. and Berman, A. (1954). The anemia of cirrhosis. *J. Lab. Clin. Med.*, **56,** 72
110. Perera, G. A. (1946). The plasma volume in Laennec's cirrhosis of the liver. *Ann. Intern. Med.*, **24,** 643
111. Hiller, G. I., Huffman, E. R. and Levey, S. (1949). Studies in cirrhosis of the liver. I. Relationship between plasma volume, plasma protein concentrations and total circulating proteins. *J. Clin. Invest.*, **23,** 322
112. Bateman, J. C., Shorr, H. M. and Elgvin, T. (1949). Hypervolemic anemia in cirrhosis. *J. Clin. Invest.*, **28,** 539
113. Hyde, G. M., Berlin, N. I., Parsons, R. J., Lawrence, J. H. and Port, S. (1952). The blood volume in portal cirrhosis as determined by P^{32} labeled red blood cells. *J. Lab. Clin. Med.*, **39,** 347
114. Eisenberg, S. (1956). Blood volume in patients with Laennec's cirrhosis of the liver as determined by radioactive chromium-tagged red cells. *Am. J. Med.*, **20,** 189
115. Adams, E. B. (1970). Anemia associated with protein deficiency. *Semin. Hematol.*, **7,** 55
116. Alfrey, C. P. and Lane, M. (1970). The effect of riboflavin deficiency on erythropoiesis. *Semin. Hematol.*, **7,** 49
117. Post, R. M. and Desforges, J. F. (1968). Thrombocytopenia and alcoholism. *Ann. Intern. Med.*, **68,** 1230
118. Heck, J. and Gehrmann, G. (1972). Alkoholische thrombozytendepression. *Deutsch Med. Wochenschr.*, **97,** 1088
119. MacLeod, E. C. and Michaels, L. (1969). Alcohol and the blood. *Lancet*, **ii,** 1198
120. Liu, Y. K. (1973). Leukopenia in alcoholics. *Am. J. Med.*, **54,** 605

121. Cowan, D. H. and Hines, J. D. (1974). Alcohol, vitamins and platelets. In N. V. Dimitrov and J. H. Nodine, eds. *Drugs and Hematologic Reactions,* p. 283. New York: Grune and Stratton
122. Sullivan, L. W. (1971). Effect of alcohol on platelet production. In J. M. Paulus, ed. *Platelet Kinetics, Radioisotopic, Cytological, Mathematical and Clinical Aspects,* p. 247. Amsterdam: North-Holland Publishing Co.
123. Ryback, R. and Desforges, J. (1970). Alcoholic thrombocytopenia in three inpatient drinking alcoholics. *Arch. Intern. Med.,* **125,** 475
124. Haut, M. J. and Cowan, D. H. (1974). The effect of ethanol on hemostatic properties of human blood platelets. *Am. J. Med.,* **56,** 22
125. Sahud, M. A. (1972). Platelet size and number in alcoholic thrombocytopenia. *N. Engl. J. Med.,* **286,** 355
126. Post, R. M. and Desforges, J. F. (1968). Thrombocytopenic effect of ethanol infusion. *Blood,* **31,** 344
127. Cowan, D. H., Shook, P. J. and Graham, R. C., Jr. (1974). Hypersomolality, effect on platelet function and ultrastructure. *Clin. Res.,* **22,** 386A
128. Cowan, D. H. (1974). Platelet metabolism in alcohol-related thrombocytopenia. *Thrombos. Diathes. Haemorrh.,* **31,** 149
129. Aster, R. H. (1966). Pooling of platelets in the spleen: role in the pathogenesis of 'hypersplenic thrombocytopenia'. *J. Clin. Invest.,* **45,** 645
130. Riedler, G. F., Straub, P. W. and Frick, P. G. (1971). Thrombocytopenia in septicemia. *Helv. Med. Acta,* **36,** 23
131. Verstraete, M., Vermylen, J. and Collen, D. (1974). Intravascular coagulation in liver disease. *Ann. Rev. Med.,* **25,** 447
132. Chanarin, I. (1969). *The Megaloblastic Anemias,* p. 344. Philadelphia: Blackwell
133. Welch, W. H. (1903). The pathological effects of alcohol. In J. S. Billings, ed. *Physiological Aspects of the Liquor Problem,* Vol. 2, p. 351. Boston and New York: Houghton Mifflin
134. Osler, W. (1927). *Modern Medicine.* Philadelphia: Lea and Febiger
135. Lyons, H. A. and Saltzman, A. (1974). Diseases of the respiratory tract in alcoholics. In B. Kissin and H. Begleiter, eds. *The Biology of Alcoholism, Volume 3, Clinical Pathology,* p. 403. New York: Plenum Press
136. Chromet, B. and Gach, B. M. (1967). Lobar pneumonia and alcoholism: an analysis of thirty-seven cases. *Am. J. Med. Sci.,* **253,** 300
137. McFarland, E. and Libre, E. P. (1963). Abnormal leucocyte response in alcoholism. *Ann. Intern. Med.,* **59,** 865
138. Craddock, C. G., Jr., Frei, E., Landy, M. and Smith, W. W. (1960). Quantitative studies of human leukocytes and febrile response to single and repeated doses of purified endotoxin. *Blood,* **15,** 840
139. Dunlap, W. M., James, G. W. and Hume, D. M. (1974). Anemia and neutropenia caused by copper deficiency. *Ann. Intern. Med.,* **80,** 470
140. Tisman, G. and Herbert, V. (1973). *In vitro* myelosuppression and immunosuppression by ethanol. *J. Clin. Invest.,* **52,** 1410
141. Beard, J. D. and Knott, D. H. (1966). Hematopoietic response to experimental chronic alcoholism. *Am. J. Med. Sci.,* **252,** 518
142. Pickrell, K. L. (1938). The effect of alcoholic intoxication and ether anesthesia on resistance to pneumococcal infection. *Bull. Johns Hopkins Hosp.,* **63,** 238
143. Brayton, R. G., Stokes, P. E., Schwartz, M. S. and Louria, D. B. (1970). Effect of alcohol and various diseases on leukocyte mobilization, phagocytosis, and intracellular bacterial killing. *N. Engl. J. Med.,* **282,** 123
144. Phelps, P. and Stanislau, D. (1969). Polymorphonuclear leukocyte motility *in vitro.* I. Effect of pH, temperature, ethyl alcohol, and caffeine, using a modified Boyden chamber technique. *Arthrit. Rheumatol.,* **12,** 181
145. DeMeo, A. N. and Anderson, B. R. (1972). Defective chemotaxis associated with a serum inhibitor in cirrhotic patients. *N. Engl. J. Med.,* **286,** 735

146. Crowley, J. P. and Abramson, N. (1971). Effect of ethanol on complement-mediated chemotaxis. *Clin. Res.*, **19**, 415
147. Craddock, P. R., Yawata, Y., Van Senten, L., Gilberstadt, S., Silvis, S. and Jacob, H. S. (1974). Acquired phagocyte dysfunction. A complication of the hypophosphatemia of parenteral hyperalimentation. *N. Engl. J. Med.*, **290**, 1403
148. Green, G. M. and Kass, E. H. (1964). Factors influencing the clearance of bacteria by the lung. *J. Clin. Invest.*, **43**, 769
149. Louria, D. B. (1963). Susceptibility to infection during experimental alcohol intoxication. *Trans. Ass. Am. Phys.*, **76**, 102
150. Guarneri, J. J. and Luarenzi, G. A. (1968). Effect of alcohol on the mobilization of alveolar macrophages. *J. Lab. Clin. Med.*, **72**, 40
151. Ali, M. V. and Nolan, J. P. (1967). Alcohol-induced depression of reticuloendothelial function in the rat. *J. Lab. Clin. Med.*, **70**, 295
152. Triger, D. R., Alp, M. H. and Wright, R. (1972). Bacterial and dietary antibodies in liver disease. *Lancet*, **i**, 60
153. Bjorneboe, M., Prytz, H. and Orskov, F. (1972). Antibodies to intestinal microbes in serum of patients with cirrhosis of the liver. *Lancet*, **i**, 58
154. Berenyi, M. R., Straus, B. and Cruz, D. (1974). *In vitro* and *in vivo* studies of cellular immunity in alcoholic cirrhosis. *Am. J. Dig. Dis.*, **19**, 199
155. Hsu, C. C. S. and Leevy, C. M. (1971). Inhibition of PHA-stimulated lymphocyte transformation by plasma from patients with advanced alcoholic cirrhosis. *Clin. Exp. Immunol.*, **8**, 749
156. Berkowitz, H., Reichel, J. and Shim, C. (1973). The effect of ethanol on the cough reflex. *Clin. Sci. Molec. Med.*, **45**, 527
157. Haltalin, K. C., Nelson, J. D., Woodman, E. B. and Allen, A. A. (1970). Fatal Shigella infection induced by folic acid deficiency in young guinea pigs. *J. Infect. Dis.*, **121**, 275

9 Metabolic Effects of Alcohol on the Endocrine System

G. G. GORDON and A. L. SOUTHREN

9.1 INTRODUCTION 250
9.2 ADRENAL GLAND 251
9.2.1 *Adrenal cortex* 251
9.2.1.1 Cortisol 251
(a) Animal studies 251
(b) Human studies 253
(i) Normal man 253
(ii) Alcoholic man 255
9.2.1.2 Aldosterone 261
9.2.1.3 Dehydroepiandrosterone (DHEA) and 17-ketosteroids (17-KS) 262
9.2.2 *Adrenal medulla—catecholamines* 262
9.2.2.1 Animal studies 262
9.2.2.2 Human studies 263
(a) Studies in normal human volunteers 263
(b) Studies in alcoholic subjects 264
9.3 THYROID FUNCTION 267
9.3.1 *Animal studies* 267
9.3.1.1 Histological studies 267
9.3.1.2 Physiological studies 267
9.3.1.3 Alcohol effect on $^{131(125)}$I thyroidal accumulation 267
9.3.1.4 Alcohol effects on the metabolism and tissue distribution of thyroid hormones 268
9.3.2 *Human studies* 269
9.4 PARATHYROID, CALCITONIN AND CALCIUM 270
9.4.1 *Hypocalcaemic effect of alcohol in the experimental animal* 270
9.4.2 *Hypocalcaemic effect of alcohol in the human* 271
9.4.3 *Calcitonin–alcohol effects* 272
9.5 GONADAL FUNCTION AND ALCOHOL 273
9.5.1 *Animal studies* 273
9.5.1.1 Histological studies in animals 273
9.5.1.2 Physiological studies in animals 273
9.5.1.3 Gonadal hormonal studies in animals 274

9.5.2 *Gonadal function in humans* 274
9.5.2.1 Histological studies 274
9.5.2.2 Hormonal studies in man 274
(a) Testosterone in plasma and urine 275
(b) Testosterone–metabolic clearance rate (MCR^T) 279
(i) Hepatic blood flow 279
(ii) Plasma-protein binding 280
(iii) Steroid metabolizing enzymes 280
(c) Plasma production rates 282
(d) Conversion ratios 282
(e) Other plasma sex steroids 282
(i) Androstenedione 282
(ii) Estradiol 283
(f) Plasma gonadotrophins 283
(g) Urinary 17-ketosteroids 284
9.6 PITUITARY GLAND 285
9.6.1 *Anterior pituitary* 285
9.6.1.1 Animal studies 285
9.6.1.2 Human studies 286
(a) Growth hormone 286
(b) Prolactin 287
(c) Gonadotrophins 287
(d) Thyrotrophin (TSH) 287
(e) Adrenocorticotrophin (ACTH) 287
9.6.2 *Posterior pituitary* 287
9.6.2.1 Antidiuretic hormone 287
9.6.2.2 Oxytocin 290
9.7 INSULIN 290
Acknowledgements 292
References 293

9.1 INTRODUCTION

Clinical observations in man, as well as histological and physiological studies in animals have suggested an important interaction between alcohol and the endocrine system. The application of radioimmunoassay and tracer methodology has made it possible to study this interaction by providing techniques for the measurement of the blood levels (in picogram amounts), plasma kinetics (including the metabolic clearance and production or secretory rates and the interconversion of precursor–product hormones) and the plasma-protein binding of the hormones. These techniques are being applied to the study of the endocrine effects of ethanol by a number of investigators.

Of some importance in carrying out studies of this type are the recent reports that hormone secretion by the endocrine glands, even in the basal state, is not constant but rather occurs in a pulsatile or staccato fashion which is related temporally to the sleep cycle[1]. Thus, single daily samples of hormones (i.e. cortisol, growth hormone, testosterone and the gonadotrophins) may not adequately reflect the mean plasma hormone concentration or detect alterations in the pattern of hormone secretion. Furthermore, random fluctuations in hormone levels may be misinterpreted as a drug effect unless an adequate number of blood samples are obtained.

Another aspect of the interaction of alcohol on the endocrine system is the effect of alcohol on increasing the activity of a variety of microsomal drug-metabolizing enzymes which may, in turn, alter the metabolism of other drugs and lead to significant changes in their pharmacological activity[2]. It has been suggested that the steroid hormones are the 'natural' substrates of the mixed function oxidases[3] (i.e. drug-metabolizing microsomal enzymes). Alcohol, by changing the activity of these enzymes, may alter the peripheral metabolism of the steroid hormones and interfere with biological activity[2]. Pharmacological agents that induce microsomal hydroxylases may shift the main pathway of steroid metabolism, in the adult human, from the A-ring reduced to the hydroxylated metabolites[4]. These metabolites, when excreted in the urine, are too polar to be extracted by the usual organic solvents and are therefore not measured in the routine procedure for urinary 17-OHCS. Thus the daily excretion of 17-OHCS would be an inadequate indicator of adrenocortical function during the administration of these enzyme-inducing agents. In addition, the hydroxylated metabolites of cortisol may have glucocorticoid activity and result in feedback effects on the hypothalamic–pituitary axis, in contrast to the common reduced metabolites which are without hormonal effect[5].

Further complicating the interpretation of reports of the effects of alcohol on endocrine function in animal studies are species differences and variability in dosage and routes of administration. In the human, the alcohol abuser has been studied most intensively. However, factors which are variable and frequently not controlled include duration and intensity of alcohol abuse, history of multi-drug abuse, nutritional factors, presence of occult liver disease and associated psychopathology. In addition, altered sleep patterns[6] found in alcoholics may in turn produce changes in hormone secretion. In this regard, the normal non-alcoholic volunteer is perhaps the most ideal subject for these studies. To date, however, studies in these individuals have been few and of short duration.

Thus, precise delineation of the endocrine effects of ethanol requires a suitable model (human or experimental animal) with proper controls, appropriate hormone measurements (including endocrine stimulation tests) and well-defined timing and frequency of sampling.

9.2 ADRENAL GLAND

9.2.1 Adrenal cortex

9.2.1.1 Cortisol

(*a*) *Animal studies*—Hion-Jon[7] studied the effects of alcohol on endocrine gland histology in rabbits. He suggested that alcohol affected the adrenal gland as evidenced by histological changes noted during acute and chronic administration of alcohol. Smith[8] evaluated the effect of alcohol on adrenal function in rats using adrenal ascorbic acid and cholesterol content as indices of adrenal activity. Alcohol was given by gavage in doses ranging from 0.6 to 2.1 ml absolute ethanol per animal and the animals were sacrificed 1 to 7 h later. A dose-related fall in adrenal ascorbic acid and cholesterol levels was noted. The non-specific effect of handling the animal and inserting the tubes was controlled by gavaging animals with saline. Only small changes were noted in adrenal ascorbic acid and cholesterol content under control conditions. In contrast, hypophysectomized rats did not show a similar response to alcohol gavage. This was confirmed by Forbes and Duncan[9]. These studies suggested that the effect of alcohol on adrenal ascorbic acid and cholesterol content was mediated via the hypothalamic–pituitary axis. Whether this was a specific alcohol effect at a discrete locus in the hypothalamic–pituitary axis or a non-specific generalized effect of alcohol as a 'stressor' could not be determined. Further studies by Forbes and Duncan[10] attempted to bypass the possible non-specific stressful effect of alcohol on the gastrointestinal tract by giving the dose intraperitoneally in dilute solutions. Adrenal ascorbic acid and cholesterol levels were depleted by this route of alcohol injection as well as by gavage. Czaja and Kalant[11] thought that the effects of alcohol on depleting adrenal ascorbic acid and cholesterol (as reported in the previously cited studies) represented effects of high (lethal or near-lethal) doses of alcohol which were administered by relatively traumatic techniques (gavage or intraperitoneal injection). They questioned whether these non-specific traumata were responsible for adrenal activation (as measured by depletion of ascorbic acid and cholesterol) rather than alcohol *per se*. Using alcohol at a 2 g/kg b.w. dose in rats, they confirmed the observation of Forbes and Duncan[10] that the intraperitoneal injection of alcohol depletes adrenal stores of the vitamin and sterol. However, alcohol, when given by gavage, at this dose, did not produce any effect. They considered the possibility that a pain-mediated response to intraperitoneal alcohol was responsible for adrenal activation. However, administration of a local anaesthetic prior to alcohol injection did not prevent the response. It was noted rather, that intraperitoneal injection of alcohol resulted in more rapid peak blood levels (300 mg/dl at 2 min) than by gavage (200 mg/dl at 90 min) at the dose range employed. They concluded that the peak level of alcohol attained was the critical factor in determining adrenocortical activation, since giving an equivalent total dose of alcohol in three injections spaced over a period of time, instead of a single i.p. dose, resulted in a decreased adrenal effect. These studies were suggestive of increased adrenocortical secretory function after alcohol exposure. Since only indirect parameters (adrenal ascorbic acid and cholesterol) of hormonal secretion were measured in these studies, they could not definitely establish that alcohol increases adrenal secretion of a glucocorticoid hormone (corticosterone in rodents and cortisol in higher mammals).

Santisteban and Swinyard[12] demonstrated that alcohol administration resulted in thymic involution in intact but not in adrenalectomized mice. Santisteban[13] showed that the degree of response to alcohol injection, as measured by thymic involution, was a function of the magnitude of the dose. Since only the 11-oxygenated steroids were known to produce this response, Santisteban[13], in effect, had demonstrated by a bioassay technique, that glucocorticoid secretion had occurred in response to alcohol. As methodology became available for quantitating glucocorticoid hormones in blood, these techniques were applied and provided further definitive evidence, in animals, for adrenocortical activation by alcohol. Ellis[14] noted a 5-fold increase in plasma corticosterone levels in rats given a large dose of alcohol (4 g/kg b.w.). Kalant *et al.*[15] studied the effect of alcohol pretreatment on steroid output from excised incubated adrenal glands. They noted that intraperitoneal alcohol treatment prior to adrenal excision was associated with significant elevations in adrenal steroid output *in vitro*. Ellis[16] measured plasma 17-hydroxycorticoids hourly during a 6-h period in dogs in response to ethanol infusions (1.0–3.0 g/kg b.w.) given over 20 min. An increase in plasma 17-hydroxysteroids was noted at all dose ranges beginning at 1 h after ethanol and persisting for 6 h. However, no definite dose–response relationship could be established. Alcohol did not appear to have any effect on the rate of removal of exogenous (non-tracer) doses of corticol from the blood. However, this technique would not be adequate to detect any but the most gross changes in metabolic clearance of cortisol. Ellis[17] was able to demonstrate a dose–response relationship in rats treated with alcohol intraperitoneally over a 0.5–4.0 g/kg b.w. range. Alcohol did not have any effect in hypophysectomized animals. Moreover, pretreatment of the animals with pentobarbitol and morphine completely obliterated the corticosterone response to alcohol. There was no adaptation (i.e. loss of response) noted on repeated daily injections of alcohol for one week. Noble[18] showed by a bioassay method that the acute injection of alcohol (1.6 g/kg b.w.) resulted in maximum pituitary ACTH depletion in mice in 10 min. A gradual increase in pituitary ACTH concentration occurred over the next 50 min, although basal levels were not attained.

The above-cited animal studies suggest that alcohol activates adrenal glucocorticoid secretory function and that the effect is mediated by ACTH release through some direct or indirect central nervous system action of alcohol. The exact locus of this alcohol effect is unknown.

(*b*) *Human studies*—(i) Normal man. Krusius *et al.*[19] studied 15 non-alcoholic subjects who received alcohol (150 ml of 88° proof whiskey) as a single dose. In five of the subjects, this initial dose was followed $\frac{1}{2}$ h later by 75 ml of whiskey. Slight decreases in plasma 17-hydroxycorticoids (17-OHCS) were noted in samples taken at $\frac{1}{2}$, 1, 2, 4 and 6 h after alcohol ingestion. Changes in eosinophil count were attributed to a non-specific 'stress' effect. Blood alcohol levels were not measured. Perman[20] gave healthy young men alcohol (as whiskey) in moderate doses (0.5 to 0.7 g/kg b.w.) and measured urinary excretion of 17-hydroxycorticoids. The output of 17-OHCS during control studies was not significantly different than after alcohol (0.50 *vs.* 0.57 mg/h). Kissin *et al.*[21] studied 15 healthy non-alcoholic volunteers. Alcohol was given in fruit juice at a dose of 1 ml/kg b.w. Urine was collected 4 h after the subjects drank either diluted alcohol or the diluent itself. There was no change noted in 17-ketosteroid excretion. However, a small increase in 17-OHCS output (0.32–0.41 mg/h) was found. The increment in urinary 17-OHCS excretion may have resulted from increased renal clearance of the steroid metabolites as a result of an alcohol-induced diuresis.

Jenkins and Connolly[22] studied eight female and seven male volunteers drawn from laboratory personnel or hospital patients without overt endocrinopathy. Intravenous alcohol was infused over a 30-min period for a total dose of 1 ml/kg b.w. in 500 ml of normal saline. Samples were taken at the end of the infusion and at $\frac{1}{2}$-h intervals for the next $2\frac{1}{2}$ h. Plasma 11-hydroxycorticoids (i.e. cortisol) were measured fluorimetrically. The male subjects attained lesser plasma ethanol levels (82–145 mg/dl) than female subjects (118–196 mg/dl). All the female subjects showed an increase in plasma cortisol with the peak response occurring at 90 min from the start of the infusion (mean increment 18.7 μg/dl). Only in the three male subjects where blood alcohol exceeded 100 mg/dl did plasma cortisol levels increase significantly. There was no change in blood glucose noted. Two female subjects exhibited a brisk cortisol response after ethanol infusion despite prior administration of morphine (which is known to block the response of the pituitary–adrenal–cortical axis to stimulation by vasopressin, but not to pyrogen). However, when four patients with hypothalamic or pituitary lesions (but with known adrenocortical competence as manifested by responsivity to exogenous ACTH) were studied, alcohol infusion produced significant increments only in patients with hypothalamic lesions but not in those with pituitary adenomas. This acute study resulted in blood alcohol levels over 100 mg/dl and was associated with increased plasma cortisol levels, presumably as a result of an increased adrenocortical secretory rate. The lack of response in patients with pituitary adenomas (i.e. damaged pituitary glands) suggests that the effect is not directly on adrenocortical release of cortisol, but is mediated via ACTH release from the pituitary gland. The cortisol response in patients with hypothalamic lesions and presumably intact pituitary glands suggests the possibility that alcohol may also directly release pituitary ACTH.

Mendelson and Stein[23] studied four non-alcoholic subjects prior to, during and after a 4-day period of ethanol intoxication. The subjects ingested 86° proof beverage alcohol in the amount of a quart per day in divided doses given every 4 h around the clock. Cortisol was measured daily at 9:30 a.m. and 4:30 p.m. by a specific ligand assay during all phases of the study (i.e. 3 days before alcohol, 4 days on alcohol and 3 days post-drinking). The subjects developed varying degrees of gastric intolerance to alcohol which prevented ingestion of the full planned dose of alcohol per day. Mean blood alcohol levels in each subject ranged from 20 to 41 mg/dl. The subjects exhibited significant increases in plasma cortisol but only when gastrointestinal symptoms occurred. Since blood alcohol apparently never exceeded 100 mg/dl, a plasma cortisol response would not have been expected (see above). The increments noted when the patients were 'ill' is an expected response to the stress of nausea and vomiting. Merry and Marks[24] studied plasma cortisol responses (fluorimetric assay) in five volunteers presumed to be normal non-alcoholic subjects; 284 ml of whiskey (70° proof) was ingested neat or diluted with water over a 15-min period and blood was sampled in the basal state and at intervals of 30 min for $2\frac{1}{2}$ h after consumption of the test dose. All subjects showed evidence of intoxication and blood alcohol levels exceeded 120 mg/dl. Three of the five 'normals' exhibited 10–30 % increments in plasma levels of cortisol. On further questioning, the two volunteers who did not respond with an increase in plasma cortisol (a 10–20 % decrement was noted) admitted to heavy prior alcohol use. This study suggested that the adrenocortical response to ethanol was altered by chronic alcohol use (see section of alcohol–adrenal effects in alcoholic subjects (9.2.1.1.(b)). Bellet and coworkers[25] administered alcohol (1.5 ml/kg b.w.) as a 20 % aqueous solution to nine normal young male volunteers. A doubling of the mean plasma cortisol was noted (15–30 mg/dl) after alcohol, compared to basal levels. Blood alcohol levels exceeded 100 mg/dl in all subjects. In a second study by the same group, similar results were noted[26].

The studies cited above have not considered, for the most part, the spontaneous variation of cortisol (diurnal variation or episodic secretion[1]). Nonetheless, they are strongly suggestive of an effect of alcohol in increasing plasma cortisol when blood levels of the intoxicant exceed 100 mg/dl. This action of alcohol is most likely the result of an alcohol-mediated activation of the hypothalamic–pituitary axis resulting in ACTH release and consequent increase in adrenocortical secretion. Since these studies show that intoxicating levels of alcohol are necessary to induce the effect, the question remains whether alcohol has a direct effect on a discrete neuroendocrine transducer or whether the increase in cortisol is part of a generalized non-specific stress reaction related to behavioural changes (i.e. at the level of the cerebral cortex). Moreover, possible effects of alcohol in altering the peripheral metabolism of the steroid by changes in protein binding or hepatic clearance have not been investigated.

(ii) Alcoholic man. Krusius[19] studied sixteen alcoholics who were admitted to the hospital in an alcohol-induced comatose state; 5 h after arousal from the coma, blood was drawn for determination of 17-OHCS; they were then given 50 ml of whiskey and blood was drawn again 1 h later. Blood was taken for 'control purposes' 3 days later. As might be expected, the plasma 17-OHCS taken 5 h after awakening from an alcohol-induced coma showed somewhat elevated levels. There was no further increase in the mean plasma 17-OHCS for the group 1 h after ingestion of the whiskey. However, in several subjects, hypoglycaemia was induced by the administered alcohol and significant increments in plasma 17-OHCS were then seen; demonstrating a normal adrenocortical response to hypoglycaemia. Since these were ill patients, it is not surprising that plasma levels of 17-OHCS taken 3 days later were still elevated. Thus patient selection in this study, i.e. subjects in a state of stress with adrenocortical activation, would tend to obscure any possible effect of alcohol on adrenal function.

Kissin *et al.*[21] studied 106 male alcoholics in a hospital setting 1 week after admission for an alcoholic episode. Alcohol was given diluted in juice in a dose of 1 ml/kg b.w. Urinary 17-ketosteroids (17-KS) and 17-OHCS and plasma 17-OHCS were measured. The first 4-h collection of urine after administration of alcohol showed no effect on the excretion of 17-ketosteroids while the 17-hydroxycorticoids increased 50 % (0.24 *vs.* 0.36 mg/h) during this same period. When 24-h urinary excretions of 17-OHCS were measured, there was no change observed between alcohol and control days. Since the 24-h urine was collected and analysed in timed fractions, it was possible to demonstrate that only in the initial 4 h after ingestion of alcohol was the 17-OHCS excretion increased. The increased 17-OHCS excretion was noted to coincide with an alcohol-induced diuresis, suggesting that it was related to changes in clearance of the cortisol metabolites rather than to increased adrenocortical secretion. When blood levels of 17-OHCS were followed over the same time-course, (0–6 h after alcohol ingestion) it was noted that plasma 17-OHCS fell 2 h after alcohol administration and then rose again to basal levels. When these studies were repeated with a large water load (1500 ml tap water) but no alcohol, similar changes in urinary and plasma 17-OHCS were noted. However, the intial fall in plasma 17-OHCS (at 2 h) persisted at 4 and 6 h, unlike the increases to baseline levels noted at 4 and 6 h after administration of alcohol. This suggested that alcohol was indeed stimulating cortisol secretion. In order to study these effects further, twelve patients received alcohol in the standard dose and drank 250 ml of water (or 0.4 % saline) every hour for four doses. Four of these patients had only a 'minor diuresis' (less than 350 mg/h) on this programme and none of them had an increase in the urinary excretion of 17-OHCS at 2 h; yet all showed a marked rise in plasma 17-OHCS. In contrast, the remaining eight patients had a 'major diuresis' and this group showed increased urinary excretion of the 17-OHCS. These data are compatible with both an increment in adrenocortical secretion, as manifested by a rise in plasma 17-OHCS, and an alteration in the renal clearance of these metabolites as a result of alcohol ingestion. It would be of interest to repeat these studies using tracer methodology, which may delineate more clearly the relative roles of renal clearance changes and altered adrenocortical secretion after alcohol ingestion.

Mendelson and Stein[22] studied the alcohol effect on adrenocortical function in four alcoholic subjects using a protocol identical to that used in their studies of normal men (see 9.2.1.1.(b)(i)). The subjects had been abstinent for 2 months prior to the study. During the drinking phase of the study, mean blood alcohol levels in the four subjects ranged from 50 to 145 mg/dl. A slight trend towards elevation of mean blood cortisol levels was noted in the drinking and post-drinking phases of the study. Inspection of individual patients' patterns of secretion is suggestive of adrenocortical activation, especially in the one patient who experienced delirium tremens. Merry and Marks[24] studied the acute effects of alcohol in male alcoholic volunteers who had been abstinent at least 3 weeks. There were no changes in plasma cortisol (fluorimetric assay) noted in the patients up to 150 min after alcohol ingestion (284 ml whiskey) although blood alcohol levels exceeded 100 mg/dl in all subjects. Indeed, they were able to detect prior heavy alcohol use in two supposed 'normal' volunteers by the lack of response of plasma cortisol. Thus, in these studies (as in Krusius'[19] earlier work), alcoholics seem to tolerate acutely intoxicating levels of alcohol without evidence of adrenocortical activation. Mendelson *et al.*[27] studied the chronic effects of alcohol in four alcoholics abstinent at least 60 days prior to study. Serum cortisol was measured daily at 9:30 a.m. by a ligand technique. Alcohol was given as bourbon (86° proof) every 4 h around the clock for 11–29 days. Serum cortisol increased during the course of the study and increments in cortisol levels tended to correlate with the higher peaks in blood alcohol or with withdrawal symptoms. Stokes[28] studied 18 alcoholic patients during an episode of chronic excess drinking of at least 2 weeks' duration. The patients were kept on their usual amount of alcohol for 4 or 5 days ('tolerant' phase), then received an increased alcohol intake for 3–6 days and lastly were tapered off alcohol over 5–10 days; 95 % ethanol diluted in fruit juice was given in divided doses every 2 h from 7:30 a.m. to 11:00 p.m. and again at 3:00 a.m. Plasma 17-OHCS were measured by a specific ligand assay at 9:00 a.m., 4:00 p.m. and 11:00 p.m. The highest blood cortisol levels were noted when the patients were ingesting their usual ration of alcohol ('tolerant' phase) or during the withdrawal period. In contrast to Mendelson's study, no significant increases in mean blood 17-OHCS were noted at the stage of highest blood alcohol levels (overt intoxication).

While the data are suggestive that alcohol mediates increased adrenocortical secretory activity, it is apparent from the above data that the effect of acute and chronic alcohol ingestion on plasma cortisol has not been consistent in all studies. Obviously, many factors were not or could not be adequately controlled for such as nutritional state, vitamin intake, sleep disturbance or occult liver disease.

Another element that may have interfered with the studies described, is that plasma cortisol fluctuates significantly during the course of the day[1]. While some of the investigators were aware of diurnal changes in cortisol, most of the investigations were carried out before the episodic nature of cortisol secretion (with wide swings between peak and nadir) became evident[1]. Studies using frequent sampling techniques should be a useful tool in further studies in this area.

Another aspect of alcohol–adrenocortical interaction is the question of primary or secondary (i.e. due to hypothalamic–pituitary dysfunction) adrenocortical insufficiency in chronic alcoholics. The occurrence in alcoholics of hypoglycaemia (Section 9.7.1) and other clinical stigmata suggested to early investigators that alcoholism may result in adrenocortical dysfunction, or conversely, adrenocortical disease may be etiologically associated with alcoholism[29]. Thus, many clinical reports of the efficacy of ACTH and other steroids in acute alcoholic states appeared in the literature[30–32]. Owen[33] pointed out that any beneficial effect of ACTH use in these disorders may have been either a result of non-specific influences associated with the therapy (i.e. more nursing attention) or due to the pharmacological effects of ACTH rather than to underlying adrenocortical insufficiency. It has been previously pointed out that patients with delirium tremens have elevated plasma cortisol levels (see above) which would suggest adequate adrenocortical function in this alcoholic state, at least.

Several investigations have been undertaken to evaluate adrenocortical function in alcoholics who were not under the influence of alcohol at the time of the study. Smith[34] studied the eosinophil response in 73 chronic alcoholics who had not been drinking for several days. Lack of eosinophilopenic response to ACTH (25 IU i.m.) and epinephrine (adrenalin) (0.3 mg s.c.) suggested the possibility of pituitary–adrenocortical insufficiency in these patients. Owen[35] using ACTH stimulation and eosinophilopenic response showed that the clinical severity of delirium tremens was unrelated to the putative 'decreased adrenocortical reserve' she found in alcoholics. It is now recognized that eosinophilopenia is not an adequate index of adrenocortical response to ACTH stimulation and the single small dose of ACTH used in this study was suboptimal. Kissin *et al.*[36] measured 24-h urinary 17-OHCS excretion in abstinent alcoholics, active alcoholics and control subjects. The active alcoholics were studied in a hospital stituation at least 5 days after stopping alcohol use. The mean urinary 17-OHCS excretion was slightly (but statistically significantly) lower in long abstinent alcoholics than in active drinkers or controls. Using the eosinophilopenic response to ACTH, an inadequate response was noted in 44 % of long-abstinent alcoholics and 38 % of active drinkers. The urinary 17-OHCS fell after ACTH (mean, 0.38–0.33 mg/h). Plasma 17-OHCS were measured in patients with delirium tremens and elevated values were noted. Plasma 17-OHCS were not measured after ACTH stimulation. These authors focused on liver disease as the most likely explanation for the 'impaired adrenocortical responsivity'. To this end, they studied the clearance of cortisol from the blood and were able to demonstrate a decreased removal of infused non-tracer steroid in 60 % of the patients studied. The authors pointed out two important areas to be considered in evaluating adrenocortical function in alcoholics. First is that underlying liver disease is quite common in alcoholics. Liver disease, *per se*, is associated with abnormal clearance of cortisol from the blood[37], and with an altered pathway of cortisol metabolism[38] so that increased 20-hydroxylated steroid metabolites are formed at the expense of A-ring reduced compounds (17-OHCS). The Porter–Silber reaction does not measure the 20-hydroxylated metabolites (cortols and cortolones) and this may account for the slightly lower basal urinary 17-OHCS excretion and perhaps for the apparent lack of response to ACTH stimulation. Secondly, the poor nutritional state and vitamin depletion seen in alcoholics rather than a direct alcohol effect *per se*, may account for decreased adrenocortical responsiveness[39] (if, indeed, it is present at all).

Magraf *et al.*[40] studied 50 alcoholic patients who had been in delirium tremens within 2 months of the study. The mean cortisol secretory rate measured in ten chronic alcoholics by an isotopic dilution technique was 17.9 mg/24 h and ranged between 11.5 and 21.2 mg/24 h. This is clearly within normal limits. Plasma cortisol (8:00 a.m.) values in alcoholics were higher (21.8 μg/%) than in controls (12.9 μg/%). Urinary 17-OHCS were lower than normal, but when 'total' 17-OHCS were estimated by measurement of 17-ketogenic steroids (which includes cortols and cortolones) it was found that this parameter was normal. These data are quite consistent with the prior observations of Kissin *et al.*[36] and with more recent observations of the effect of liver disease on cortisol metabolism[38]. In 50 alcoholic patients, the 17-ketosteroids were significantly decreased both in male (18 *vs.* 10 mg/24 h) and in female (16 *vs.* 10 mg/24 h) alcoholics compared to controls (See Section 9.5.2.2.(g) for further discussion of 17-ketosteroids). These investigators also carried out ACTH stimulation studies and showed a poor response in urinary 17-OHCS after 1 day, with an improved response after 3 days of ACTH stimulation. This type of response is more characteristic of secondary than primary adrenocortical insufficiency. In this study, the plasma cortisol levels increased in response to 1 day of ACTH stimulation, again demonstrating adrenocortical responsiveness, although at a slightly lower level than normal. It is again emphasized that the 'abnormal' urinary 17-OHCS are most likely a result of delayed and divergent cortisol metabolism rather than adrenocortical deficiency. If 17-ketogenic steroids had been measured after ACTH stimulation, a response might well have been found. Although diurnal studies were carried out in three patients the small number precluded significant conclusions concerning alterations in this parameter. Using a non-isotopic technique, the authors showed decreased clearance of cortisol. Measurement of blood levels of 'free' and conjugated steroids suggested that a defect in conjugation was present, but again the number of studies was small. The authors concluded that basal adrenocortical function was 'normal' in their 50 alcoholic subjects 2 months off alcohol. While the authors believed that the responsiveness of the alcoholic to ACTH was diminished (based on urinary 17-

OHCS, although plasma 17-OHCS were responsive) it is more likely, that the lack of response reflected alterations in the rate and pathway of cortisol metabolism, rather than adrenocortical disease *per se*. Consistent with this is their observation that in three patients in whom cortols and cortolones were measured these metabolites accounted for 80 % of the difference between 17-OHCS and 17-ketogenic steroids.

Shaver *et al.*[41] studied adrenocortical function in alcoholics who were abstinent for at least 2 years. The long interval of abstinence was chosen to remove the possibility of nutritional impairment influencing adrenocortical function[39]; sixteen fully rehabilitated male alcoholic and thirteen normal male volunteers were evaluated. Duration of abstinence ranged from 2 to 21 years with a median duration of 4 years. The extensive studies carried out included measurements of 24-h urinary excretions of 17-KS and 17-OCHS, diurnal plasma cortisol levels, isotopic tracer studies of cortisol metabolism (half-life, volume of distribution, secretory rate, and isolation and quantification of specific urinary metabolites) and response to ACTH. These sophisticated studies yielded normal results. This study strongly dispels any doubt as to the basic normality of the adrenocortical status in alcoholics *per se* (aside from the direct and indirect effects of alcohol).

The possibility of secondary adrenocortical insufficiency, due to abnormal hypothalamic–pituitary function in alcoholics has been investigated. Merry and Marks[42] studied 30 chronic alcoholic males admitted in an intoxicated state. On the morning of admission, patients were given 284 ml whiskey and they were then allowed free access to alcohol. On succeeding mornings, patients were treated with amylobarbitone (400–450 mg) or diazepam (30–40 mg) but did not receive alcohol until the midday. Plasma cortisol was studied while on alcohol and during the a.m. alcohol withdrawal periods, at which time the barbiturate or diazepam was given. Plasma cortisol was measured at $\frac{1}{2}$ h intervals for 2 h. Fasting (9:00 a.m.) cortisol levels were higher in alcoholic than in 30 control subjects. Alcohol or amylobarbitone administration resulted in a significant decrease of plasma cortisol, while diazepam administration did not have this effect. The authors felt that in naive subjects, alcohol ingestion activates the hypothalamic–pituitary axis, while conversely, in alcoholics, withdrawal of alcohol results in a similar activation which is then suppressible by alcohol or barbiturate use (but not by diazepam). These studies suggest a basic difference in CNS–adrenocortical response to alcohol between normal subjects and those chronically using the intoxicant. Consistent with this concept are a series of observations from this group[43,44] on hypothalamic–pituitary–adrenocortical response to stress tests in alcoholics abstinent for varying periods of time. They[43] initially reported seven alcoholic males who had been abstinent for 3–6 weeks before study. Adrenocortical function was stimulated by intramuscular injection of a synthetic ACTH preparation (Synacthen). Two subjects had slightly subnormal responses in plasma cortisol. In our experience, this is a useful screening test, but no definitive statement concerning adrenocortical reserve can be made in an individual with an abnormal Synacthen test unless confirmed by standard i.v. ACTH testing. Insulin tolerance tests were carried out in eight abstinent alcoholics. All subjects developed significant decreases in blood sugar and five of the eight experienced normal increments in plasma cortisol. Three of the eight had subnormal increments in plasma cortisol in response to the hypoglycaemic challenge and one of these subjects had a flat plasma cortisol curve despite marked persistent hypoglycaemia. One patient with poor cortisol response to hypoglycaemia was retested after 6 months' abstinence and a normal response was evoked[42]. More recently, this group[44] reported on eleven patients who had been drinking heavily up to the time of admission and were tested within 48 or 72 hours of hospitalization. In this group, Synacthen testing showed adequate adrenocortical reserve and nine of the eleven had normal plasma cortisol response to insulin-induced hypoglycaemia. However, in two subjects, no plasma cortisol response to hypoglycaemia was detected, although release of growth hormone occurred. These studies raise the question of an isolated ACTH defect in some alcoholics (which apparently is reversible by abstinence from alcohol). Further studies in this area would be of interest.

9.2.1.2 Aldosterone

The findings of Ogata *et al.*[45] and Sereny *et al.*[46] that alcohol administration to alcoholics results in decreased urinary sodium excretion and increased serum sodium levels led to investigations of the effect of alcohol on aldosterone secretion.

Fabre *et al.*[47] showed that a high dose of alcohol, with blood alcohol levels of 300 mg/dl or higher, was associated with a 50 % or greater inhibition of the aldosterone secretory response to haemorrhage in dogs. Lower blood alcohol levels were associated with a variable increase in aldosterone secretion[47]. Human subjects exposed to alcohol (bourbon) showed a biphasic increase in aldosterone excretion and secretory rates[48]. On day 2 of the study period in four alcoholic patients, the aldosterone excretion rate was increased 4-fold compared to the basal state. In some studies, a biphasic increase in aldosterone excretion was noted with an early and late peak. Blood alcohol levels of 100–200 mg/dl were associated with increments in aldosterone secretion while higher levels of blood alcohol appeared to inhibit aldosterone secretion.

Further studies in alcoholic subjects were reported by Farmer *et al.*[49], who measured plasma aldosterone and renin, and urinary aldosterone excretion. Again, urinary aldosterone excretion was greatest on the first day of drinking and no systematic change in plasma levels of the hormone was noted. There was no relation noted between plasma renin activity and urinary aldosterone excretion. In addition, in five normal men studied during acute alcohol ingestion, there was no change in plasma renin or aldosterone noted until blood alcohol levels declined and the patients experienced 'considerable distress'. At this time the plasma levels of renin and aldosterone increased, suggesting a non-specific stress response.

Saruta *et al.*[50] noted that alcohol has an inhibitory effect on aldosterone synthesis in minced adrenal tissue. There was no effect noted at an alcohol concentration of 0.1 %, but a 10- and 20-fold increase in alcohol concentration significantly inhibited aldosterone biosynthesis in these *in vitro* studies. The 1 % concentration of alcohol (equivalent to blood alcohol levels of 1000 mg/dl) necessary to inhibit aldosterone biosynthesis in these preparations is beyond the levels obtained in the studies cited above (dog and human) by a factor of two or more. However, no intermediate concentrations between 0.1 and 1 % were evaluated and the aldosterone-inhibitory effect might occur at more usual levels of blood alcohol. The site of action of alcohol in inhibiting aldosterone biosynthesis was at the level of conversion of corticosterone to aldosterone. The exact step was undefined. Until further studies at appropriate blood levels are reported, this mechanism for the decrease in aldosterone noted in dog and human studies must be speculative.

9.2.1.3 Dehydroepiandrosterone (DHEA) and 17-ketosteroids (17-KS)

See Section 9.5.2.2 (g) for DHEA.
See Section 9.2.1.1 and 9.5.2.2 (g) for 17-KS.

9.2.2 Adrenal medulla—catecholamines

9.2.2.1 Animal studies

Matunaga[51], in 1942, noting that interruption of splanchnic nerves prevented the hyperglycaemic (see Section 9.7) response to alcohol administration, suggested that the sympathetic nervous system mediated this response. Klingman and Goodall[52] studied the participation of the sympathetic nervous system in mediating the hyperglycaemic response to alcohol by quantitating by bioassay the urinary excretion of epinephrine (adrenalin) and norepinephrine (noradrenalin) in dogs. The animals were conditioned not to show excitement during passage or use of stomach tubes or urinary catheters and alcohol was given in high, but usually sublethal, doses. Urine was collected in baseline periods, after passage of the feeding tubes but before alcohol administration and these samples served as controls. Additional control data were obtained by studying catecholamine excretion in untreated intact and adrenalectomized dogs. There was a marked increase in bioassayable epinephrine and norepinephrine excretion after alcohol administration. The peak excretion was found 3–6 h after administration of the intoxicant and both catecholamines increased markedly in the urine (more than 30-fold increase for epinephrine and 15-fold for norepinephrine). In adrenalectomized dogs, no change in epinephrine excretion was noted and only minimal increases were detected in norepinephrine output after alcohol. Moreover, the time sequence of the norepinephrine peak excretion in adrenalectomized animals was noted 18–24 h after alcohol gavage, during the 'recovery phase' from intoxication, a time when the animal would be excited. In studies of adrenal gland catecholamine content (using colorometric and chromatographic assays), it was found that alcohol administration decreased the adrenal content of epinephrine by more than a half compared to control animals, but no changes in adrenal norepinephrine were detected. At the time of maximal urinary excretion of catecholamines (3–6 h post-alcohol) in intact animals, the blood alcohol levels approached 600 mg/dl. This study demonstrated that large doses of alcohol activated the sympathetic–adrenal–medullary system and led to the release of epinephrine and norepinephrine from the adrenal gland. Studies in adrenalectomized animals showing no epinephrine excretion and only a minimal and delayed release of noreprinephrine (presumably from peripheral nerve endings) are compatible with the adrenal origin of excreted catecholamines after alcohol ingestion. Whether the alcohol-mediated release of catecholamines was due to a specific effect on the adrenal medulla or the CNS or a non-specific response could not be determined.

Permin[53], using relatively lower alcohol doses than Klingman and Goodall[52], measured the release of epinephrine and norepinephrine (bioassay) in the adrenal venous effluent of nembutal-anaesthetized cats. Alcohol was administered intravenously over a dose range of 0.3 to 1.1 g/kg b.w. and catecholamine release was noted at doses above 0.6 g/kg. The author suggested that the use of an anaesthetized animal ruled out non-specific stress release of catecholamines by alcohol and suggested a direct CNS activating effect. Direct adrenal effects of alcohol were not considered. Further studies by Perman[54] in the rat again showed release of catecholamines in response to alcohol.

9.2.2.2 Human studies

(*a*) *Studies in normal human volunteers*—Kinzius[55] reported transient elevations in blood epinephrine levels 15–30 min after alcohol ingestion. Abelin *et al.*[56] had normal men ingest whiskey diluted in mineral water and noted that the urinary excretion of epinephrine increased 12-fold and norepinephrine increased by a factor of three or four during the first hour after alcohol ingestion. A decline to below normal levels was noted in some subjects at 3–4 h after drinking the alcohol. Perman[57] gave healthy young men whiskey (86° proof) or wine (10°–24° proof) in doses of 0.27–0.54 g/kg b.w. (as ethanol) and noted that the rate of urinary catecholamine excretion increased compared to baseline values. He noted augmentation of epinephrine excretion, but not of norepinephrine. Similar results were reported by Perman[20] in another study using a slightly lower dose range. Anton[58], in carefully controlled studies of the effects of alcohol in normal subjects, measured urinary dopamine, epinephrine, norepinephrine and their methylated (metanephrine and normetanephrine) and oxidized (vanilmandelic acid—VMA) metabolites using colorometric techniques. He found that the administration of the diluent (orange juice) itself altered the excretion of these biogenic amines in a statistically significant fashion. However, by the use of analysis of variance, he was able to show that alcohol (0.7 g/kg b.w.) significantly increased urinary dopamine, norepinephrine and metanephrine. Since the subjects were not at rest when studied, the predominate norepinephrine response may have been related to their moderate activity[59]. Anton[58] discusses a wide variety of possible ethanol-mediated events that could lead to increased urinary excretion of the catecholamines, their precursors or metabolites.

Davis *et al.*[60,61] showed that alcohol can significantly alter the peripheral metabolism of norepinephrine. They studied two normal men after ingestion of 60 ml of alcohol and found a decrease in VMA (3-methoxy-4-hydroxymandelic acid) and an increased MHPG (3-methoxy-4-hydrophenylglycol). Studies[60] with [^{14}C]norepinephrine showed that this was due to an alcohol-mediated effect on the peripheral metabolism of norepinephrine tracer and studies[61] of the pattern of excretion of endogenous VMA and MHPG showed a similar effect. This change in metabolism reflects an increase in the reductive (MHPG) at the expense of the oxidative pathway (VMA). The increase in reduction could reflect increased availability of reducing equivalents in the form of NADH (which occurs as alcohol is metabolized by alcohol dehydrogenase[2]); however, competitive inhibition of oxidative enzymes, by acetaldehyde perhaps, could produce a similar effect[62].

Garlind *et al.*[59] could not demonstrate any effect of alcohol on catecholamine excretion in exercising subjects. They noted markedly elevated urinary norepinephrine excretion as a result of the vigorous exercise in their subjects with no further increase with administration of alcohol. In contrast to studies which show an increase in catecholamine excretion after alcohol, Goddard[63] showed than 50 ml of brandy given to student pilots before stressful training obliterated the expected increase in urinary norepinephrine. It was suggested that the sedative effect of alcohol suppressed the perception of stress and prevented the stress-related increase in norepinephrine excretion. Thus, in normal subjects, alcohol in large doses can activate the sympathetic–adrenal–medullary system. The site of activation is unknown and could be either at the periphery (i.e. adrenal) directly, or perhaps at a central locus (hypothalamus) as a specific effect. In addition, alcohol could produce this effect by virtue of a generalized, non-specific stressor action. At lower doses, alcohol can decrease catecholamine excretion by altering the perception of stressful stimuli (a cortical sedative effect). Moreover, alcohol alters the peripheral metabolism of endogenous and exogenous catecholamines by increasing reductive metabolism.

(*b*) *Studies in alcoholic subjects*—Giacobini *et al.*[64] noting that certain clinical findings during alcohol withdrawal (i.e. changes in blood pressure, pulse, temperature, and pupil diameter) could represent endogenous catecholamine effects and, being aware of the alcohol-mediated release of these biogenic amines in normal subjects and in experimental animals, undertook a study of the effects of alcohol withdrawal on catecholamine excretion. These investigators studied a large group of alcoholics hospitalized after chronic alcohol abuse and suffering from delirium tremens, pure alcoholic hallucinosis or other withdrawal syndromes. Some of the subjects had elevated blood alcohol at the time of study and all were treated with sedatives and vitamins. Twelve normal subjects were studied as a control group. All alcoholics studied had significantly elevated urinary excretion of epinephrine and norepinephrine as determined by a fluorimetric technique. There were no control studies of the effects of the sedative agent or vitamins (potentially interfering compounds in a fluorimetric assay) carried out. Those patients with maximal clinical disturbance had the greatest elevations of urinary catecholamines and there was some correlation with the clinical manifestations of sympathetic overstimulation (i.e. increase in blood pressure and pulse rate) and urinary catecholamine excretion. The decrease in clinical symptoms was accompanied by a corresponding fall in the elevated urinary catecholamines towards normal. However, the onset of delirium did not coincide with elevations in catecholamine excretion. During convalescent states, the catecholamine excretion was normal. The authors state that several patients with high excretion values had 'low muscular activity and weak tremor'. The mechanism of the increase in catecholamine excretion is unknown and may be related more to anxiety[65] and the muscular work[59] associated with tremor and hyperactivity than to a specific alcohol effect. However, some specific event in the CNS or possibly in the peripheral metabolism or synthesis of the catecholamines may occur during alcohol withdrawal.

In a further study, Giacobini *et al.*[66] studied 16 male alcoholic patients 'showing no acute alcoholic syndromes for at least one week'. Urinary catecholamines were determined in 24-h urinary collections before, during and after alcohol exposure. Eight patients consumed brandy or wine and the others received intravenous alcohol infusions (2.3 g/kg b.w.) over 5 h. Despite markedly elevated blood alcohol levels, no change in excretion of urinary catecholamines was observed. The lack of adrenal medullary activation by alcohol in alcoholic subjects (in a convalescent phase) in contrast to the response seen in acute studies in normal non-alcoholic volunteers or experimental animals may be a manifestation of the 'tolerance' to alcohol seen in alcoholics (see Section 9.2.1).

Carlsson and Häggendal[67] noted increased arterial norepinephrine levels by a fluorimetric technique in 36 alcoholics studied at intervals from 6 h to 21 days after alcohol withdrawal. Abstinence symptoms developed at about 12 h and elevated norepinephrine levels were noted between 13 and 24 h. The more striking withdrawal symptoms were associated with the highest levels of norepinephrine. Treatment with a sedative ameliorated the severity of the withdrawal state, and in these sedated patients the arterial norepinephrine levels were normal despite the presence of hallucinations. The authors suggest that the sympathetic nervous system is activated upon withdrawal of alcohol analogous to the findings upon withdrawal of narcotic drugs.

Ogata *et al.*[68] studied four alcoholic subjects who had abstained from alcohol for at least 7 days prior to study. Daily 24-h urines for catecholamines (epinephrine and norepinephrine), dopamine, metanephrine and normetanephrine, VMA and MHPG were collected. Fluorometric and spectrophotometric methods were used. Subjects imbibed alcohol on a free-choice programme (*ad lib*) and a programmed dose protocol. Higher blood alcohol levels were obtained in the free-choice protocol (mean 190 mg/dl) compared to the programmed studies (mean 86 mg/dl). During *ad lib* alcohol ingestion, but not during programmed alcohol use, there was a significant increase in epinephrine values. During the post-alcohol phase of the free-choice study, the epinephrine levels reached the highest mean levels; however, a high degree of variability in excretion levels did not permit attainment of statistical significance. Metanephrine values were highest during the alcohol ingesting phase of the free-choice alcohol study and were also significantly elevated in the withdrawal phase. There were no significant changes in norepinephrine excretion during the alcohol phase of the programmed study, although a small increase was observed. Normetanephrine increased significantly during the alcohol use phase of the free-choice study. VMA levels fell during the alcohol phase of both programmed and free-choice alcohol studies and then returned to basal levels during the post-alcohol phase. MHPG increased as VMA decreased. The data confirm the observation of Davis *et al.*[60,61]. The authors noted that in the free-choice study, the progressive increase in epinephrine, norepinephrine, metanephrine and normetanephrine values paralleled the upward movement of blood alcohol levels, and that during the post-withdrawal period in a subject who experienced a symptomatically significant withdrawal syndrome, the epinephrine and norepinephrine levels were maximally elevated. These studies suggest that enhanced urinary catecholamines occur throughout the course of long-term ethanol intake in alcoholics without any adaptational response (i.e. sympathetic–adrenal–medullary tolerance). There were no significant changes in dopamine excretion.

The studies in normal volunteers and alcoholics suggest adrenal medullary activation by alcohol. There is a suggestion that the chronic alcoholic may be more tolerant of alcohol acutely than naive subjects (note the similarity to acute effects of alcohol on cortisol, Section 9.2.1.1. (b)). Chronic administration of alcohol also results in adrenal medullary activation in alcoholics. The effects may be mediated by a non-specific stress response, although direct effects on the adrenal medulla, nerve endings or in the CNS must be considered. There is evidence from several groups that alcohol (or a metabolite) can alter the peripheral metabolism of the catecholamines. Alcohol also may have significant effects on catecholamine metabolism in the central nervous system[69] and these would not necessarily be reflected as changes in the peripheral hormone levels (blood and urine) which were the subject of this review.

9.3 THYROID FUNCTION

9.3.1 Animal studies

9.3.1.1 Histological studies

Sanchez-Calvo[70] and Hion-Jon[7] suggested on the basis of histologic studies in rabbits, that alcohol altered the functional state of the thyroid gland. Üprus[71] claimed that thyroidal changes could be detected in the offspring of alcohol-treated rabbits. Aschkenasy-Lelu and Guérin[72] studied rats whose sole fluid intake was 10 % alcohol or red wine for 6 months and found that relative thyroid weights and iodine fixation was not altered in these studies.

9.3.1.2 Physiological studies

Richter[73] related thyroid function to alcohol preference in rats. He showed that feeding thyroid powder or purified thyroid hormones led to a decrease in alcohol intake. Thyroid hypofunction, on the other hand, increased ethanol intake[74]. The changes in level of thyroid function induced by these treatments, however, were not monitored. In contrast, Prieto *et al.*[75] found that thyroid feeding (0.5 % powder) for 3 weeks did not reduce, but actually increased, alcohol intake in a 'non-drinking' substrain of rats. Although several authors[76–78] have shown that an increase in thyroid function leads to death with smaller doses of alcohol than that required in the euthyroid state, the mechanism of the mortality did not correlate with the occurrence of hypoglycaemia, acid–base changes or enhancement of respiratory depression. The mechanism of this thyroid hormone–ethanol interaction is unclear and its relation to voluntary alcohol intake in rats with altered thyroid function remains to be investigated more fully. Thyroid hormone inhibits alcohol dehydrogenase[79], an enzyme which is important in ethanol metabolism[2], which may play a role in the sensitization to alcohol. This should be investigated more fully.

9.3.1.3 Alcohol effect on $^{131(125)}I$ thyroidal accumulation

Murdock[80] showed an increased thyroidal accumulation of isotopic iodide (^{125}I and ^{131}I) in rats fed a 20 % solution of alcohol for 2–3 weeks, compared to control animals. In these animals, there were significant increases in nuclide uptake at 6, 24, 48 and 72 h after the i.p. administration of the tracer dose. However, no difference was noted in tracer uptake in rats treated with alcohol i.p. or by gavage. Although Murdock[80] showed that dehydration of control animals (by omitting fluids for 48 h) leads to an increased thyroidal radioiodide uptake, presumably by decreasing renal clearance of the tracer, this mechanism did not appear to account for the alcohol effect since blood volume and haematocrit determinations did not support the presence of dehydration in the alcohol-treated rats. However, the alcohol-treated animals had a significant (one-third) fall in food intake, which could have led to a relatively decreased iodide pool. The increase in thyroidal uptake probably reflects this phenomenon rather than a direct pituitary effect of alcohol, which was suggested by the authors. Measurement of inorganic iodide levels would have been important in this study.

9.3.1.4 Alcohol effects on the metabolism and tissue distribution of thyroid hormones

Bleecker *et al.*[81] studied the acute effect of alcohol given i.p. (20 % solution) on the tissue uptake of a tracer dose of [^{131}I]l-triiodothyronine. The tissue distribution of the compound was expressed as the ratio of counts in tissue to plasma (organ/plasma ratio) and was found to be increased by alcohol in anterior pituitary, thyroid, adrenal, kidney and liver tissue. However, this ratio was not altered in skeletal muscle, posterior pituitary, cerebral cortex (white and grey matter) diencephalon, cerebellum, pineal or brain stem. The functional significance of the alcohol-mediated increase in the endocrine tissue uptake of l-triiodothyronine is uncertain, although it has been suggested that an increase in the organ/plasma ratio in other tissues such as the liver, may be important in mediating some of the metabolic effects of alcohol. It was shown that chronic administration of ethanol decreases the phosphorylation potential and increases the respiratory rate in liver slices[82–84]. The activity of both the Na^+ and K^+-dependent ATPase system[83] and mitochondrial alpha-glycerophosphate dehydrogenase activity[84] were increased. Urea synthesis was increased 52 % and mitochondrial cross-sectional area (measured by electron microphotography) was increased 80 % by alcohol treatment[84]. The hepatic uptake of [^{131}I]thyroxine was increased 30 % and 55 % by ethanol in doses of 4 and 6 g/kg b.w. respectively[84]. These effects of alcohol mimic those of thyroxine itself[84]. Furthermore, the response to ouabain is similar in alcohol- and thyroxine-treated rats. The authors[84] suggest that alcohol, by altering the binding of thyroxine in blood as a result of pH changes and/or alterations in non-esterified fatty acids, leads to increased hepatic uptake of thyroxine and to a 'hyperthyroid hepatic state'. Studies in animals whose thyroid function was ablated would be appropriate controls for this hypothesis as the effects reported may be mediated directly by alcohol and the increase uptake of thyroxine might represent an enzyme-mediated alcohol effect since phenobarbitol[85] (enzyme inducer) increases thyroxine retention in the liver.

9.3.2 Human studies

Gross[86] and Goldfarb and Berman[87] suggested that alcoholism and endocrine dysfunction were possibly interconnected. Goldberg[88] undertook a systematic study of thyroid function in 33 alcoholics (military personnel and dependents in the Paris area) partly as a result of Richter's[74] observation relating the intensity of alcohol intake to the level of thyroid function in rats. He reported a 64 and 45 % incidence of thyroid deficiency in the military population[88] and in a group of 100 civilian alcoholics respectively[89]. Goldberg based his diagnosis of hypothyroidism on the PBI measurements (below 4.0 μg/%), failure of the PBI to rise more than 1.0 μg/% after treatment with 10 IU of thyrotrophin (TSH), elevated serum cholesterol and achilles reflex contraction time exceeding 240 to 280 msec. Furthermore, he reported good clinical response to treatment with triidothyronine or thyroxine in these studies. The incidence of hypothyroidism reported by Goldberg[88,89] is astonishingly high and led several investigators to carry out more detailed studies in alcoholics. Satterfield and Guze[90] treated 24 male alcoholics with triiodothyronine or placebo and found no difference in response to treatment between groups. However, thyroid function was not investigated in these patients. Selzer and Van Houten[91], in a letter to the editor, reported on 22 male alcoholics and a control group of 21 non-alcoholic men studied after admission to a psychiatric ward. They found no clinical evidence of hypothyroidism and the PBIs were all within the normal range. They also reported on the level of PBI in a group of 21 intoxicated patients admitted to a private hospital. PBIs were drawn on admission and again 1 week later. Three subjects had PBIs below 4.0 μg/%, but these levels rose to within the normal range by time of discharge 1 week later. They concluded that no thyroid abnormality was present in their alcoholic patients. Augustine[92] studied the PBI in 102, and the resin T_3 uptake in 103 alcoholic patients admitted to a general hospital. Eight patients had low (less than 4 μg/%) PBIs, and eight had elevated PBIs (over 8.0 μg/%). Thirteen abnormalities of the resin T_3 uptake were noted, but only two were depressed below 25 % as would be seen in hypothyroidism. The author reports only one patient in whom both the PBI and resin T_3 uptake were abnormal but in this patient the tests were discordant. The low PBI and elevated resin uptake in this patient suggests an alteration in protein binding of thyroxine rather than a primary hormonal abnormality. This author reported that his survey did not show any consistent thyroid functional abnormalities. Murdock[80] states that alcoholic patients on admission to the hospital had elevated radioiodine uptakes and after being denied alcohol, the uptakes, when repeated a week later, decreased to 'low euthyroid or hypothyroid ranges'. Stokes[93] found no correlation between the PBI, resin T_3 uptake, radioiodine uptake or cholesterol levels and length of alcoholism, or time since the last drink. Wright *et al.*[44], in a recent study, noted 'diminished TSH response to TSHRH' (thyrotrophin releasing hormone) in only two of thirteen alcoholic subjects studied in the hospital within 72 h of 'heavy' drinking. It is also stated that the T_4 and T_3 levels were normal in all subjects.

It is apparent that definitive studies in animals or humans have not been carried out to date. Using current methodology, it should be possible to clearly define thyroid function and to definitively exclude thyroid hormonal abnormalities in alcoholics. It should also be possible to demonstrate the direct effects of alcohol in animals and/or human volunteers on thyroid function and to separate these effects from those of dietary iodide depletion and protein abnormalities (which may alter the PBI, T_4 and resin T_3 uptake tests) in alcoholic patients with occult liver disease or disturbed nutrition. Basal measurement of TSH and response to TSH releasing factor would be the most definitive method of excluding the presence of hypothyroidism. The preliminary report of Wright *et al.*[44] suggests the occurrence of hypothyroidism in alcoholic patients is indeed infrequent. The use of thyroid hormone in the treatment of alcohol intoxication[94] or chronic alcoholism[88,89] seems to be without solid clinical support at present[90,95]. Moreover, large oral or intravenous doses of thyroid hormones are not without potential hazard.

9.4 PARATHYROID, CALCITONIN AND CALCIUM

9.4.1 Hypocalcaemic effect of alcohol in the experimental animal

Peng *et al.*[96] noted an acute dose related hypocalcaemic effect of alcohol in male rats 30 min after oral administration of alcohol (2 to 8 g/kg b.w.). The effect persisted for 5 h after administration of alcohol and was not associated with changes in blood levels of phosphate. Pyrazole, an inhibitor of alcohol dehydrogenase, prolonged the duration of both the hypocalcaemia and the period of alcohol intoxication. Pyrazole or acetaldehyde administration in control studies had no hypocalcaemic effect. Nephrectomized animals also exhibited a hypocalcaemic reaction to alcohol administration. In another group of animals, alcohol led to a 20 % fall in urinary calcium excretion compared to control animals. Phosphate, sodium and potassium were retained (i.e. decreased excretion) in the alcohol-treated animals although urinary volume was not altered significantly. It is apparent that alcohol does not produce hypocalcaemia by a renal effect. Moreover, the hypocalcaemia was not mediated by the thyroid or parathyroid glands since in thyroparathyroidectomized rats, alcohol was able to produce hypocalcaemia 1 h after surgery. Thyroparathyroidectomized controls not given alcohol were able to maintain their serum calcium at normal levels at this time. Studies of ethanol effect on serum proteins and blood pH failed to reveal any alterations 30 min after alcohol administration. There were no data reported at later time intervals. Investigations using ^{45}Ca failed to show alterations in specific activity as hypocalcaemia developed, suggesting that the fall in calcium was due to a shift of the electrolyte out of the serum. Both conscious and anaesthetized dogs experienced hypocalcaemia after oral alcohol administration (2–4 g/kg). In another study, Peng *et al.*[97] noted that alcohol administration decreased the ionized fraction of plasma calcium and parathormone administration could not prevent the ethanol-induced hypocalcaemia (in thyroparathyroidectomized rats). Significant increments in serum magnesium were not noted until 3½ h after alcohol administration; the hypocalcaemic effects preceded this event by 3 h.

It is apparent that alcohol does not produce hypocalcaemia by suppressing parathormone secretion, by a renal effect, or by changes in pH or serum proteins. The ^{45}Ca studies suggest that alcohol may decrease the serum level of calcium by shifting it into bone or other tissues. That this effect is not due to an alcohol-mediated release of calcitonin was suggested by the constant specific activity of ^{45}Ca noted while total serum calcium fell. The author further suggests that the increase in magnesium seen at 3½ h after alcohol administration may interfere with release of parathormone and thus delay resolution of the hypocalcaemia.

In confirmation of Peng's finding, Hillbom and Pöso[78] found a significant fall of serum calcium in euthyroid rats treated with 3 g/kg b.w. of ethanol as a single oral dose. In rats previously made hyperthyroid with triiodothyronine falls in serum calcium also occurred although the fall was not statistically significant.

9.4.2 Human studies—hypocalcaemia in alcoholics

Studies in several laboratories, in normal and alcoholic subjects[98,99], demonstrate that alcohol administration is associated with an increased loss of calcium and magnesium in the urine. Indeed, hypocalcaemia is not an unusual clinical event in hospitalized alcoholics[100,101]. Hypocalcaemia may be a manifestation of pancreatitis, intestinal malabsorption, or malnutrition with hypoalbuminaemia. However, in many alcoholics, none of these mechanisms apply and the low serum calcium resolves after a short period in the hospital usually associated with adequate food and vitamin intake and with cessation of alcohol intake. The studies of Peng[96,97] suggest one possible mechanism (i.e. some direct effect of alcohol on the distribution of calcium in the blood) for the hypocalcaemia. However, the hypocalcaemia seen in Peng's animal studies seems of shorter duration (hours) than the hypocalcaemia noted during the early phase of alcoholic admissions (days) to the hospital. The effect of alcohol on magnesium and calcium homeostasis may be of more significance in these patients, since many alcoholics are magnesium deficient and this electrolyte seems to be important for regulating the secretion of parathormone in response to hypocalcaemia[102] or, as suggested by Estep *et al.*[103], may mediate the peripheral action of parathormone. These investigators[103] showed that their alcoholic patients tended to correct the hypocalcaemia spontaneously a few days after hospitalization. However, if they were treated with parathormone extract, of proven potency, a bimodal response was noted in that in five of thirteen patients, the serum calcium and urinary hydroxyproline excretion increased and the tubular resorption of phosphate decreased in a quantitively normal fashion. The rest of the patients so tested, at the same dosage, were resistant to the effects of parathormone extract. The parathormone-resistant group had reduced serum magnesium (0.8 mEq/l) levels as opposed to normal values (1.8 mEq/l) in the responsive group. When the parathormone-resistant patients were repleted with magnesium for 3 days, they then responded to parathormone injection. The authors suggest a significant role for hypomagnesaemia and subsequent parathormone resistance in the hypocalcaemia of alcoholism. Another possible mechanism for the hypocalcaemia in hypomagnesaemic states may be related to decreased secretion of parathormone, i.e. an acquired hypoparathyroidism, since it has been suggested that magnesium is necessary for the secretion of parathormone in response to hypocalcaemia[102]. Measurement of parathormone levels in these patients would be most useful.

9.4.3 Calcitonin–alcohol effects

Cohen *et al.*[104] in a study of a patient with documented medullary carcinoma of the thyroid with episodes of flushing and watery diarrhea, reported that alcohol stimulated the release of calcitonin. Since the episodes of flushing and diarrhea were provoked by alcohol, the patient was studied before and after the administration of 45 ml (80° proof) of whiskey. Calcitonin levels increased in arterial blood (728 to 4590 ng/ml) 3 min after the administration of the whiskey and remained elevated for 15 min, while prostaglandins ($F_{2\alpha}$) were not elevated until 15 min (0.04–4.2 ng/ml). The authors point out that the flushing noted by the patient was not related temporally to the elevation of the prostaglandin. They suggested that the increase in calcitonin could be mediated by either gastrin release or a direct effect of alcohol. Wells and coworkers[105] further studied alcohol–calcitonin effects in five patients with medullary carcinoma of the thyroid. Ethanol was given either orally (0.4 ml/kg b.w. as a 20 % solution (v/v) over a 5-min period, or intravenously (0.3 ml/kg b.w. as a 10 % solution (v/v) in 0.15 M NaCl) over 30 min. In both studies, two baseline bloods were drawn and blood was sampled at 5, 15, 30, 60 and 90 min after the beginning of each administration of alcohol. Oral administration of alcohol resulted in a rise in serum thyrocalcitonin in four of the five patients studied with a mean increase of 216 % over baseline values. Serum gastrin increased to mean peak levels of 236 pg/ml at 5 to 30 min after alcohol ingestion; IV alcohol, in contrast to Becker's observation[106], did not increase gastrin levels which remained below 50 pg/ml in all patients during the infusion, while the calcitonin level rose 97 %. Serum calcium was monitored during the study and no significant changes were noted. Since alcohol, both by the oral and intravenous routes, increased gastrin levels and gastrin is known to release calcitonin[107], it was postulated that alcohol would release gastrin which, in turn, would increase calcitonin. The oral studies are consistent with this effect and showed the greatest increments in calcitonin levels. However, intravenous alcohol did not alter gastrin levels within the sensitivity of the assay (50 pg/ml), but did increase calcitonin, although the increment was more modest than that provoked by the oral route. These studies suggest that alcohol has a direct effect on the C cells in causing release of calcitonin and the effect is not mediated by changes in calcium levels (also known to significantly affect calcitonin secretion[107]). It is also worth noting that at the non-intoxicating doses used here, there was no change in calcium levels, in contrast to Peng's[96] study in animals. The possible use of alcohol as a provocative test for calcitonin release in patients suspected of medullary carcinoma of the thyroid was suggested by these studies.

9.5 GONADAL FUNCTION AND ALCOHOL

9.5.1 Animal studies

9.5.1.1 Histological studies in animals

Alcohol administration to rabbits has been reported to cause significant alterations in testicular histology, including atrophy and abnormal spermatogenesis[108–111]. The sperm count of dogs was decreased by large doses of alcohol[112,113]. Van Thiel *et al.*[114] studied rats fed 36 % of total calories as alcohol for 41 days and isocalorically maintained controls for a similar time period. There was a decreased growth curve (body weight) in both alcohol-treated and control animals compared with rats fed *ad lib.* After correction for body weight, atrophy of the testes and accessory sex glands (prostate and seminal vesicles) was noted in the alcohol-treated animals. The testicular weight of isocalorically fed controls was twice that of the alcohol-treated group. The loss of testicular weight was related to reduction of mean seminiferous tubular diameter and to a decrease in the amount of germinal epithelium within the tubules. The pituitary glands did not show any histological changes in this study.

9.5.1.2 Physiological studies in animals

Studies in male rats[115–117] and dogs[118,119] showed that alcohol interferes with copulatory behaviour. Estrous cycles in female mice[120] were interfered with by alcohol feeding (10 % solution). Higher doses (20 % solution) almost completely abolished the cycles. Feeding of wine, but not pure alcohol, caused alterations in the estrous cycle of rats[121]. Reproduction and lactation in rats was not affected by wine or alcohol feeding, although neonatal mortality was increased[122].

9.5.1.3 Gonadal hormonal studies in animals

Badr and Bartke[123] treated CBA/J mice with alcohol in doses ranging from 1.24 to 0.16 g ethanol/kg b.w. for 5 days. Control groups were fed water. No change in relative testicular weight was noted. Plasma testosterone, measured by radioimmunoassay, fell from control levels of 8.5 ng/ml to 0.49 ng/ml at the highest alcohol dose. The fall in plasma testosterone was proportional to the dose of alcohol administered. The effect of caloric intake was not controlled in these studies (i.e. isocaloric feeding in alcohol-treated animals and controls was not maintained). In addition, data on body weight changes in alcohol-treated and control groups were not given. Van Thiel *et al.*[114] showed significant decreases in plasma testosterone in alcohol-fed rats relative to isocaloric controls (29 ng/dl *vs.* 162 ng/dl). Rats on an *ad lib.* diet had testosterone levels of 159 ng/dl. It was suggested that alcohol had toxic effects both on Leydig cell and germinal epithelium.

9.5.2 Gonadal function in humans

9.5.2.1 Histological studies

Testicular atrophy and abnormal testicular histology has been documented in men with cirrhosis[124–126]. However, studies in alcoholic men without overt liver disease have not been reported to our knowledge. Early reports, cited by Arlitt and Wells[111] dating back to 1837, suggested a relationship between testicular atrophy (with fatty degeneration of seminal epithelium and decrease in numbers of spermatozoa) and alcoholism. However, these studies were complicated by coexistent chronic disease, nutritional impairment and/or cirrhosis. Von Thiel *et al.*[127] have presented data suggesting that alcohol may impair vitamin A metabolism in the testes, and thus alter spermatogenesis.

9.5.2.2 Hormonal studies in man

While it has been well established on a clinical basis, that overt alcoholic liver disease is associated with a syndrome of hypogonadism and feminization[124,125], it became apparent as well, in the past 10 years, that significant hormonal abnormalities in the plasma concentration of the sex steroids[128–136] and in such parameters of hormone metabolism as metabolic clearance and production rate[129,134,135], interconversion of precursor–product hormones[129,134,135] and hormone binding by specific high-affinity plasma proteins[130–133,136,137] occur with considerable frequency in this group of patients. However, the relative contribution of the altered liver function and that of direct alcohol effects has not been clearly settled. Thus, in order to separate the direct or early effects of alcohol itself from those of liver disease, plasma testosterone levels, urinary testosterone glucuronide and other parameters of hormone metabolism have been studied both in normal volunteers and alcoholic subjects.

(*a*) *Testosterone in plasma and urine*—Fabre *et al.*[138] studied ten alcoholic men, aged 25 to 45 years, who were admitted to a metabolic ward after 2 weeks of enforced abstinence in penal custody. No clinical evidence of liver disease was noted. After urine was collected during a baseline (pre-drinking) period, the subject were allowed alcohol *ad lib.* for 6 days while urine collections were continued daily. Baseline urinary testosterone glucuronide (TG) ranged between 17.6 and 52.3 μg/24 h (mean 36.7 μg/24 h) in the controls. In contrast, the alcoholic men had elevated excretion of TG in the baseline period. The values ranged from 37.5 to 497.6 μg/24 h (mean 153 μg/24 h). During the alcohol ingestion period TG 'seemed to increase slightly' and further increases were noted in the post-alcohol period (3 days after cessation of drinking). However, the variance of the TG measurement was so large that significant differences could not be established. Blood testosterone was not studied in these subjects. Liegel *et al.*[139] measured plasma testosterone in abstaining alcoholics before and during alcohol ingestion and after withdrawal. They found normal basal testosterone levels 557 ± 50 (SD) ng/dl) which decreased during imbibition of alcohol.

Mendelson and Mello[140] studied nine male alcoholics before, during and after a drinking period of 11 or 12 consecutive days. Subjects ranged in age from 28 to 48 years and were volunteers from an alcoholic rehabilitation programme. They had abstained from alcohol for at least 6 days prior to admission to a clinical research ward. No clinical or laboratory evidence of liver disease was noted. Plasma testosterone was measured once daily at 8 a.m. They noted suppression of plasma testosterone in eight of nine subjects during chronic alcohol intoxication. The one subject who failed to suppress his plasma testosterone drank very little alcohol. Several subjects had baseline testosterone levels in the low or high range. The authors comment on the 'erratic' patterns in some patients (see below). In some of the subjects who had initial 'suppression' of plasma testosterone, this was followed by a gradual return to the pre-drinking baseline range, despite continued ingestion of alcohol. A 'rebound' increase above baseline levels was seen in the post-drinking period in some patients. Plasma testosterone also was studied in sober alcoholics using single or repeat samples both in hospitalized subjects (eight men, aged 27 to 52 years) and in residents of correctional or rehabilitation institutions (34 male subjects aged 20 to 36 years). They noted 'elevated' plasma testosterone levels in seven of the eight patients studied during hospitalization. However, they had to be discharged because of medical or emotional factors which precluded their being placed on alcohol. Plasma testosterone ranged from 550 to 1224 ng/dl in these subjects. The 34 subjects in institutions had a wide range of testosterone levels but most clustered in the normal range. In essence, this study showed a suppressive effect of alcohol on plasma testosterone in alcoholics with a rebound in the post-drinking period.

Wright *et al.*[44] noted slightly elevated 17β-hydroxyandrogens in a group of thirteen male alcoholics hospitalized and then studied 40–72 h after cessation of drinking. This group of androgens would include testosterone, dihydrotestosterone and androstane (or-ene-) diol *en masse*. This is somewhat similar to the report of Mendelson and Mello[140] in that alcoholics in a post-drinking period had elevated testosterone levels ('rebound effect'?). The increase in 17β-hydroxyandrogens may also be related to an alteration in the peripheral metabolism of testosterone due to enzymatic changes in the liver (Section 9.5.2.2.b.iii).

However, in normal subjects, Toro *et al.*[141] failed to note any acute change in plasma testosterone in fourteen normal men and sixteen normal females after the oral administration of alcohol (1.0 g/kg b.w.). Blood was assayed at $\frac{1}{2}$ h intervals for 2 h and again at 3 h after alcohol ingestion. Blood alcohol levels were in the 100 mg/dl range. Ylikahri *et al.*[142] studied plasma testosterone in ten healthy male (non-alcoholic) volunteers. They each ingested ethanol at a dose of 1.5 g/kg b.w., as a 20 % aqueous solution, over a 3-h period. The subjects served as their own controls in another experiment in which they drank only water. Blood was taken at the start of drinking and at 4, 8, 12, 15 and 20 h intervals. Plasma testosterone was unchanged during the period of intoxication, i.e. the first 12 h, but fell by 50 % at the 12th and 20th h of the study (hangover period). In contrast, Farmer and Fabre[49] state that in an acute study of alcohol ingestion in normal subjects, no significant changes in plasma testosterone were noted during the drinking or withdrawal phases. Blood alcohol reached the 100 mg/dl range. Dotson *et al.*[143] showed a small fall in mean plasma testosterone (424 ± 167 ng/dl to 387 ± 164 ng/dl) during a social drinking situation.

Since plasma testosterone has a diurnal fall[144] and an episodic pattern of secretion[1], studies utilizing single daily samples or $\frac{1}{2}$-h specimens taken over a period of only several hours may not detect changes in hormone concentration of a magnitude that falls within the variation due to episodic secretion. Similarly, random sampling errors (i.e. sampling at episodic secretory peaks or nadirs) could lead to erroneous conclusions as to the presence or absence of changes in plasma concentration of testosterone after alcohol. Studies by our group[145] in normal male volunteers have shown significant changes in the episodic pattern of plasma testosterone secretion (Figure 9.1) during the first day of alcohol ingestion. Alcohol was begun at 6 a.m. at a dose of 3 g/kg b.w. divided into eight daily doses. More chronic exposure to alcohol leads to a more marked loss of secretory episodes and a fall in mean plasma concentration of the steroid (Figure 9.2). Although control subjects exposed to a similar feeding programme, i.e. eight equal doses given every 3 h

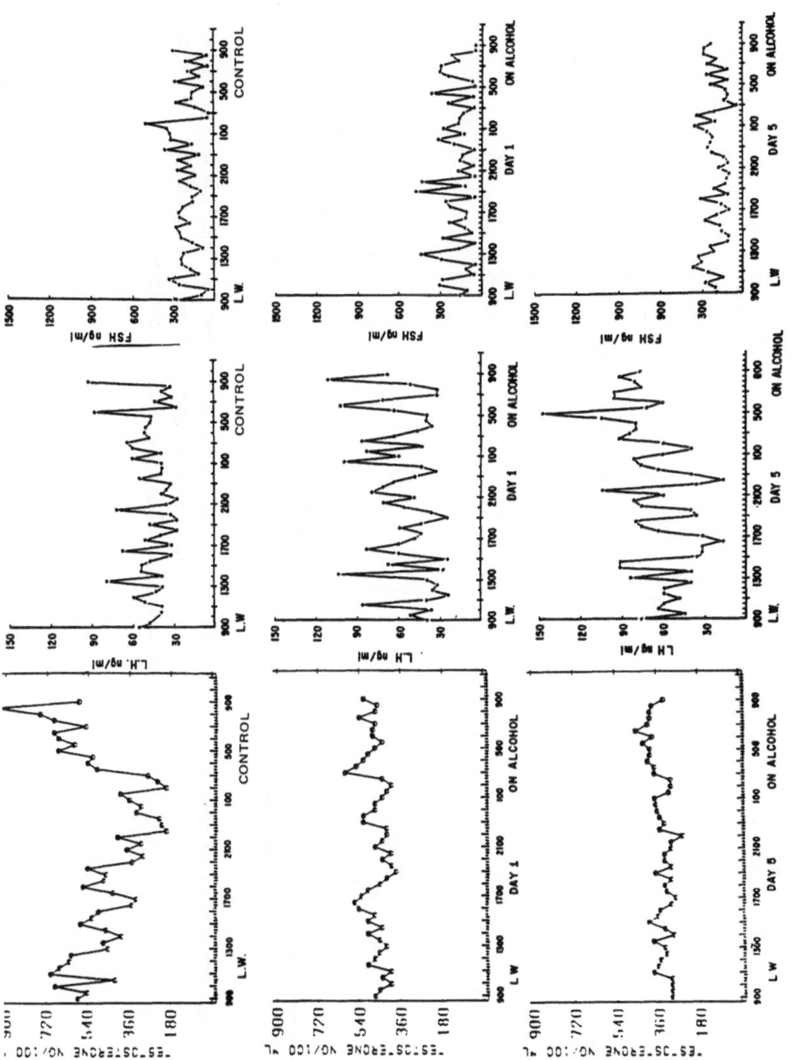

Figure 9.1 The acute effect of alcohol on the episodic secretion of plasma testosterone, LH and FSH in a normal male volunteer. (L.W.). Samples were obtained at 30-min intervals for 24 h in each study period. A marked change in the episodic pattern of testosterone secretion is seen on day 1 of alcohol administration. By day 5, there is a significant fall in the mean plasma concentration of the steroid. The lack of LH suppression suggests a direct gonadal effect

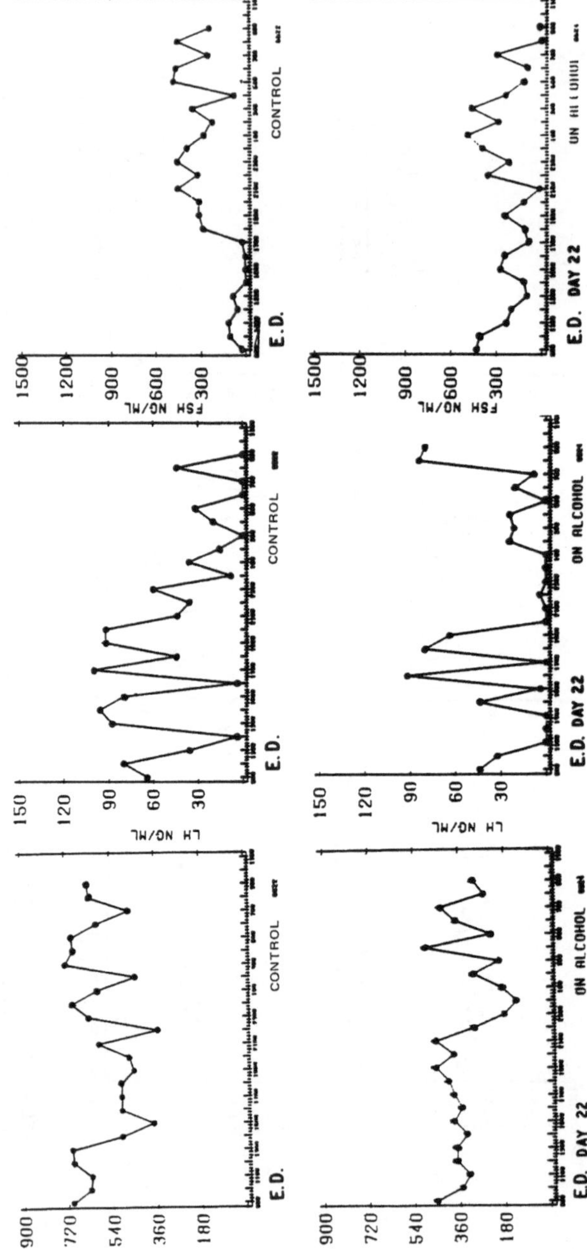

Figure 9.2 The chronic effect of alcohol on the episodic secretion of plasma testosterone, LH and FSH in a normal male volunteer (E.D.). Samples were obtained at 60-min intervals for 24 h in each study period. There is a significant fall in both the mean plasma concentration of testosterone and LH suggesting a central as well as a gonadal effect of alcohol

around the clock, but without alcohol, showed a slight fall in mean plasma concentration of testosterone, the decrease was significantly less than with alcohol. Further control studies are being carried out to evaluate the effect of such factors as hospitalization, and sleep disturbance on plasma testosterone levels.

(*b*) *Testosterone — metabolic clearance rate* (MCR^T) — Measurement of the metabolic clearance rate of testosterone by a constant infusion technique[146,147] in eight normal male volunteers showed increases (up to 40 %) in a majority of patients (Figure 9.3) after 4 weeks of alcohol ingestion[145]. Alcohol was discontinued 12 h before the clearances were determined so that essentially no alcohol was in the circulation at that time.

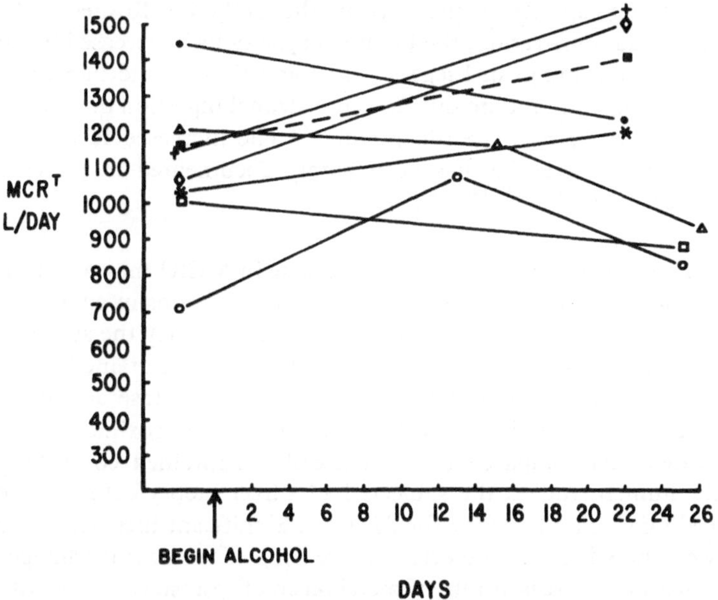

Figure 9.3 The effect of alcohol on the metabolic clearance rate of testosterone (MCR^T) in eight normal male volunteers. Five of the eight subjects showed an increase in the MCR^T. Two of the three subjects demonstrated minor decreases. In only one subject was there a significant decrease in this parameter

(i) Hepatic blood flow. Increases in hepatic blood flow could account for the increases seen in the MCR^T. Childs *et al.*[148] and Mendeloff[149] have shown that acute alcohol infusion increases hepatic blood flow about 50 % with blood alcohol levels in the 50 to 130 mg/dl range. Since the metabolic clearance rate of a steroid equals its hepatic extraction multiplied by the hepatic blood flow, a significant increase in blood flow could account for the clearance changes. However, the clearance was measured 12 h after cessation of the alcohol, and any alcohol effect on blood flow should have abated by that time. Moreover, Castenfors *et al.*[150] showed that low alcohol concentrations in the blood do not alter hepatic blood flow.

(ii) Plasma-protein binding. A decrease in binding of testosterone to the specific binding proteins in the blood also could account for the increase in the clearance rate of the hormone. The binding of testosterone to specific high-affinity plasma proteins is known to influence the metabolism of the steroid[151]. The level of the binding protein is decreased by androgens[152] and increased by estrogens[152]. Liegel *et al.*[139] and Farmer and Fabre[49] reported elevated levels of sex hormone binding protein in chronically alcoholic men and noted decreases in *in vitro* binding when alcohol was added to normal sera. During our study of the MCR^T in normal male volunteers, we noted a gradual and progressive fall in the binding capacity as measured by the method of Rosner[153]. After 24 days of alcohol administration, the binding capacity had decreased by 40 %[145]. In contrast to the findings of Liegel *et al.*[139] and Farmer and Fabre[49], we did not find any change in binding during acute alcohol ingestion or when alcohol was added to sera *in vitro* (~100 mg/dl)[145]. The increased level of plasma binding for the sex steroids has been amply documented in patients with alcoholic liver disease[130–133,135–137].

(iii) Steroid metabolizing enzymes. The increase in MCR^T may also be related to an increased hepatic extraction as a result of alterations in enzymes which are rate-limiting for the metabolism of testosterone, namely the steroid A-ring reductases. Studies in animals and normal humans maintained on alcohol show a marked increase in hepatic steroid A-ring reductase activity[154]. The animals were pair-fed and the level of activity was approximately 2-fold in alcohol-treated rats compared to isocalorically maintained controls (Figure 9.4). In the human studies, the subjects had a liver biopsy before and during alcohol feeding (3 g/kg b.w./day for 28 days). Significant increases in enzyme activity were noted in all subjects (Figure 9.5). The enzyme changes were associated with an increased rate of metabolism of testosterone (i.e. MCR^T) *in vivo* in five of the eight subjects studied[145]. The increased clearance may be related to the increased enzyme activity, although other factors such as plasma protein binding of the steroid and hepatic blood flow changes must be considered (see above). It should be pointed out that the assay for steroid A-ring reductase activity was carried out with excess amounts of NADPH, and thus, the increase in enzyme activity was not due to altered endogenous NADPH. Fabre *et al.*[138] noted slight increases in urinary $5\alpha/5\beta$ androgen metabolites, which would be consistent with increased 5α reductase activity. Dioguardi *et al.*[155] has reported that ethanol treatment in rats increases uridine diphosphate glucuronyl-transferase (UDPGT) activity 50 % above base levels. This enzyme is important in the conjugation of steroid metabolites. Lieber[2] has pointed out similarities in the effects of alcohol and other drugs on in-

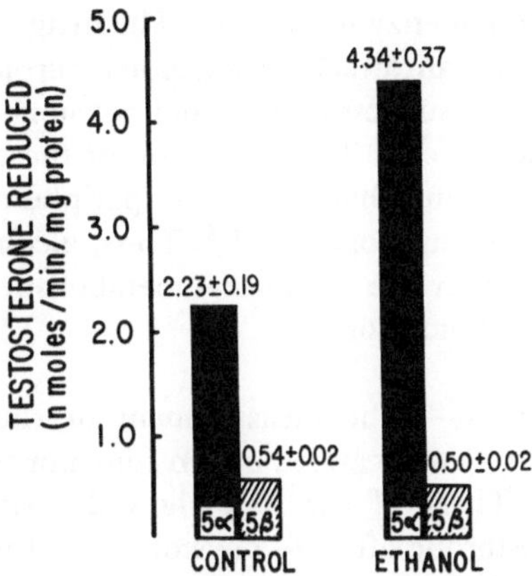

Figure 9.4 Testosterone A-ring reductase activity (mean ± SD) in microsomal (5α) (solid bars) and cytosolic (5β) (hatched bars) fractions obtained from livers of isocalorically fed control and ethanol-treated rats. It can be seen that alcohol markedly increases the activity of hepatic 5α-reductase

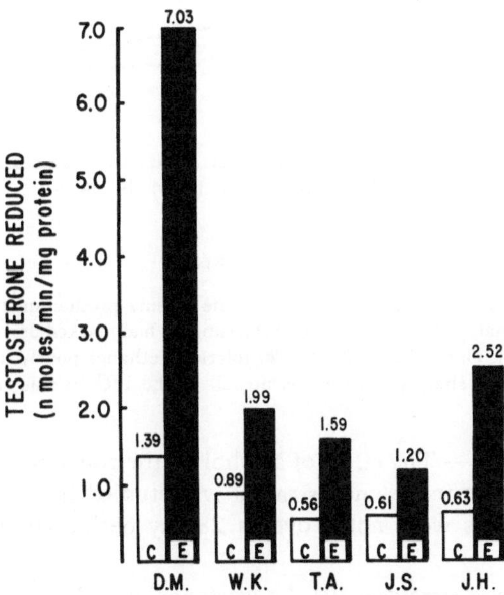

Figure 9.5 Hepatic testosterone A-ring reductase activity (whole homogenates) in liver biopsy specimens obtained from normal human male volunteers before (clear bars) and after (solid bars) 28 days of ethanol administration. Alcohol administration resulted in significant increases in the hepatic enzyme. C = Control and E = Ethanol

creasing hepatic microsomal enzyme activity. The drug metabolizing enzymes (mixed function oxidases) can attack endogenous steroid hormones. Indeed, studies by Kuntzman *et al.*[3] suggest that steroid hormones are the natural substrates for these enzyme systems. The activation of these enzymes by various drugs can produce significant changes in the peripheral metabolism of the glucocorticords[4,156] and the androgens[157,158]. Thus, alcohol, as an enzyme inducer, may significantly alter the peripheral metabolism of the sex hormones and possibly other steroid hormones.

(*c*) *Plasma production rates* — The measurement of the production rate of testosterone ($MCR^T \times PC^T$) was carried out in four normal volunteers during ingestion of alcohol[145]. Three of the four showed a significant decrease in production rate of testosterone after 24 days of alcohol ingestion. The fourth subject had minimal alcohol intake because of gastric complaints and did not demonstrate any change in his plasma level or production rate of the steroid (Figure 9.6).

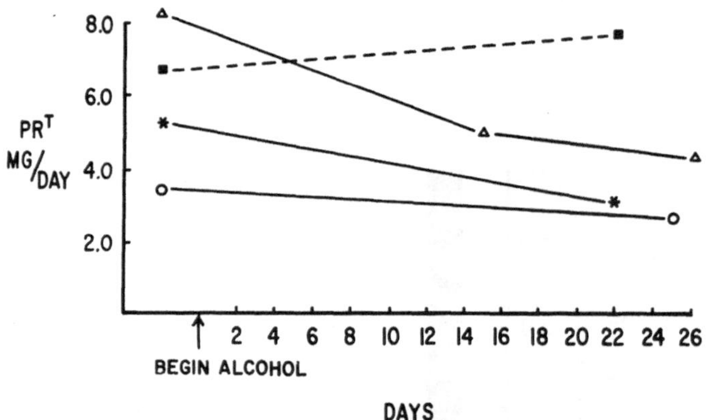

Figure 9.6 The effect of ethanol (ETOH) on the plasma production rate of testosterone (PR^T) in four normal male volunteers. Three of the subjects had marked decreases in their PR^T's after alcohol ingestion. One subject (■ - - - - ■) tolerated ethanol poorly and the dose of the agent had to be reduced sharply. There was no fall in the PR^T in this subject

(*d*) *Conversion ratios* — The effect of alcohol on the conversion of testosterone to androstenedione, estrone and estradiol was studied in normal men[145]. No significant alterations were noted over a 28-day period (Figure 9.7).

(*e*) *Other plasma sex steroids* — (i) Androstenedione (PC^A). There were no changes in plasma levels of androstenedione noted during alcohol administration in our normal volunteers[145]. The hormone was measured every $\frac{1}{2}$ h during a 24-h period at varying time intervals during alcohol ingestion (up to 24 days) (Figure 9.8).

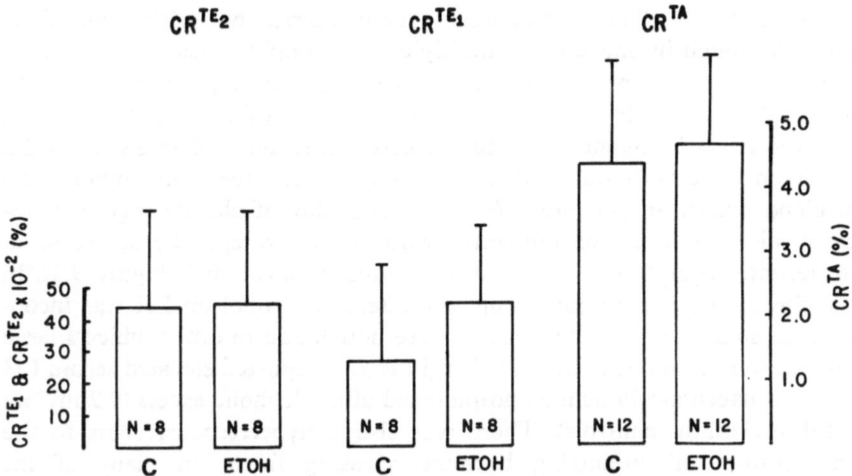

Figure 9.7 The conversion ratio (CR) of testosterone (T) to estradiol (E_2), estrone (E_1) and androstenedione (A) in eight normal male volunteers before (C) and during ethanol (ETOH) administration. There were no changes noted in these parameters

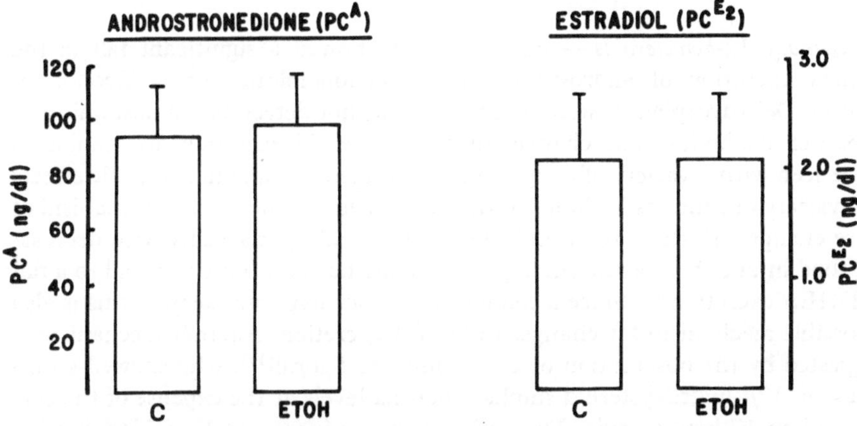

Figure 9.8 The mean of the daily plasma concentrations and standard deviations of androstenedione (PC^A) and estradiol (PC^{E_2}) in six male volunteers studied before (C) and during ethanol (ETOH) administration. There were no changes noted in the plasma levels of these sex steroids

(ii) Estradiol (PC^{E_2}). Similarly, there were no changes in plasma estradiol noted in our study[145] (Figure 9.8).

(f) Plasma gonadotrophins — The plasma gonadrotrophins (FSH/LH) have been evaluated by radioimmunoassay procedures in patients with alcoholic

liver disease[128–134]. The studies were usually carried out with single daily samples although in one study[134] multiple daily sampling was used. The level of serum LH was generally within normal limits or slightly elevated. The effect of alcohol on LH in normal subjects has been evaluated. In the study of 'hangover effects' Ylikahri[142] noted increases in serum LH levels (6.0–12.2 IU/l) in ten subjects. In our study in normal male volunteers, one subject, who had blood drawn at $\frac{1}{2}$-h intervals on the first day of alcohol ingestion, increased his LH level concomitantly with decreased episodic secretion of testosterone, suggesting a direct gonadal effect of alcohol[145] (Figure 9.1). In more chronic studies by our group, the effect of alcohol on LH was inconsistent, in some cases small increases were noted, and in other subjects large decreases were found (Figure 9.2). Wright *et al.*[44] reported elevated serum LH levels in thirteen alcoholic men hospitalized after alcoholic excess (9.2 mU/ml *vs.* 5.4 mU/ml in controls). There was also a hyperresponsiveness to the administration of luteinizing hormone-releasing factor in many of the alcoholic men they studied. This is similar in a sense, to the hyperresponsiveness to TSH-releasing hormone seen in primary hypothyroidism. Serum FSH response to alcohol was studied in our subjects[145] and no consistent changes were noted. Thus, alcohol may alter gonadotrophin activity by gonadal and/or central effects.

(*g*) *Urinary 17-ketosteroids* — Fabre *et al.*[138] showed a significant fall in the urinary excretion of androsterone and etiocholanolone during alcohol ingestion. Dehydroepiandrosterone (DHEA) was not detectable in abstaining or imbibing alcoholics. The changes in 17-ketosteroid excretion are similar to those seen with a variety of enzyme inducing agents[156] and non-specific effects of a variety of illnesses[159]. More studies are needed to clarify the mechanism of these changes. DHEA excretion is quite labile, falling markedly with decreasing food intake[160]. In addition, hyperuricaemia has been noted to lead to a fall in DHEA excretion[161]. Since alcohol can produce hyperuricaemia[2], this is also a possible mechanism for changes in DHEA excretion. Another mechanism is suggested by the observation of Cronholm and Sgörall[162], who showed an increase in 17β-hydroxysteroid sulphate plasma levels at the expense of the corresponding 17-ketosteroids. They related this to increased 17-oxidoreduction as a result of increased hepatic NADH. The changes in 17-KS excretion may thus be non-specific (see also Section 9.2.1).

In summary, alcohol ingestion can alter certain aspects of the metabolism of testosterone independent of cirrhosis. The acute and subacute studies cited above suggest that alcohol feeding and plasma alcohol levels in the 100 mg/dl range can alter the episodic pattern of plasma testosterone acutely and in the 'hangover' period; more chronic administration of alcohol to normals and alcoholics leads to a decrease in the mean plasma concentration of the steroid. The lack of consistent plasma LH suppression in the face of decreased episodic secretion of plasma testosterone in our acute studies is compatible with a direct gonadal effect. In addition, however, a central effect as evidenced by falls in LH in some of our more chronically treated patients, is probable. This is compatible with the 'dual effect' of alcohol postulated by Von Thiel *et al.*[133] in their study of patients with alcoholic liver disease. In addition to the gonadal and CNS (hypothalamic–pituitary?) effects, alcohol alters the peripheral metabolism of testosterone by changing plasma binding parameters, increasing hepatic blood flow, co-factor concentrations (NADH) and hepatic steroid metabolizing enzymes which use testosterone as an endogenous substrate. The changes in the peripheral metabolism of testosterone are reflected as changes in its rate of clearance from the blood (MCR^T)[145].

The low plasma concentration and production rates of testosterone seen in normal men on alcohol are similar to that found in cirrhosis. However, in contrast to the findings in established liver disease, there were no changes noted, within the time constraints of our study, on circulating estradiol or androstenedione or the conversion ratios of testosterone to product steroids. The fall in plasma binding during alcohol administration to normal subjects is opposite to the elevated levels found in cirrhosis. Moreover, the MCR^T is decreased in cirrhosis as compared to the increases noted during alcohol administration to normal subjects. Thus, alcohol ingestion, for periods up to 24 days, cannot account for the entire pattern of altered sex steroid metabolism as seen in cirrhosis. Possibly more chronic exposure to alcohol for a period of months to years would be necessary to produce these changes. In this regard, the baboon might be a suitable model[163] to study the effects of chronic alcohol ingestion on sex hormone metabolism, since this animal develops sequential hepatic changes eventuating in cirrhosis, similar to the human. This model may be useful in tracing the exact sequence of events in the interaction of alcohol, sex steroid hormone metabolism and evolving liver disease.

9.6 PITUITARY GLAND

9.6.1 Anterior pituitary

9.6.1.1 Animal studies

Histological studies by early investigators suggested that alcohol results in degenerative changes in the hypophysis[70,71]. The inhibition of growth in young animals treated with alcohol has been attributed to suppression of growth hormone[164–167] because of the 'retarded but harmonious growth pattern' and normal body composition. Growth hormone however, was not measured in these studies and the alcohol-treated animals were not isocalorically matched with controls. However, less growth was also noted in animals fed ethanol as compared to an isocaloric carbohydrate diet[168]. The growth retardation has been attributed to energy wastage since microsomal ethanol metabolism is inefficient in that no high energy chemical bonds are produced and the heat generated by this reaction is in excess of that necessary for temperature homeostasis[2]. Measurements of growth hormone in growth retardation in young alcohol-treated rats and pair-fed isocaloric controls have not been reported to our knowledge.

9.6.1.2 Human studies

(*a*) *Growth hormone* — Arky and Freinkel[169] used ethanol to induce hypoglycaemia in two patients with alcohol hypoglycaemia and 'isolated adrenocorticotrophin defect'. They found that 1 litre of a 15 % solution of alcohol given intravenously over an 8-h period, after an overnight fast, was associated with the slow development of hypoglycaemia and increased release of growth hormone. However, in one normal female volunteer who fasted for 3 days prior to the study, alcohol infusion, as above, produced hypoglycaemia and an 86 % fall in the level of growth hormone.

Growth hormone secretion in response to the ingestion of alcohol was studied in eleven healthy, normal males, ages 20 to 25 years, by Bellet *et al.*[26]. Blood for growth hormone was obtained before and at 30, 60, 90, 120 and 180 min after the ingestion of a dose of 1.5 ml/kg b.w. of alcohol given as a 20 % aqueous solution. Subjects also were studied in a similar fashion after ingestion of an equal volume of water without alcohol. In eight out of eleven subjects, growth hormone rose above control levels. The maximal mean growth hormone value was noted at 90 min (5.94 *vs.* 1.32 ng/ml). Blood alcohol levels peaked between 90 and 120 min after ingestion and did not exceed 140 mg/dl. Changes in growth hormone were not associated with alterations in free fatty acids or glucose. A non-specific stress-related response was suggested, as well as other possible factors, as the cause of the increased growth hormone.

Toro *et al.*[141] administered oral alcohol (1 g/kg b.w.) to fourteen normal men and sixteen normal women. Blood was drawn for radioimmunoassay of a variety of steroid and peptide hormones at 0, 30, 60, 120 and 180 min after ingestion of either alcohol or an equal volume of water. Patients were studied at both 9:00 a.m. and 7:00 p.m. No significant differences were noted between maximal increments over baseline levels for growth hormone in men or women, in morning or evening hours, using ethanol or commercial liquor. Blood alcohol levels achieved were in the 110 mg/dl range. This study is in conflict with that of Bellet *et al.*[26]. Wright and co-workers[44] measured growth hormone responses during insulin hypoglycaemia in eleven hospitalized alcoholics who had been drinking heavily up to the time of admission. They were studied within 48–72 h after hospitalization. Most of these patients showed severe prolonged hypoglycaemia and all responded well with normal growth hormone release.

(*b*) *Prolactin* (*12*) — Toro *et al.*[141] reported that prolactin levels do not increase in normal men or women after ingestion of alcohol (see GH section for details of study).

(*c*) *Gonadotropins* — See Section 9.5.2.2 (f) on gonads for studies of alcohol effects on FSH/LH in normal and alcoholic subjects.

(*d*) *TSH* — See Section 9.3.

(*e*) *ACTH* — See Section 9.2.

9.6.2 Posterior pituitary

9.6.2.1 Antidiuretic hormone

It is well known that alcoholic beverages produce a diuresis. In 1886, this was shown experimentally by Simonowsky[170], who noted that beer produced a greater diuretic response than an equivalent amount of water. Although several subsequent investigators[171,172] could not confirm this finding, there has since been extensive confirmation of alcohol or beverage alcohol-induced water diuresis[173–182]. Murray[176] suggested that alcohol itself, rather than some other substance in alcoholic beverages, was the diuretic substance and demonstrated that pituitrin (pituitary extract) could abolish the diuresis. This investigator concluded that the mechanism of the alcohol diuresis was of the same nature as that of water diuresis. Haggard *et al.*[177] and Eggleton[178] further showed that the diuretic effect of alcohol was related to the duration of the increasing blood alcohol levels rather than the absolute concentrations attained. The diuretic effect was not maintained at steady state concentrations of alcohol. Eggleton[178] confirmed Murray's observation of inhibition of the alcohol-induced water diuresis by pituitary extract. She also noted that the height of the diuresis was unrelated to the peak level in blood alcohol concentration and the degree of diuresis, from a given dose of alcohol, varied widely in given subjects depending on the rate of alcohol and water absorption during the study. However, in one subject, there was some correlation between dose of alcohol and diuretic response. In other subjects, repeated doses of alcohol, at short intervals, resulted in additional smaller diuretic episodes. Eggleton suggested that alcohol serves to inhibit the posterior hypophysis and that part of the variation in diuretic response depended on a 'variation in the sensitivity of the pituitary mechanism'. Van Dyke and Ames[179] studied the diuretic effect of repeated doses of alcohol in dogs (0.6 g alcohol/kg b.w. given four times in 5 h) and noted that each succeeding diuretic event had a lesser magnitude compared with the initial diuresis until the fourth dose when no diuresis was noted.

Although earlier investigations postulated direct renal effects of alcohol, the studies of Murray[176] and Eggleton[178] suggested a hormonal mechanism for the alcohol diuresis (i.e. an alcohol effect on antidiuretic hormone (ADH) secretion from the posterior hypophysis). Strauss *et al.*[180] carried out further studies of the mechanism of the diuretic effect of alcohol. They showed that alcohol administration did not change endogenous creatinine clearance suggesting that the alcohol-stimulated diuresis was not due to an increase in glomerular filtration rate, but rather, was due to a decreased tubular reabsorption of water. They indicated that a diuresis of this type is usually due to a decreased ADH effect. These investigators were able to confirm the earlier observations of Murray[176] and Eggleton[178], that ADH (pitressin) given at the time of alcohol ingestion inhibits the diuretic effect of alcohol. Furthermore, they suggested that since alcohol does not inhibit the action of exogenous ADH, its effect is most likely on the release of ADH, rather than its peripheral action in the renal tubules. In the study of Strauss *et al.*[180], the effect of alcohol on the response of ADH release to hypertonic and hypotonic stimuli was evaluated. They demonstrated that a sufficient hypertonic stimulus (ingestion of 200 mEq NaCl crystals on celery stalks) was able to override the inhibitory effect of alcohol (50 g as bourbon) on ADH release as shown by an antidiuresis. Similarly, a hypotonic stimulus (ingestion of 850 ml H_2O 20 min. after alcohol) did not summate with the diuresis of alcohol by increasing the flow rate, but did prolong the diuretic phase. Since the total diuresis effected was greater than that effected by the water load alone, the authors suggested that alcohol may have quantitatively altered reactivity to this class of stimuli. It was considered that all of the effects of alcohol were consistent with an effect on the supraoptico-hypophyseal area rather than on the kidney tubules. Van Dyke and Ames[179] showed that alcohol diuresis occurs in intact dogs, but not in dogs with surgically induced chronic diabetes insipidus. It was also shown by these investigators that the intracarotid injection of alcohol to intact dogs produced a diuretic effect similar in magnitude to that seen with an oral dose 10-fold larger. This again suggests a CNS-mediated diuretic effect of alcohol.

Studies by Rubini *et al.*[181] and Kleeman *et al.*[182] defined the effect of alcohol on free water clearance in human subjects. Rubini showed a marked rise in free water clearance (from negative 2 ml/min pre-alcohol, to positive 4 ml/min maximum) in the period 60 to 120 min after ingesting alcohol (48 g as bourbon). The rise in free water clearance accounted for 60–80 % of the observed urine flow and was associated with a decrease in osmolar clearance. There was no change in endogenous creatinine clearance and thus no change in GFR as noted earlier by Strauss[183]. These observations are consistent with a diuresis due to decreased ADH activity. Kleeman *et al.*[182] studied the effect of alcohol in physiological states where perturbations of ADH secretion have been demonstrated. They studied subjects in states of minimal ADH activity produced by sustained positive water loading; during increased ADH activity produced by infusions of hypertonic sodium chloride solution both in patients with the high urine flow (10–15 ml/min) of water diuresis and in subjects with low flow rates (1–2 ml/min); and in patients with increased ADH activity due to diminished effective blood volume produced by inducing venous stasis in the limbs with inflated blood pressure cuffs. They again found that in patients with positive water balance that alcohol did not induce a further increase in urine flow of free water clearance. Since large positive water loads completely inhibit ADH release (in the recumbent or semi-recumbent positions, the conditions under which these studies were carried out) this result is again consistent with alcohol effect being mediated via ADH. In studies in water-loaded subjects with high urine flow rates, administration of sufficient quantities of hypertonic saline can provoke ADH release and an ensuing antidiuresis. However, in subjects receiving alcohol simultaneously with hypertonic saline, the antidiuretic effect of the hypertonic stimulus was obliterated, showing that alcohol could block the ADH releasing effect of the hypertonic saline if appropriate time relationships are maintained. In two subjects, the saline was infused 30 min after alcohol ingestion, and in these subjects, antidiuresis occurred. Presumably, ADH had been released by the saline infusion and, since alcohol does not block ADH peripherally, antidiuresis rather than diuresis occurred. This is consistent with the prevention of alcohol-induced diuresis by injected pitressin[176,178] or the inhibition of diuresis noted in patients who ingested dry sodium chloride before drinking bourbon. Seemingly discordant with these observations is the antidiuresis noted by Strauss[180] when the dry sodium chloride was given 20 min after alcohol ingestion. Several possible explanations for this discrepancy can be suggested. Alcohol absorption may have been delayed or sufficient time did not elapse to permit full hypothalamic suppression. In addition, the patients may have been in the upright position while ingesting the dry NaCl and tonic ADH release may have overridden the alcohol effect[182]. Administration of alcohol prior to producing venous congestion with blood pressure cuffs on the limbs prevented the expected antidiuresis. These observations taken in conjunction with the finding that alcohol prevents the antidiuresis of acetylcholine administration[179] constitute strong evidence that alcohol has an inhibiting action on the supraoptico-hypophyseal system leading to diuresis as a result of inhibition of ADH release. Consistent with a hypothalamic locus of alcohol activity is the observation of Räihä[183] that alcohol administration prevented histological changes in supraoptic nuclei after large doses of NaCl to animals. Furthermore, Miller and Mill[184] demonstrated that ethanol decreased the sensitivity of supraoptic nuclear neurosecretory cells to direct electrical stimulation.

The inhibition of ADH release by alcohol may be restricted to osmotic stimuli, since, in rats, pain or haemorrhage causes an antidiuresis that cannot be overcome by alcohol[185]. Although the antidiuresis associated with surgery is not inhibited by alcohol[186], the antidiuresis after exercise can be blocked by alcohol use[187]. Studies of ADH levels during alcohol ingestion by direct measurements have not yet been reported.

Alcohol administration has been used clinically in situations of ADH excess. However, the results have been less than satisfactory since the inhibitory effect is of short duration and, as discussed previously, obtains only during the period of increasing blood levels of the agent[188].

9.6.2.2 Oxytocin

It has been suggested by indirect evidence in human and animal studies, that alcohol inhibits the release of oxytocin from the posterior pituitary. Chaudhury and Matthews[189], using milk ejection after suckling, found that alcohol (3 to 4 g/kg b.w.) inhibited oxytocin release in rats. A dose-related response in oxytocin inhibition by alcohol has been shown in rabbits[190]. Fuchs[191] has demonstrated during parturition in rabbits that alcohol inhibits oxytocin release and delays the onset of labour. Wagner and Fuchs[192] studied oxytocin release (as measured by uterine contractions in response to nursing in post-partum women) and suggested it was decreased by alcohol. The alcohol-mediated inhibition of oxytocin has been applied therapeutically to control of premature labour[193,194]. The definitive proof of alcohol inhibition of posterior lobe function must await the application of radioimmunoassay and the direct measurement of oxytocin in normal and alcoholic human subjects.

In summary, posterior hypophyseal function is determined by 'biologic assay' of ADH and oxytocin release is inhibited by alcohol use.

9.7 INSULIN

Studies by Bleicher *et al.*[195], in the dog, suggest that alcohol does not increase insulin secretion. In acute studies, using orally administered alcohol, Bellet *et al.*[26] did not note any effect on plasma insulin levels in normal volunteers. Nikkila and Taskinen[196] fed normal volunteers 25 % of their daily caloric intake as alcohol for 1 week and were unable to demonstrate any change in the mean fasting plasma insulin levels. However, Metz and co-workers[197] reported that giving alcohol intravenously, or orally, from 8:00 p.m. to 6:00 a.m., potentiated, by 50 %, the plasma insulin response to a glucose load. An augmented insulin secretory response was also found by Dornhorst and Onyang[198], who gave normal volunteers ethanol and glucose simultaneously. Friedenberg *et al.*[199] noted alcohol-induced augmentation of plasma insulin after a glucose load both in normal and in non-insulin requiring diabetic subjects. Phillips and Sofrit[200] also found that alcohol pretreatment increased the insulin secretory response after a glucose load in diabetics and in patients with a 'strong family history' of diabetes. In contrast, Nikkilä and Taskinen[196] noted that intravenous alcohol potentiated the first (early) and second (late) phases of insulin secretion after a glucose load in normal subjects. In obese non-diabetic subjects, only the second phase of insulin release was augmented and little or no effect was noted in their newly discovered non-ketotic, untreated diabetic subjects. Farmer *et al.*[201] studied insulin response during an oral glucose tolerance test in 29 chronically alcoholic subjects who abstained from alcohol for at least 2 weeks prior to the study. Twenty-one of these subjects showed increased plasma insulin levels. McMonagle and Felig[202] studied normal subjects and non-insulin-requiring diabetics by administering whiskey (60 ml ethanol) in divided doses over a 4-h period followed by a glucose tolerance test beginning at 5:00 p.m. They, too, noted a significant increase in the first phase of insulin release, and found glucagon levels significantly higher than control values at the 45, 75 and 90 min time points. The diabetics, in their study, also reponded with insulin levels higher than controls. Ethanol pretreatment also increases insulin response to other releasers of insulin, such as tolbutamide[203] and arginine[204] but not to glucagon[199] or cyclic AMP[205]. The refractoriness to glucagon (a cyclic AMP-mediated hormone) and cyclic AMP suggests that the alcohol effect on the beta cell (if that is the locus of action) may be mediated by the second messenger. Alcohol has been reported to increase adenyl cyclase activity in islet cell homogenates at concentrations similar to those reached in blood after moderate alcohol intake[206]. However, another locus of action may be the gastrointestinal tract with release of intestinal insulin secretagogues. Moreover, until insulin tracer studies are carried out, the increase in circulating insulin levels noted after alcohol and a secretory stimulus is only putatively due to increased secretion. The increased insulin levels could reflect decreased degradation, although the normal second phase of insulin secretion and the lack of effect of glucagon and cyclic AMP point to the beta cell as the site of action. The normal basal insulin levels noted in all the above-cited studies also suggests that the effect is not mediated via alterations in insulin clearance from the blood, although Farmer's[201] study in chronic alcoholics who were not pretreated with alcohol, and indeed had not imbibed for 2 weeks, may reflect altered insulin degradation as a result of underlying liver disease.

The significance of the alcohol-mediated augmentation of plasma insulin levels on glucose homeostasis is unclear. In many, but not all of the above-cited studies, glucose tolerance was reported as being improved in conjunction with the increased insulin secretion. It is uncertain whether this apparent improved glucose tolerance represents hormonal action of the increased circulating insulin and/or altered glucose absorption from the gastrointestinal tract or other mechanisms entirely. Oral and i.v. alcohol delays gastric emplying[207] and inhibits glucose absorption in the isolated small intestine[208]. In one study[196] more chronic administration of alcohol (1 week) did not result in potentiation of insulin secretion. The well-known alcohol hypoglycaemia syndrome is apparently not related to this accentuation of plasma insulin. In several other studies, plasma insulin was measured, in a patient in coma[209] or during the experimental induction of hypoglycaemia[210], and was found to be depressed as is appropriate in response to hypoglycaemia. Alcohol impairment of gluconeogenesis is the mechanism for the hypoglycaemia observed in most, if not all, of these hypoglycaemias[210] which usually occur in malnourished individuals after alcohol excess. However, the hypoglycaemic reaction to alcohol is occasionally seen in well-nourished individuals after a single acute exposure to alcohol and it could be postulated that in at least some of these hypoglycaemic situations, alcohol consumption in association with carbohydrate intake leads to augmented circulating plasma insulin and thence to hypoglycaemia. The presence of low plasma insulin levels at the time of hospitalization for hypoglycaemia does not necessarily exclude this hypothesis since, in some studies, the second phase of insulin secretion is not augmented and/or counter-regulatory hormonal events may have arrested further insulin secretion. Indeed, several studies have shown augmented peripheral glucose utilization after ethanol[211,212], although Frienkel *et al.*[209,210] did not note enhanced peripheral glucose utilization in their studies. Perhaps further studies of insulin levels in some alcohol hypoglycaemias may be useful in further delineating the pathophysiology of this syndrome.

In contrast to the above-cited studies, hyperglycaemia has also been described in alcoholism, although its mechanism is uncertain. Tennent[213] showed that lethal doses of alcohol are associated with hyperglycaemia. The increment in blood sugar depends on the level of hepatic glycogen stores[51,213] and on an intact adrenal medullary-sympathetic nervous system[51]. The hyperglycaemia can be blocked by adrenalectomy[214] or by β-adrenergic blockade[215]. Alcohol may also augment gluconeogenesis in well-nourished subjects[216]. The role of other alcohol-mediated humoral control mechanisms remains to be investigated. Liver disease, as such, may also decrease glucose tolerance and lead to hyperglycaemia[217,218].

In summary, alcohol does not affect basal insulin levels, but potentiates the release of insulin after appropriate stimuli. Depending on the clinical or experimental situation, alcohol use may be associated with severe hypoglycaemia as a result of impaired gluconeogenesis or hyperglycaemia as a result of adrenergic-mediated glycogenolysis.

Acknowledgements

We would like to acknowledge the able and cheerful assistance of librarians Judy Myers and Nadine DeCosta in obtaining the literature reviewed here and the diligent efforts of Elizabeth Johnstone and Selma Polsky in their typing of the manuscript.

References

1. Weitzman, E. D., Boyar, R. M., Kapen, S. and Hellman, L. (1975). The relationship of sleep and sleep stages to neuroendocrine secretion and biological rhythms in man. In *Recent Progress in Hormone Research,* Vol. 31, pp. 399–466. New York: Academic Press
2. Lieber, C. S. (1973). Liver adaptation and injury in alcoholism. *N. Engl. J. Med.,* **288,** 356
3. Kuntzman, R., Jacobson, M., Schneidman, K. and Conney, A. H. (1964). Similarities between oxidative drug-metabolizing enzymes and steroid hydroxylases in liver microsomes. *J. Pharmacol. Exp. Ther.,* **146,** 280
4. Southren, A. L., Tochimoto, S., Strom, L., Ratuschni, A., Ross, H. and Gordon, G. G. (1966). Remission in Cushing's syndrome with *o,p*[1]-DDD. *J. Clin. Endocrinol. Metab.,* **26,** 268
5. Gordon, G. G., Altman, K. and Southren, A. L. (1968). The effect of 6α, 6β-hydroxycortisol and *o,p*[1]-DDD on the induction of rat hepatic tryptophanpyrrolase. *Endocrinology,* **83,** 384
6. Gross, M. M., Goodenough, D. R., Hastey, J. and Lewis, E. (1973). Experimental study of sleep in chronic alcoholics before, during and after four days of heavy drinking with a non-drinking comparison. *Ann. N.Y. Acad. Sci.,* **215,** 254
7. Hion-Jon, V. (1928). The influence of alcohol on the endocrine glands. *Fol. Neuropathol. Eston.,* **3,** 288
8. Smith, J. J. (1951). The effect of alcohol on the adrenal ascorbic acid and cholesterol of the rat. *J. Clin. Endocrinol. Metab.,* **11,** 792
9. Forges, J. C. and Duncan, G. M. (1951). The effect of acute alcohol intoxication on the adrenal glands of rats and guinea pigs. *Q. J. Stud. Alc.,* **12,** 355
10. Forbes, J. C. and Duncan, G. M. (1953). Effect of intraperitoneal administration of alcohol on the adrenal levels of cholesterol and ascorbic acid in rats and guinea pigs. *Q. J. Stud. Alc.,* **14,** 19
11. Czaja, C. and Kalant, H. (1961). The effect of acute alcoholic intoxication on adrenal ascorbic acid and cholesterol in the rat. *Can. J. Biochem. Physiol.,* **39,** 327
12. Santisteban, G. A. and Swinyard, C. A. (1956). The effect of ethyl alcohol on adrenal cortical activity in mice. *Endocrinology,* **59,** 391
13. Santisteban, G. A. (1961). The response of the thymolymphatic system to graded doses of ethyl alcohol and its relationship to adrenocortical activity. *Q. J. Stud. Alc.,* **22,** 1
14. Ellis, F. W. (1962). Effect of ethanol on plasma corticosterone concentration in rats. *Fed. Proc.,* **21,** 339
15. Kalant, H., Hawkins, R. D. and Czaja, C. (1963). Effect of acute alcohol intoxication on steroid output of rat adrenals *in vitro. Am. J. Physiol.,* **204,** 849
16. Ellis, F. W. (1965). Adrenal cortical function in experimental alcoholism in dogs. *Proc. Soc. Exp. Biol. Med.,* **120,** 740
17. Ellis, F. W. (1966). Effect of ethanol on plasma corticosterone levels. *J. Pharmacol. Exp. Ther.,* **153,** 121
18. Noble, E. P. (1971). Ethanol and adrenocortical stimulation in inbred mouse strains. In N. K. Mello and J. H. Mendelson, eds. *Recent Advances in Studies of Alcoholism,* pp. 77–79. Washington, D.C.: U.S. Government Printing Office
19. Krusius, F. E., Vartia, K. O. and Forsander, O. (1958). Experimentelle Studien über die biologische Wirkung von Alkohol. *Ann. Med. Exp. Biol. Fenn.,* **36,** 424
20. Perman, E. S. (1960). Observations on the effect of ethanol on the urinary excretion of histamine, 5-hydroxyindolacetic acid, catecholamines and 17-hydroxycorticosteroids in man. *Acta Physiol. Scand.,* **51,** 62
21. Kissin, B., Schenker, V. and Schenker, A. C. (1960). The acute effect of alcohol ingestion on plasma and urinary 17-hydroxycorticoids in alcoholic subjects. *Am. J. Med. Sci.,* **239,** 690
22. Jenkins, J. S. and Connolly, J. (1968). Adrenocortical response to alcohol in man. *Br. Med. J.,* **ii,** 804

23. Mendelson, J. H. and Stein, S. (1966). Serum cortisol levels in alcoholic and non-alcoholic subjects during experimentally induced ethanol intoxication. *Psychosomat. Med.*, **28**, 616
24. Merry, J. and Marks, V. (1969). Plasma-hydrocortisone response to ethanol in chronic alcoholics. *Lancet*, **i**, 921
25. Bellet, S., Roman, L., DeCastro, O. A. P. and Herrera, M. (1970). Effect of acute ethanol intake on plasma 11-hydroxycorticosteroid levels. *Metabolism*, **19**, 664
26. Bellet, S., Yoshimine, N., DeCastro, O. A. P., Roman, L., Parmar, S. S. and Sandberg, H. (1971). Effect of alcohol ingestion on growth hormone levels: Their relation to 11-hydroxycorticoid levels and serum FFA. *Metabolism*, **20**, 762
27. Mendelson, J. H., Ogata, M. and Mello, N. K. (1971). Adrenal function and alcoholism. I. Serum cortisol. *Psychosomat. Med.*, **33**, 145
28. Stokes, P. E. (1973). Adrenocortical activation in alcoholics during chronic drinking. *Ann. N.Y. Acad. Sci.*, **215**, 77
29. Smith, J. J. (1950). The endocrine basis and hormonal therapy of alcoholism. *N.Y.S.J. Med.*, **50**, 1704
30. Smith, J. J. (1950). The treatment of acute alcoholic states with ACTH and adrenocortical hormones. *Q. J. Stud. Alc.*, **11**, 190
31. Fischbach, K., Simmons, E. M. and Pollard, R. E. (1952). Delirium tremens treated with intravenously administered corticotropin (ACTH). *J. Am. Med. Ass.*, **149**, 927
32. Bettencourt-Gomes, S. C. (1953). ACTH in delirium tremens. *Br. Med. J.*, **2**, 339
33. Owen, M. (1954). A study of the rationale of the treatment of delirium tremens with adrenocorticotropic hormone. *Q. J. Stud. Alc.*, **15**, 387
34. Smith, J. J. (1951). The blood eosinophil responses of the alcoholic to epinephrine and to ACTH, with a note on the treatment of chronic alcoholism with ACTH. In *Proceedings of the Second Clinical ACTH Conference*, Vol. 2, pp. 161–171. New York: The Blakiston Co.
35. Owen, M. (1954). A study of the rationale of the treatment of delirium tremens with adrenocorticotropic hormone. I. The eosinophil response of patients with delirium tremens, after a test with ACTH. *Q. J. Stud. Alc.*, **15**, 384
36. Kissin, B., Schenker, V. and Schenker, A. C. (1969). Adrenal cortical function and liver disease in alcoholics. *Am. J. Med. Sci.*, **238**, 344
37. Peterson, R. F. (1960). Adrenocortical steroid metabolism and adrenal cortical function in liver disease. *J. Clin. Invest.*, **39**, 320
38. Zumoff, B., Bradlow, H. L., Gallagher, T. F. and Hellman, L. (1967). Cortisol metabolism in cirrhosis. *J. Clin. Invest.*, **46**, 1735
39. Eisenstein, A. B. (1967). Nutritional factors and the adrenal cortex. In A. B. Eisenstein, ed. *The Adrenal Cortex*, pp. 315–349. Boston: Little, Brown and Co.
40. Magraf, H. W., Moyer, C. A., Ashford, L. E. and Lavalle, L. W. (1967). Adrenocortical function in alcoholics. *J. Surg. Res.*, **7**, 55
41. Shaver, J. C., Roy, S., Killian, P., Frantz, A. G., Christy, N. P. and Bissell, L. (1974). Endocrine function in long-abstinent alcoholic males. *Report of the International Conference on Alcoholism and Drug Abuse.* Lausanne: International Council on Alcohol and Addiction
42. Merry, J. and Marks, V. (1972). The effect of alcohol, barbiturate and diazepam on hypothalamic pituitary-adrenal function in chronic alcoholics. *Lancet*, **ii**, 990
43. Merry, J. and Marks, V. (1971). Ethanol and cortisol release in man. In G. A. Martini and C. Bode, eds. *Metabolic Changes Induced by Alcohol*, pp. 199–206. Berlin: Springer-Verlag
44. Wright, J., Merry, J., Fry, D. and Marks, V. (1976). Pituitary function in chronic alcoholism. In M. M. Gross, ed. *Alcohol Intoxication and Withdrawal. Adv. Exp. Med. Biol.*, Vol. 59, pp. 253–256. New York: Plenum Press
45. Ogata, M., Mendelson, J. H. and Mello, N. K. (1968). Electrolyte and osmolality in alcoholics during experimentally induced intoxication. *Psychosomat. Med.*, **30**, 463
46. Sereny, G., Rapoport, A. and Husdare, H. (1966). The effect of alcohol withdrawal on electrolyte and acid–base balance. *Metabolism*, **15**, 896

47. Fabre, L. F., Jr., Farmer, R. W., Pellizzari, E. D. and Farrell, G. (1972). Aldosterone secretion in phenobarbital anesthetized ethanol-infused dogs. *Q. J. Stud. Alc.*, **33,** 476
48. Fabre, L. F., Jr., Farmer, R. W., Pellizzari, E. D. and Mendelson, J. H. (1971). Adrenal response to alcohol: mineralocorticoid metabolism. In N. K. Mello and J. H. Mendelson, eds. *Recent Advances in Studies of Alcoholism,* pp. 173–187. Washington, D.C.: U.S. Government Printing Office
49. Farmer, R. W. and Fabre, L. F., Jr. (1975). Some endocrine aspects of alcoholism. In E. Majchrowitz, ed. *Biochemical Pharmacology of Ethanol. Adv. Exp. Med. and Biol.,* Vol. 56, pp. 277–289. New York: Plenum Press
50. Saruta, T. R., Cook, R. and Kaplan, N. M. (1971). Inhibitory effect of ethanol on aldosterone synthesis by beef adrenal tissue. *Proc. Soc. Exp. Biol. Med.,* **138,** 353
51. Matununga, H. (1942). Experimentelle Untersuchungen über den Einfluss des Alkohols und den Kohlenhydratstoffwechsel. I. Über die Wirkung des Alkohols auf den Blutzuckerspiegel und den Glykogengehalt der Leber mit besonderer Berücksightigung seines Wirkungsmechanismus. *Tohoku J. Exp. Med.,* **44,** 130
52. Klingman, G. I. and Goodall, McC. (1957). Urinary epinephrine and levarterenol excretion during acute sublethal intoxication in dogs. *J. Pharmacol. Exp. Ther.,* **121,** 313
53. Perman, E. S. (1960). The effect of ethyl alcohol on the secretion from the adrenal medulla of the cat. *Acta Physiol. Scand.,* **48,** 323
54. Perman, E. S. (1961). Effect of ethanol and hydration on the urinary excretion of adrenaline and noradrenaline and on the blood sugar of rats. *Acta Physiol. Scand.,* **51,** 68
55. Kinzius, H. (1950). Adrenalin und Arbeit, die Beeinfluss und des Blutadrenalin Spiegels durch Pervitin, Luminal und Alkohol. *Arbeits Physiol.,* **14,** 243
56. Abelin, V. I., Herren, C. and Berli, W. (1958). Über die erregende Wirkung des Alkohols auf den Adrenalin und Noradrenalinhaushalt des menschlichen Organismus. *Helvet. Med. Acta,* **25,** 591
57. Perman, E. S. (1958). The effect of ethyl alcohol on the secretion from the adrenal medulla in man. *Acta Physiol. Scand.,* **44,** 241
58. Anton, A. H. (1965). Ethanol and urinary catecholamines in man. *Clin. Pharmacol. Ther.,* **6,** 462
59. Garlind, T., Goldberg, L., Graf, K., Perman, E. S., Strandell, T. and Strom, G. (1960). Effect of ethanol on circulatory, metabolic and neurohormonal function during muscular work in man. *Acta Pharmacol. Toxicol.,* **17,** 106
60. Davis, V. E., Brown, H., Huff, J. A. and Cashaw, J. L. (1967). Ethanol induced alterations of norepinephrine metabolism in man. *J. Lab. Clin. Med.,* **69,** 787
61. Davis, V. E., Cashaw, J. L., Huff, J. A., Brown, H. and Nicholas, L. (1967). Alteration of endogenous catecholamine metabolism by ethanol ingestion. *Proc. Soc. Exp. Biol. Med.,* **125,** 1140
62. Smith, A. A. and Gitlow, S. (1967). Effect of disulfiram and ethanol on the catabolism of norepinephrine in man. In R. P. Maickel, ed. *Biochemical Factors in Alcoholism,* pp. 53–59. New York: Pergamon Press
63. Goddard, P. J. (1958). Effect of alcohol on excretion of catecholamines in conditions giving rise to anxiety. *J. Appl. Physiol.,* **13,** 118
64. Giacobini, E., Izekowitz, S. and Wegmann, A. (1960). Urinary norepinephrine and epinephrine excretion in delirium tremens. *Arch. Gen. Psychol.,* **3,** 289
65. Elmadjian, F., Hope, J. M. and Lamson, E. T. (1957). Excretion of epinephrine and norepinephrine in various emotional states. *J. Clin. Endocrinol. Metab.,* **17,** 608
66. Giacobini, E., Izekowitz, S. and Wegmann, A. (1960). The urinary excretion of noradrenaline and adrenaline during acute alcohol intoxication in alcoholic subjects. *Experientia,* **16,** 467
67. Carlsson, C. and Häggendal, J. (1967). Arterial noradrenaline levels after ethanol withdrawal, *Lancet,* **ii,** 889

68. Ogata, M., Mendelson, J. H., Mello, N. K. and Majchrowicz, E. (1971). Adrenal function and alcoholism. II. Catecholamines, *Psychosomat. Med.*, **33,** 159
69. Majchowicz, E. (1973). Alcohol aldehydes and biogenic amines. *Ann. N.Y. Acad. Sci.*, **215,** 84
70. Sanchez-Calvo, R. (1941). Die Alkoholvergiftung und ihre Folgen für das Ernahrungs-System. *Virchows Arch.*, **308,** 14
71. Üprus, V. (1931). Die Theoretischen Grundlagen der wissenschaftlichen Untersuchungen über die Wirkung des alkohols auf den Organismus und die Ergebnisse der letzteren in der Neuenklinik der Universität Tartu-Dorjat in Laufe von 10 Jahren (1921–1931). *Folia Neuropathol. Eston.*, **11,** 82
72. Aschkenasy-Lelu, P. and Guérin, M. T. (1960). Action de boissons alcoolisées sur l'activité physiologique de la thyroïde du rat. *C. R. Biol.*, **154,** 1409
73. Richter, C. P. (1956). Loss of appetite in alcohol and alcoholic beverages produced in rats by treatment with thyroid preparations. *Endocrinology*, **59,** 472
74. Richter, C. P. (1957). Production and control of alcoholic cravings in rats. In H. A. Abramson, ed. *Neuropharmacology*, Vol. III, pp. 39–146. Princeton, N.J.: Josiah Macy Foundation
75. Prieto, R., Varela, A. and Mardones, J. (1958). Influence of oral administration of thyroid powder on the voluntary alcohol intake by rats. *Acta Physiol. Lat. Am.*, **8,** 203 (abs.)
76. Ylikahri, R. H. (1970). Ethanol-induced hypoglycemia in thyroxine-treated animals. *Metab. Clin. Exp.*, **19,** 518
77. Hilbom, M. E. (1971). Thyroid state and voluntary alcohol consumption of albino rats. *Acta Pharmacol. Toxicol.*, **29,** 95
78. Hillbom, M. E. and Pöso, A. R. (1975). Effects of ethanol on serum electrolytes and respiration in euthyroid and hyperthyroid rats. *Toxicol. Appl. Pharmacol.*, **32,** 168
79. Von Wartburg, J. P., Bethune, J. L. and Vallee, B. L. (1964). The mechanism of inhibition of horse liver alcohol dehydrogenase by thyroxine and related compounds. *Biochemistry*, **3,** 1775
80. Murdock, H. R. (1967). Thyroidal effects of alcohol. *Q. J. Stud. Alc.*, **28,** 419
81. Bleecker, M., Ford, D. H. and Rhines, R. K. (1969). A comparison of ^{131}I-triiodothyronine accumulation and degradation in ethanol-treated and control rats. *Life Sci.*, **8,** 267
82. Videla, L., Bernstein, J. and Israel, Y. (1973). Metabolic alterations produced in the liver by chronic ethanol administration. Increased oxidative capacity. *Biochem. J.*, **134,** 507
83. Bernstein, J., Videla, L. and Israel, Y. (1973). Metabolic alterations produced in the liver by chronic ethanol administration. Changes related to energetic parameters of the cell. *Biochem. J.*, **134,** 515
84. Israel, Y., Videla, L., MacDonald, A. and Bernstein, J. (1973). Metabolic alterations produced in the liver by chronic ethanol administration. Comparison between the effects produced by ethanol and by thyroid hormones. *Biochem. J.*, **134,** 523
85. Bernstein, G., Artz, S. A., Hasen, J. and Oppenheimer, J. H. (1968). Hepatic accumulation of ^{125}I-thyroxine in the rat: augmentation by phenobarbital and chlordane. *Endocrinology*, **82,** 406
86. Gross, M. (1945). The relationship of the pituitary gland to some symptoms of alcoholic intoxication and chronic alcoholism. *Q. J. Stud. Alc.*, **6,** 25
87. Goldfarb, A. T. and Berman, S. (1949). Alcoholism as a psychosomatic disorder. I. Endocrine pathology of animals and man excessively exposed to alcohol; its possible relation to behavioral pathology. *Q. J. Stud. Alc.*, **10,** 415
88. Goldberg, M. (1960). The occurrence and treatment of hypothyroidism among alcoholics. *J. Clin. Endocrinol. Metab.*, **20,** 609
89. Goldberg, M. (1962). Thyroid function in chronic alcoholism. *Lancet*, **ii,** 746
90. Satterfield, J. H. and Guze, S. B. (1961). Treatment of alcoholic patients with triiodothyronine. *Dis. Nerv. Syst.*, **22,** 227

91. Selzer, M. L. and Van Houten, N. H. (1964). Normal thyroid function in chronic alcoholism. *J. Clin. Endocrinol. Metab.*, **24,** 380
92. Augustine, J. R. (1967). Laboratory studies in acute alcoholics. *Can. Med. Ass. J.*, **96,** 1367
93. Stokes, P. E. (1971). Alcohol–endocrine interrelationships. In B. Kissin and H. Bergleiter, eds. *The Biology of Alcoholism: Biochemistry,* Vol. I, p. 427. New York: Plenum Press
94. Goldberg, M., Hehir, R. and Hurowitz, M. (1960). Intravenous triiodothyronine in acute alcoholic intoxication. *N. Engl. J. Med.*, **263,** 1336
95. Kalant, H., Sereny, G. and Charlebois, R. (1962). Evaluation of triiodothyronine in the treatment of acute alcoholic intoxication. *N. Engl. J. Med.*, **267,** 1
96. Peng, T., Cooper, C. W. and Munson, P. L. (1972). The hypocalcemic effect of ethyl alcohol in rats and dogs. *Endocrinology,* **91,** 586
97. Peng, T. and Gitelman, H. J. (1974). Ethanol-induced hypocalcemia, hypermagnesemia and inhibition of the serum calcium raising effects of parathyroid hormone in rats. *Endocrinology,* **94,** 608
98. Kalbfleisch, J. M., Lindeman, R. D., Ginn, H. E. and Smith, W. O. (1963). Effects of ethanol administration in urinary excretion of magnesium and other electrolytes in alcoholic and normal subjects. *J. Clin. Invest.*, **42,** 1471
99. Jones, J. E., Shane, S. R., Jacobs, W. H. and Flink, E. B. (1969). Magnesium balance studies in chronic alcoholism. *Ann. N.Y. Acad. Sci.*, **162,** 934
100. Martin, H. E., McCuskey, C., Jr. and Tupikova, N. (1959). Electrolyte disturbances in acute alcoholism with particular reference to magnesium. *Am. J. Clin. Nutrition,* **7,** 191
101. Fankushen, D., Raskin, D., Dimick, A. and Wallach, S. (1964). The significance of hypomagnesemia in alcoholic patients. *Am. J. Med.*, **27,** 802
102. Rasmussen, H. (1974). Parathyroid hormone calcitonin and the calciferols. In R. H. Williams, ed. *Textbook of Endocrinology,* 5th ed., p. 686. Philadelphia: W. B. Saunders Co.
103. Estep, H., Shaw, W. A., Watlington, C., Hobe, R., Holland, W. and Tucker, S. (1969). Hypocalcemia due to hypomagnesemia and reversible parathyroid hormone unresponsiveness. *J. Clin. Endocrinol. Metab.*, **29,** 847
104. Cohen, S. L., Grahame-Smith, D., MacIntyre, I. and Walker, J. G. (1973). Alcohol-stimulated calcitonin release in medullary carcinoma of the thyroid. *Lancet,* **ii,** 1172
105. Wells, S. A., Jr., Cooper, C. W. and Ontjes, D. A. (1975). Stimulation of thyrocalcitonin secretion by ethanol in patients with medullary thyroid carcinoma—an effect apparently not mediated by gastrin. *Metabolism,* **24,** 1215
106. Becker, H. D., Reeder, D. D. and Thompson, J. C. (1974). Gastrin release by ethanol in man and dogs. *Ann. Surg.*, **179,** 906
107. Hennessy, J. F., Wells, S. A., Jr., Ontjes, D. A. and Cooper, C. W. (1974). A comparison of pentagastrin injection and calcium infusion as provocative agents for the detection of medullary carcinoma of the thyroid. *J. Clin. Endocrinol. Metab.*, **39,** 487
108. Kyle, J. and Schopper, K. J. (1914). Untersuchungen über den Einfluss des Alkohols auf Leber und Hoden des Kaninchens. *Virchows Arch.*, **215,** 309
109. Weichselbaum, A. and Kyle, J. (1912). Über die Veränderungen des Hoden bei chronischem alkoholismus. *S.B. Mayer, Akad. Wiss.*, **121,** 51
110. Kostoff, D. and Hadjidimitroff, P. (1931). Spermatogenesis der Alkoholisierten Kaninchen. *Z. Zell Forsch. Mikros. Anat.*, **14,** 194
111. Arlitt, A. and Wells, H. G. (1917). Effect of alcohol on the reproductive tissues. *J. Exp. Med.*, **26,** 769
112. Doepfmer, R. and Hinchers, H. J. (1965). Zur Frage der Keimschadigung im abuten Rausch. *Z. Haut-u. Geschlechtskr.*, **39,** 94
113. Teitlebaum, H. A. and Gantt, W. H. (1958). The effect of alcohol on sexual reflexes and sperm count in the dog. *Q. J. Stud. Alc.*, **19,** 394
114. Van Theil, D. H., Gavaler, J. S., Lester, R. and Goodman, M. D. (1975). Alcohol-induced testicular atrophy. *Gastroenterology,* **69,** 326

115. Rasmussen, E. W. (1953). Alkoholproblemet belust ved eksperimentelde dyreforsak. *Forhandlingar Nordiska Psykologmotet i Helsingfors*, pp. 244–256
116. Hart, B. L. (1969). Effects of alcohol on sexual reflexes and mating behavior in the male dog. *Q. J. Stud. Alc.*, **29**, 839
117. Dewsburg, P. A. (1967). Effects of alcohol ingestion on copulatory behavior of male rats. *Psychopharmacologia*, **11**, 276
118. Hart, B. L. (1968). Effects of alcohol on sexual reflexes and mating behavior in the male dog. *Q. J. Stud. Alc.*, **29**, 839
119. Gantt, W. H. (1957). Acute effect of alcohol on autonomic (sexual, secretory, cardiac) and somatic responses. In Himwich, ed. *Alcoholism, Basic Aspects and Treatment*, pp. 73–89. Washington, D.C.: Am. Ass. Adv. Sci.
120. Cranston, E. M. (1958). Effects of tranquilizers and other agents on sexual cycle of mice. *Proc. Soc. Exp. Biol. Med.*, **98**, 320
121. Aron, E., Flanzy, M., Combescot, C., Puisas, J., Demaret, J., Reynouard-Brandt F. and Igert, C. (1965). L'alcool est-il dans le vin l'element qui perturbe chez la ralle, le cycle vaginale? *Bull. Acad. Nat. Med. (Paris)*, **149**, 112; *Abst. Q. J. Stud. Alc.*, **27**, 746, 1966
122. Aschkenasy-Lelu, P. (1958). Action des boissons alcoolisées sur le rendement reproducteur du rat. *C. R. Acad. Sci.*, **246**, 1275
123. Badr, F. M. and Bartke, A. (1974). Effect of ethyl alcohol on plasma testosterone levels in mice. *Steroids*, **23**, 921
124. Corda, L. and Sulla, E. D. (1925). Reviviscenza della mammella maschile nella cirrosi epatica. *Minerva Medica*, **5**, 1067
125. Lloyd, C. E. and Williams, R. H. (1948). Endocrine changes associated with Laennec's cirrhosis of the liver. *Am. J. Med.*, **4**, 315
126. van Thiel, D. H., Sherins, R. J. and Lester, R. (1973). Mechanism of hypogonadism in alcoholic liver disease: evidence for a double defect. *Gastroenterology*, **65**, 574 (Abs. 50)
127. Van Thiel, D. H., Gavaler, J. and Lester, R. (1974). Ethanol inhibition of vitamin A metabolism in the testes: possible mechanism for sterility in alcoholics. *Science*, **186**, 941
128. Coppage, W. S., Jr. and Cooner, A. E. (1965). Testosterone in human plasma. *N. Engl. J. Med.*, **273**, 902
129. Southren, A. L., Gordon, G. G., Olivo, J., Rafii, F. and Rosenthal, W. S. (1973). Androgen metabolism in cirrhosis of the liver. *Metabolism*, **22**, 695
130. Galvo-Teles, A., Anderson, D. C., Burke, C. W., Marshall, J. C., Corker, C. S., Brown, R. C. and Clark, M. L. (1973). Biologically active androgens and oestradiol in men with chronic liver disease. *Lancet*, **i**, 173
131. Kent, J. R., Scaramuzzi, R. I. and Lauwers, W. (1973). Plasma testosterone, estradiol and gonadotrophins in hepatic insufficiency. *Gastroenterology*, **64**, 111
132. Chopra, I. J., Tulchinsky, D. and Greenway, F. L. (1973). Estrogen-androgen imbalance in hepatic cirrhosis. *Ann. Intern. Med.*, **79**, 198
133. van Thiel, D. H., Lester, R. and Sherins, R. J. (1974). Hypogonadism in alcoholic liver disease: evidence for a double defect. *Gastroenterology*, **67**, 1188
134. Gordon, G. G., Olivo, J., Rafii, F. and Southren, A. L. (1975). Conversion of androgens to estrogens in cirrhosis of the liver. *J. Clin. Endocrinol. Metab.*, **40**, 1018
135. Olivo, J., Gordon, G. G., Rafii, F. and Southren, A. L. (1975). Estrogen metabolism in hyperthyroidism and in cirrhosis of the liver. *Steroids*, **26**, 47
136. van Thiel, D. H., Gavaler, J. S., Lester, R., Loriaux, D. L. and Braunstein, G. D. (1975). Plasma estrone prolactin neurophysin and sex steroid-binding globulin in chronic alcoholic men. *Metabolism*, **24**, 105
137. Tavernetti, R. R., Rosenbaum, W., Kelly, W. G., Christy, N. P. and Roginsky, M. S. (1967). Evidence for the presence in human plasma of an estrogen-binding factor other than albumin: abnormal binding of estradiol in men with hepatic cirrhosis. *J. Clin. Endocrinol. Metab.*, **27**, 920

138. Fabre, L. F., Pasco, P. J., Liegel, J. M. and Farmer, R. W. (1973). Abnormal testosterone excretion in men alcoholics. *Q. J. Stud. Alc.*, **34**, 57
139. Liegel, J., Fabre, L. F., Jr., Howard, P. Y. and Farmer, R. W. (1972). Plasma testosterone binding globulin (SBG) in alcoholic subjects. *Physiologist*, **15**, 198 (abs.)
140. Mendelson, J. H. and Mello, N. K. (1974). Alcohol, aggression and androgens. In S. H. Frazier, ed. *Aggression*, pp. 225–247. Baltimore: Williams and Wilkins
141. Toro, G., Kolodny, R. C., Jacobs, L. S., Masters, W. H. and Daughaday, W. H. (1973). *Clin. Res.*, **21**, 505 (abs.)
142. Ylikahri, R., Huttumen, M., Harkonen and Adlercreutz, H. (1974). Letter to the editor: Hangover and testosterone. *Br. Med. J.*, **ii**, 445
143. Dotson, L. E., Robertson, L. S. and Tuchfeld, B. (1975). Plasma alcohol, smoking, hormone concentrations, and self-reported aggression. *J. Stud. Alc.*, **36**, 578
144. Southren, A. L., Tochimoto, S., Carmody, N. C. and Isurugi, K. (1965). Plasma production rates of testosterone in normal adult men and women and in patients with the syndrome of feminizing testes. *J. Clin. Endocrinol. Metab.*, **25**, 1441
145. Gordon, G. G., Southren, A. L., Altman, K., Rubin, E. and Lieber, C. S. (1976). The effect of alcohol (ethanol) administration on sex hormone metabolism in normal men. *N. Engl. J. Med.* (in press)
146. Southren, A. L., Gordon, G. G., Tochimoto, S., Pinzon, G., Lane, D. and Stypulkowski, W. (1967). Mean plasma concentration, metabolic clearance and basal plasma production rates of testosterone in normal young men and women using a constant infusion procedure: effect of time of day and plasma concentration on the metabolic clearance rate of testosterone. *J. Clin. Endocrinol. Metab.*, **27**, 686
147. Southren, A. L., Gordon, G. G. and Tochimoto, S. (1968). Further study of factors affecting the metabolic clearance rate of testosterone in man. *J. Clin. Endocrinol. Metab.*, **28**, 1105
148. Childs, A. W., Kivel, R. M. and Lieberman, A. (1963). Effect of ethyl alcohol on hepatic circulation, sulfobromophthalein clearance and hepatic glutamic-oxalacetic transaminase production in man. *Gastroenterology*, **45**, 176
149. Mendeloff, A. I. (1954). Effect of intravenous infusions of ethanol upon estimated hepatic blood flow in man. *J. Clin. Invest.*, **32**, 1298
150. Castenfors, H., Hultman, E. and Josephson, B. (1960). Effect of intravenous infusions of ethyl alcohol on estimated hepatic blood flow in man. *J. Clin. Invest.*, **39**, 776
151. Vermeulen, A., Verdonck, L., van der Straeten, M. and Orle, N. (1969). Capacity of the testosterone-binding globulin in human plasma and influence of specific binding of testosterone on its metabolic clearance rate. *J. Clin. Endocrinol. Metab.*, **29**, 1470
152. Southren, A. L. and Gordon, G. G. (1970). Studies in androgen metabolism. *Mt. Sinai J. Med.*, **37**, 516
153. Rosner, W. (1972). A simplified method for the quantitative determination of testosterone-estradiol-binding globulin activity in human plasma. *J. Clin. Endocrinol Metab.*, **34**, 983
154. Rubin, E., Lieber, C. S., Altman, K., Gordon, G. G. and Southren, A. L. (1976). Prolonged ethanol consumption increases testosterone metabolism in the liver. *Science*, **191**, 563
155. Dioguardi, N., Idéo, G., Delninno, E. and DeFranchis, R. (1970). Letter to the editor: Induction of liver UDPGT by ethanol. *Lancet*, **i**, 1063
156. Bradlow, H. L., Zumoff, B., Fukushima, D. K. and Hellman, L. (1973). Drug-induced alterations of steroid hormone metabolism in man. *Ann. N.Y. Acad. Sci.*, **212**, 148
157. Resan, T. K., Shahidi, N. T. and Korst, D. R. (1972). The effect of phenobarbital on testosterone-induced erythroporesis. *J. Lab. Clin. Med.*, **79**, 187
158. Lipsett, M. B. (1971). Factors influencing the rate of metabolism of steroid hormones in man. *Ann. N.Y. Acad. Sci.*, **179**, 442
159. Zumoff, B., Bradlow, H. L., Gallagher, T. F. and Hellman, L. (1971). Decreased conver-

sion of androgens to normal 17-ketosteroid metabolites: a non-specific consequence of illness. *J. Clin. Endocrinol. Metab.*, **32,** 824

160. Hendrikx, A., Heyns, W., Steeno, O. and DeMoor, P. (1966). Influence of body size, changes in body weight, and/or food intake on urinary excretion of 11-desoxy-17-ketosteroids. In A. Vermeulen and D. Exley, eds. *Androgens in Normal and Pathological Conditions.* Proceedings Second Symposium on Steroid Hormones, Ghent, 1965, pp. 63–70. Amsterdam: Excerpta Medica Foundation
161. Casey, J. H., Hoffman, M. M. and Solomon, S. (1968). The excretion of urinary dehydroepiandrosterone in gout. *Arthr. Rheum.*, **11,** 444
162. Cronholm, T. and Sjövall, J. (1970). Effect of ethanol metabolism on redox state of steroid sulfates in man. *Eur. J. Biochem.*, **13,** 124
163. Lieber, C. S. and DeCarli, L. M. (1974). An experimental model of alcohol feeding and liver injury in the baboon. *J. Med. Prim.*, **3,** 153
164. MacDowell, E. C. (1922). Alcoholism and the growth of white rats. *Genetics,* **7,** 427
165. Hanson, F. B. and Heys, F. (1924). Correlations of body weight, body length and tail length of normal and alcoholic albino rats. *Genetics,* **9,** 368
166. Sollman, T. (1920). Studies of chronic intoxications on albino rats. II. Alcohols (ethyl, methyl and 'wood') and acetone. *J. Pharmacol. Exp. Ther.*, **16,** 291
167. Ratcliff, F. (1972). The effect of chronic ethanol administration on the growth of rats. *Arch. Intern. Pharmacodyn.*, **197,** 19
168. Lieber, C. S., Jones, D. P. and DeCarli, L. M. (1965). Effects of prolonged ethanol intake: production of fatty liver despite adequate diets. *J. Clin. Invest.*, **44,** 1009
169. Arky, R. A. and Freinkel, N. (1964). The response of plasma growth hormone to insulin and ethanol-induced hypoglycemia in two patients with 'isolated adrenocorticotrophic defect'. *Metabolism,* **13,** 547
170. Simanowsky, N. P. (1886). Über die Gesundheits-Schädlichkeit hefetruber Biere und über den Ablauf der knorstlichen Verdauung bei Burzusatz. *Arch. Hyg.*, **4,** 1
171. Raphael, A. (1894). Über die diuretische Wirkung einiger Mittel auf den Menschen. *Arb. Pharmakol. Inst. Zu Dorpat. Stuttg.*, **10,** 81
172. Mendel, L. B. and Hilditch, W. W. (1910). The influence of alcohol upon nitrogenous metabolism in men and animals. *Am. J. Physiol.*, **27,** 1
173. Miles, W. R. (1922). The comparative concentrations of alcohol in human blood and urine at intervals after ingestion. *J. Pharm. Exp. Therap.*, **20,** 265
174. Nicholson, W. M. and Taylor, H. M. (1938). The effect of alcohol on the water and electrolyte balance in man. *J. Clin. Invest.*, **17,** 279
175. Brieger, M. (1940). The effects of alcohol on the normal and pathologic kidney: a review. *Q. J. Stud. Alc.*, **1,** 85
176. Murray, M. M. (1932). The diuretic action of alcohol and its relations to pituitarism. *J. Physiol.*, **76,** 379
177. Haggard, H. W., Greenberg, L. A. and Carroll, R. P. (1941). Studies on the absorption, distribution and elimination of alcohol VIII. The diuresis from alcohol and its influence on the elimination of alcohol in urine. *J. Pharmacol. Exp. Therap.*, **71,** 349
178. Eggleton, M. G. (1942). The diuretic action of alcohol in man. *J. Physiol.*, **101,** 172
179. Van Dyke, H. B. and Ames, R. G. (1951). Alcohol diuresis. *Acta Endocrinol.*, **7,** 110
180. Strauss, M. B., Rosenbaum, J. D. and Nelson, W. P. III (1950). The effect of alcohol on the renal excretion of water and electrolyte. *J. Clin. Invest.*, **29,** 1053
181. Rubini, M. E., Keeman, C. R. and Landin, E. (1955). Studies on alcohol diuresis. I. The effect of ethyl alcohol ingestion on water electrolyte and acid base metabolism. *J. Clin. Invest.*, **34,** 439
182. Kleeman, C. R., Rubini, M. E., Landin, E. and Epstein, F. H. (1955). Studies on alcohol as an inhibitor of the neurohypophysis. *J. Clin. Invest.*, **34,** 448
183. Räihä, N. (1960). Effect of ethanol on cytological changes induced by salt load in nucleus supraopticus of rat. *Proc. Soc. Exp. Biol. Med.*, **103,** 387

184. Miller, D. A. and Mill, J. A., Jr. (1967). Interactions among ethanol, hypothermia and asphyxia in guinea pigs. *Cryobiology,* **3,** 400
185. Tata, P. S. and Byzalkov, R. (1966). Vasopressin studies in the rat. III. Inability of ethanol anesthesia to prevent ADH secretion due to pain and hemorrhage. *Arch. Ges. Physiol.,* **290,** 294
186. Bennett, N. B., Mackay, W. D. and Matheson, N. A. (1964). The effect of alcohol on postoperative diuresis. *Lancet,* **i,** 1073
187. Kazlowski, S., Szczepanska, E. and Zielinski, A. (1967). The hypothalamohypophyseal antidiuretic system in physical exercises. *Arch. Intern. Physiol. Biochem.,* **75,** 218
188. Kleeman, C. R. (1972). Water metabolism. In M. H. Maxwell and C. R. Kleeman, eds. *Clinical Disorders of Fluid and Electrolyte Metabolism,* 2nd ed., p. 243. New York: McGraw Hill
189. Chaudhury, R. R. and Matthews, M. (1960). Effect of alcohol on the fertility of female rabbits. *J. Endocrinol.,* **34,** 275
190. Fuchs, A. R. and Wagner, G. (1963). Effect of alcohol on release of oxytocin. *Nature (London),* **198,** 92
191. Fuchs, A. R. (1966). The inhibitory effect of ethanol on the release of oxytocin during parturition in the rabbit. *J. Endocrinol.,* **35,** 125
192. Wagner, G. and Fuchs, A. R. (1968). Effect of ethanol on uterine activity during suckling in post-partum women. *Acta Endocrinol.,* **58,** 131
193. Fuchs, F., Fuchs, A. R., Pobete, V. F. and Risk, A. (1967). Effects of alcohol on threatened premature labor. *Am. J. Obstet. Gynecol.,* **99,** 627
194. Luukainen, T., Vaisto, L. and Jarvinen, P. A. (1967). The effect of oral intake of ethyl alcohol on the activity of pregnant human uterus. *Acta Obstet. Gynecol. Scand.,* **46,** 486
195. Bleicher, S. J., Freinkel, N., Byrne, J. J. and Seifert, D. (1964). Effect of ethanol on plasma glucose and insulin in the fasted dog. *Proc. Soc. Exp. Biol. Med.,* **115,** 369
196. Nikkilä, E. A. and Taskinen, M. R. (1975). Ethanol-induced alterations in glucose tolerance, post-glucose hypoglycemia, and insulin secretion in normal obese and diabetic subjects. *Diabetes,* **24,** 933
197. Metz, R., Berger, S. and Mako, M. (1969). Potentiation of plasma response to glucose by prior administration of alcohol. *Diabetes,* **18,** 517
198. Dornhorst, A. and Onyang, A. (1971). Effect of alcohol on glucose tolerance. *Lancet,* **ii,** 957
199. Friedenberg, R., Metz, R., Mako, M. and Surmaczynska, B. (1971). Differential plasma insulin response to glucose and glucagon stimulation following ethanol priming. *Diabetes,* **20,** 397
200. Phillips, G. and Sofrit, H. (1971). Alcoholic diabetes. Induction of glucose intolerance with alcohol. *J. Am. Med. Ass.,* **217,** 1513
201. Farmer, R. W., Farrell, G., Pellizzari, E. D. and Fabre, L. F. (1971). Serum insulin levels during oral GTT in chronic alcoholics. *Fed. Proc.,* **30,** 250 (abs.)
202. McMonagle, J. and Felig, P. (1975). Effects of ethanol ingestion on glucose tolerance and insulin secretion in normal and diabetic subjects. *Metabolism,* **24,** 625
203. Kühl, C. and Anderson, O. (1974). Glucose and tolbutamide mediated insulin response after preinfusion with ethanol. *Diabetes,* **23,** 821
204. Andreani, D., Tamburrano, G., Tamburrano, S. and Gambardella, S. (1974). Hormonal changes in alcohol hypoglycemia. *Diabetalogia,* **10,** 357
205. Colwell, A. R., Feingimer, M., Cooper, D. and Zuckerman, L. (1973). Alcohol inhibition of cyclic AMP-induced insulin release. *Diabetes,* **22,** 854
206. Kuo, W. N., Hodgins, S. and Kuo, J. F. (1973). Adenylate cyclase in islets of Langerhans. Isolation of islet and regulation of adenylate cyclase activity by various hormones and agents. *J. Biol. Chem.,* **248,** 2705
207. Schapiro, H., Cummins, A. and Ludey, J. (1965). Dissociation between gastric secretion and motility. *Am. J. Dig. Dis.,* **10,** 751

208. Panowicz, H. (1967). Wplyn alkoholu etylowego na wchlanianie glukozy w izolowanym odcinku jaclita crenkiego szczura. *Rocznicki Pomorskiej Akad. Med. Szecinie,* **13,** 385
209. Freinkel, N., Singer, D. L., Arky, R. A., Bleicher, S. J., Anderson, J. B. and Silbert, C. K. (1963). Alcohol hypoglycemia in carbohydrate metabolism of patients with clinical alcohol hypoglycemia and the experimental reproduction of the syndrome with pure ethanol. *J. Clin. Invest.,* **42,** 1152
210. Freinkel, N., Arky, R. A., Singer, D. L., Cohen, A. K., Bleicher, S. J., Anderson, J. B., Silbert, C. K. and Foster, A. E. (1965). Alcohol hypoglycemia. IV. Current concepts of its pathogenesis. *Diabetes,* **14,** 350
211. Lindquist, F., Sestoft, L., Damgard, S. E., Clausen, J. P. and Trap-Jensen, J. (1973). Utilization of acetate in human forearm during exercise after ethanol ingestion. *J. Clin. Invest.,* **52,** 3231
212. Searle, G. L., Shames, D., Cavalieri, R. R., Bagerde, J. D. and Poste, D., Jr. (1974). Evaluation of ethanol hypoglycemia in men: turnover studies with C-6^{14}C glucose. *Metabolism,* **23,** 1023
213. Tennent, D. M. (1941). Factors influencing the effects of alcohol on blood sugar and liver glycogen. *Q. J. Stud. Alc.,* **2,** 263
214. Klingman, G. I., Bane, R. and Haag, H. B. (1959). Studies on severe alcohol intoxication in dogs. III. Effect of adrenalectomy. *Q. J. Stud. Alc.,* **20,** 13
215. Ammon, H. P. T. and Estler, C. J. (1968). Inhibition of ethanol-induced glycogenolysis in brain and liver by adrenergic β-blockade. *J. Pharm. Pharmacol.,* **20,** 164
216. Freinkel, N., Cohen, A. K., Arky, R. A. and Foster, A. E. (1965). Alcohol hypoglycemia. II. A postulated mechanism of action based on experiments with rat liver slices. *J. Clin. Endocrinol. Metab.,* **25,** 76
217. Lundquist, G. A. R. (1965). Glucose tolerance in alcoholism. *Br. J. Addict.,* **61,** 51
218. Rehfeld, J. F., Juhi, E. and Hilden, M. (1973). Carbohydrate metabolism in alcohol-induced fatty liver. *Gastroenterology,* **64,** 445

Index

Acanthocytosis 229, 230
Acatalasaemic mice 8
Acetaldehyde 37, 264, 270
  pathways of metabolism 9–10, 16–21
Acetate 37
Acetylcholine 159–61
Acquired hypoparathyroidism 272
ACTH,
  pituitary 253
  release of 255
  stimulation 258, 259
Adenosine triphosphatase (ATPase) activity 12, 64, 169–72
  [Na^+ + K^+]-activated 95, 169–72
ADP 10
  : O ratio 10
Adrenal ascorbic acid 252
Adrenal cortex 251–62
Adrenal gland catecholamine content 263
Adrenal medulla — catecholamines 262–7
Adrenal venous effluent 263
Aldehyde dehydrogenase 10
Alcohol dehydrogenase 2, 267
Alcohol diuresis 288
Alcohol hypoglycaemia 292
Alcohol effect on [$^{131(125)}I$] thyroidal accumulation 267–8
Alcoholic cardiomyopathy 119, 188–96
Alcoholic fatty liver 46–52
Alcoholic hyaline 61
Alcoholic hyperlipaemia 41–4
Aldosterone 261–2
  plasma 261
  secretion 261
  urinary excretion 261
Alkaloids, catecholamine-derived 157–9
Amines, biogenic 264
Amino acid 84, 163–6
Aminotriazole 6
Aminopyrine demethylase 36
Anabolic steroids 64
Anaemia,
  iron deficiency 232
  megaloblastic 216
  sideroblastic 220
Anaesthesia, theories of 168–9
Androgen metabolites, $5\alpha/5\beta$ 280
Aniline hydroxylase 36
Antabuse 37
Antidiuretic hormone (ADH) 187–8
  'atypical' 11
Arginine 291
Arterial norepinephrine levels 265
Ascorbic acid, adrenal 252
Atrophy 198
Australian antigen 58
Azide 6

β-adrenergic blockage 292
Bile-acid 40
Bile salt secretion 90
Biogenic amines 264
'Biological Freudianism' 136
Blood epinephrine levels 263
Blood ethanol clearance 11
Blood lactic acid 197
Bone density, changes in 136–9
Bone marrow 217, 225
Butanol 8

C cells 273
Calcitonin 271
  levels 272
  parathyroid and calcium 270–3
Calcium 84
  dietary 139
  homeostasis 271
  loss of in urine 271
  parathyroid, calcitonin and 270–3
  plasma 271
  transport 139
  urinary excretion of 270
Carbohydrate absorption 88
Carcinoma of the thyroid, medullary 272
Cardiac contractility 127
Cardiac metabolism 124–30

Cardiac output 191
Cardiac triglycerides 194
Cardiomyopathy, alcoholic 119, 188–96
Cardiomegaly 190
Carotene 82
Catecholamines 154–7, 262, 267
  content of adrenal gland, 263
  excretion of 262, 263
  24-hour urines for 266
Catecholamine-derived alkaloids 157–9
Catheterization 191
Cation metabolism 169–72
Cells,
  C 273
  Leydig 274
  life span of red 227
  'spur' 229
  target 228
Cell populations 102
Charcot's feet 139, 144
Chemotaxis 239
Chlorpromazine 64
Cholesterol 97, 252
  metabolism 40
  synthesis 40
Choline oxidase 51
Chronic ethanol consumption 11–21
Chronotropic effect 195
Chylomicrons 42
Cirrhosis 59, 108
Citric acid cycle 5
Collagen 33
Conversion ratios 282
Copulatory behaviour 273
Coronary flow 121–4
Corticosteroid metabolism 140
Cortisol 251–61
  metabolism 259
  secretory rate 259
Cortols and cortolones 259
Creatine phosphokinase (CPK) 197–8
Cyanide 8
Cyclic 3′,5′-adenosine monophosphate (cyclic AMP) 172–3, 291
Cytochrome P-450 8

DEAE-cellulose column chromatography 7
D-glucose 85
Dehydroepiandrosterone (DHEA) 262
Dehydrogenase,
  alcohol 2, 267
  acetaldehyde 10
  isocitric 191
  lactic 191, 197
  malic 191
  succinic 191
Diurnal fall of plasma testosterone 276
Dopamine, urinary 263
  24-hour urines for 266
d-penicillamine therapy 65
Diarrhea 82
Dietary calcium 139
Dietary factors 50
Dietary fat 36
Dietary phosphorus 139
Disaccharidase activity 103
Disaccharides 82
Diuresis, magnesium 139
Drugs 36
  metabolism of 12, 37
  tolerance to 38–9
d-xylose 82, 103

Electronmicroscopy 61
Emboli, fat 144
Embolization, fat 144
Endoplasmic reticulum 201
Energy metabolism 151–2
Energy wastage 16
Enzyme inducer 268
Enzymes,
  hepatic microsomal activity of 282
  microsomal drug-detoxifying 36
  steroid metabolizing 280
Eosinophil count 253
Eosinophil response 258
Epinephrine 263
  blood levels, 263
  24-hour urines for 266
  urinary excretion of 262
Episodic pattern of secretion 276
Estradiol (PC^{E_2}) 283
Estrous cycles 273
Ethanol,
  blood clearance 11
  concentrations 93
  consumption, chronic 10–21
  drug interaction 37
  effects on intestinal motility 90
  oxidation 1, 91
Ethyl fatty acid esters 97
Export proteins 53

Fat,
  absorption 86
  emboli and embolization 144
  malabsorption 83

Fatty acids 5, 35, 96
  ethyl esters 97
  oxidation 98
Fatty liver, alcoholic 46–52
  prevention and treatment of 64
Fecal excretion of nitrogen 83
Feminization, and hypogonadism syndrome 274
Femoral neck fractures 137
Fibrosis 192
Folate deficiency 221
Folic acid 82, 84
  deficiency 216
Fractures 135, 136, 137, 138
  femoral neck 137
  hip 138
  humerus 138
  metabolic 137
  spine 138
  wrist 138
Free water clearance 288
Fructose 45

γ-aminobutyric acid 161–2
Gastrin levels 272
Gastric emptying, effects of ethanol on 89–90
Gastric lesions 99
Germinal epithelium 274
Glucagon levels 291
Gluconeogenesis 292
Glucose tolerance test, oral 291
Golgi apparatus 41
Gout 33
Granulocyte mobilization 238–9
Granulocytopenia 236
Growth and development, of skeletal system 135–6
Growth hormone 285, 286–7
  retardation of 285

Haemodynamic changes 123–4
Haemolysis of liver disease 227, 231–2
Heart failure 190
Hepatic blood flow 279–80
Hepatic extraction 279
Hepatic microsomal enzyme activity 282
Hepatic microtubulin 53
Hepatic uptake of [^{131}I]thyroxine 268
Hepatitis, alcoholic 59
Hip,
  fracture 138
  osteoarthritis of 143
Hormone binding 274

H_2O_2 6, 7
Humerus fracture 138
Hyaline, alcoholic 61
Hydrogen 3
Hydroxyproline urinary excretion 272
Hyperglycaemia 292
Hyperglycaemic response 262
Hyperkalaemia 198
Hyperlactacidaemia 33
Hyperlipaemia, alcoholic 41–4
Hyperosmolality 235
Hypertrophy 192
Hyperuricaemia 33
Hypocalcaemia 271
  alcoholic 292
Hypocalcaemic effect of alcohol 270
Hypoglycaemia 256
Hypogonadism, and feminization syndrome 274
Hypomagnesaemia 272
Hypoparathyroidism, acquired 272
Hypophosphataemia 231–2
Hypothyroidism 269

Immune system 58
Inclusion bodies 192
Insulin levels, plasma 290
Insulin tolerance tests 261
Infections 236
Intestinal motility 205
  effects of ethanol on 90
Intestinal triglyceride synthesis 96
Intestine 43
Iodine fixation 267
Ionotropic effect 195
Iron 84
Iron deficiency anaemia 232

Ketosis 33
K_m 6

Lactate 33
Lactic acid, blood 197
Lactic dehydrogenase isoenzyme-5 (LDH-5) 197
Lactose 82
  intolerance to 103
L-α-glycerophosphate acyltransferase 41
Leydig cell 274
Lipids 21
  oxidation 33
  peroxidation 40
Lipogenesis 33, 35

Lipoproteins, low density 42
lipase 195
Lipuria 143
Lymph lipid 104
Lymphocyte function 239

Macrocytosis of liver disease 228
Macrophase function 239
Magnesium,
depletion 191
diuresis 139
homeostasis 271
loss of in urine 271
Malabsorption 82
of fat 83
of folic acid 219
Malnutrition 63, 106, 107
Manganese 86
Medullary carcinoma of the thyroid 272
Megaloblastic anaemia 216
Membrane,
neural 167–73
permeability 202
potential 202
Mental deficiency 136
Meprobamate 39
Mesenteric lymph 104
Metabolites, androgen $5\alpha/5\beta$ 280
20-hydroxylated 259
Metabolic clearance rate 279
Metabolic fractures 137
Metabolism,
cardiac 124–30
cation 169–72
energy 151–2
Metanephrine, methylated 263
24-hour urines for 266
Methanol 8
Microsomal drug-detoxifying enzymes 36
Microsomal ethanol-oxidizing system (MEOS) 6–7, 12
Microsomes 37
Mineral mass 138
Mitochondria 4, 192, 201
myocardial 125
Mitochondrial inclusions 201
Mitochondrial injury 55
Mixed function oxidases 282
MHPG (3-methoxy-4-hydrophenylglycol) 264
24-hour urines for 266
Mural thrombosis 192
Muscle action potentials 197
Muscle cramps 197
Myocardial, infarction 189
Myocardial mitochondria 125
Myofibrils 201
Myoglobin 198
Myoglobinuria 198
Myopathy 199

[Na^+ + K^+]-activated ATPase activity 95
NADH 3, 32, 264
NADP 3
NADPH 3, 280
oxidase-dependent H_2O_2 7
Neural membranes 167–73
Neurohypophysis 204
Neurotransmitter systems 152–62, 173–4
Neutropenia 236
Nicotinamide adenine dinucleotide (NAD) 3
Nitrogen, fecal excretion of 83
Norepinephrine 263, 264
arterial levels of 265
24-hour urines for 266
Normetanephrine, methylated 263
24-hour urines for 266

Oral glucose tolerance test 291
Organ/plasma ratio 268
Osteoarthritis of the hip 143
Osteoclastic bone resorption 140
Osteonecrosis, non-traumatic 135, 141–6
Osteoporosis 136
Oxidases, mixed function 282
Oxidation,
ethanol 1
fatty acid 98
lipid 33
Oxidative phosphorylation 16, 56
Oxygen 9, 16
consumption 95
Oxytocin 204, 290

Pancreatic secretion 90
Pancreatic disease 108
Paralysis 198
Parathormone administration 271
Parathormone resistance 272
Parathormone secretion 271
Parathyroid, calcitonin and calcium 270–3
PBI 269
Pentobarbital 39
Perfused liver 35
Peripheral metabolism of norepinephrine 264

Peroxidation, lipid 40
pH 6
Phosphate,
  deficiency 198
  depletion 139
  pyridoxal 221
  tubular resorption of 272
Phospholipids 8, 43
Phosphorus, dietary 139
Pituitary ACTH 253
Pituitary activity 204
Pituitary, posterior 287–8
Plasma,
  aldosterone 261
  amino acid 52
  calcium 271
  gonadotrophins (FSH/LH) 283–4
  insulin levels 290
  production rates 282
  17-hydroxycorticoids 253
  testosterone 274, 276
  urinary excretion of 254
Plasma protein binding 280
Platelet lifespan 234
Platelet function, abnormal 235
Posterior pituitary 287–8
Prevention and treatment of alcoholic fatty liver 64
Prolactin 287
Proline hydroxylase 33
Propanol 8
Protein 163–6
  constituent 53
  deficiency 51
  export 53
  malnutrition 106
  plasma binding 280
  retinol-binding 82
  synthesis 54
Pyrazole 5, 64, 270
Pyridoxal phosphate 221
Pyridoxine deficiency 221

Radioimmunoassay 274
Red cell life span 227
Redox state 3
Reductase,
  steroid A-ring 280
  5α 280
Renin 261
Retinol-binding protein 82
Respiratory capacity 56
Rhabdomyolysis 198, 199
Ribonucleic acids 166–7
'Ringed sideroblasts' 220
Rotenone 10

Sarcolemmal nuclei 199
Sarcoplasmic reticulum (SR) 125, 126, 127, 192
Secretion,
  aldosterone 261
  biliary 90
  episodic pattern of 276
  pancreatic 90
  parathormone 271
Serotonin 152–4
Serum,
  enzymes 57
  folate 217
  immunoglobulins 58
  iron 221
  magnesium 271, 272
  sodium levels 261
17β-hydroxyandrogens 276
17-hydroxycorticoids, urinary excretion of 254
17-ketosteroids (17-KS) 262, 284–5
17-ketogenic steroids 259
'Shuttle' mechanisms 35
Sideroblastic anaemia 220
Sideroblasts, 'ringed' 220
Smooth endoplasmic reticulum 6
Smooth muscle 204
Sodium,
  absorption 84
  serum levels 261
  urinary excretion of 261
  water transport 83
Sperm count (of dogs) 273
Spermatogenesis 274
Spermatozoa 274
Spine fracture 138
Splanchnic circulation 103
'Spur cells' 229–30
Steatorrhea 82, 109
Steroids 5
  anabolic 64
  A-ring reductases 280
  metabolites, conjugation of 280
  metabolizing enzymes 280
  17-ketogenic 259
Stomatocytosis 231
Sucrose 45
Supra optico-hypophyseal system 289
Sympathetic nervous system 262

Target cells 228
Testicular atrophy 274
Testicular histology 273, 274
Testicular weight 273
Testosterone,
  in plasma and urine 275
  metabolic clearance rate (MRC^T) 279–82
  plasma 274, 276
  urinary glucuronide 275
Thiamine 82
Thrombocytopenia 232–5
Thrombophlebitis 198
Thrombosis, mural, 192
Thyroid function 267–70
  animal studies in 267–68
  histological studies in 267
  human studies in 269–70
  physiological studies in 267
Thyroid, medullary carcinoma of the 272
Thyroid weights 267
Thyroidal accumulation [$^{131(125)}$I], alcohol effect on 267–8
Thyroidal radioiodide uptake 268
Thyroxine, [^{131}I]
  binding of 268
  protein binding of 269
  treatment with 269
Tissue uptake, of [^{131}I]-1-tri-iodothyronine 268
Tolbutamide 291
Transaminase 191
Triglyceride,
  accumulation 33
  cardiac 195
  synthesis, intestinal 96, 98
  uptake 191
Tri-iodothyronine, [^{131}I]-1- 268
  treatment with 269
TSH response to TSHRH (Thyrotropin Releasing Hormone) 269
Tubular resorption of phosphate 272
Tubular resorption of water 288
20-hydroxylated steroid metabolites 259
2,4-dinitrophenol 10

Uric acid 33
Uridine diphosphate glucuronyl-transferase (UDPGT) 280
Urinary excretion of,
  aldosterone 261
  calcium 270
  catecholamine 263
  epinephrine 262
  hydroxyproline 272
  17-hydroxycorticoids 254
  17-ketosteroids 284-5
  sodium 261
Urinary testosterone glucuronide 275
Uterine contractility 204

Vacuolization 224
Vanilmandelic acid, oxidized (VMA) 263, 264
  24-hour urines for 266
Vitamins 63
  A 82, 84
  B_{12} 82
  metabolism 274

Wrist fracture 138

Xylose 82, 103

Zieve's syndrome 231